Concepts of Health-Related Fitness

Thomas M. Adams, II
Arkansas State University

KENDALL/HUNT PUBLISHING COMPANY
4050 Westmark Drive   Dubuque, Iowa 52002

Tables from *Guidelines for Exercise Testing and Prescription,* 6th Edition, are used with permission of Lippincott Williams & Wilkins.

The illustrations in this publication which are © VHI Inc. are used with permission.

Copyright © 2002 by Thomás M. Adams, II

ISBN 13: 978-0-7575-3191-0
ISBN 10: 0-7575-3191-1

Kendall/Hunt Publishing Company has the exclusive rights to reproduce this work, to prepare derivative works from this work, to publicly distribute this work, to publicly perform this work and to publicly display this work.

All rights reserved. No part of this publication may be reproduced, stored in a retrieval system, or transmitted, in any form or by any means, electronic, mechanical, photocopying, recording, or otherwise, without the prior written permission of Kendall/Hunt Publishing Company.

Printed in the United States of America
10 9 8 7 6 5 4

Dedication

To my parents who taught me all the important things in life. Mom, I miss you dearly. I wish that you could be here to see the completion of this work. Dad, I know you discovered the power of exercise late in life. I hope that you will always benefit from it. Even though this manuscript was written as a text for college students, if it helps you in any way to live a better and healthier life, then all the late nights and lost weekends have been worth it.

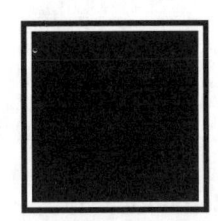

Contents

Chapter 1: Concepts of Health and Wellness *1*

    Introduction: 24-7 *3*
    The Power of Choice *4*
        Causes of Death *4*
        Cardiovascular Disease *4*
        Smoking *5*
        Obesity *5*
        Diabetes *5*
        Physical Inactivity/Sedentary Lifestyle *5*
        Serum Cholesterol *5*
        Hypertension *6*
    Exercise Is Power *6*
    What Is Health? *6*
    Components of Health *7*
        Physical Health *7*
        Mental Health *7*
        Social Health *7*
        Intellectual Health *7*
        Spiritual Health *8*
    What Is Wellness? *8*
        Differences between Health and Wellness *8*
        The Health Field Concept *8*
    Why Physical Fitness? *9*
    U.S. Surgeon General's Report *10*
    Physical Fitness, Physical Exercise, and Physical Activity *10*
    Benefits of Being Physically Fit *10*
    Economic Benefits of Being Physically Fit *11*

Chapter 2: Understanding and Changing Human Behavior *35*

    Understanding Our Behaviors *37*
    Determinants of Behavior *37*
        Predisposing Factors *37*
        Reinforcing Factors *38*
        Enabling Factors *38*
        Levels of Prevention *38*
    Developing a Behavior Change Plan *39*
        Locus of Control *40*
        Transtheoretical Model *40*
        Six Stages of Change *41*
            Precontemplation *41*
            Contemplation *41*

Preparation *42*
Action *42*
Maintenance *42*
Termination *43*
Making the Change *43*
Step 1: Choose a Problem Behavior *43*
Step 2: Learn Your Actions and Behaviors *43*
Step 3: Establish Personal Goals and Objectives *44*
Step 4: Prepare a Plan of Action *44*
Step 5: Implement Your Plan *45*
Step 6: Revaluate and Modify Your Plan *45*

Chapter 3: Beginning a Health-Related Fitness Program 53

Basic Considerations When Beginning a Fitness Program *55*
Beginning a Fitness Program: Basic Training Principles *55*
Principle of Adaptation *55*
Principle of Overload *56*
Principle of Progressive Overload *56*
Principle of Reversibility (Disuse) *57*
Principle of Consistency *57*
Principle of Specificity *57*
Principle of Individuality *58*
Principle of Hard and Easy *58*
Principle of Safety *58*
Three Basic Elements of a Daily Exercise Session *59*
Warm-Up *59*
Conditioning (Workout) *59*
Cool-Down *59*
Exercise Precautions *59*
Overtraining *59*

Chapter 4: Understanding the Cardiovascular System 75

Cardiorespiratory System: Function *77*
Anatomical Considerations of the Cardiovascular System *77*
Exercise and Cardiovascular Disease *77*
Understanding Cardiovascular Risk: Coronary Risk Factors *78*
Smoking *79*
Blood Pressure and Hypertension *79*
Measurement of Blood Pressure *80*
Hypercholesterolemia/Hyperlipidemia *80*
Physical Inactivity *81*
Diabetes Mellitus and Glucose Intolerance *82*
Obesity *82*
Stress *82*
Age *82*
Family History *82*
Gender *82*
Physical Activity and Coronary Risk *83*

Chapter 5: Principles of Cardiorespiratory Endurance   93

    Purpose of the Cardiorespiratory Endurance Exercise Program   95
    Health vs. Fitness: Program Considerations   95
    Benefits of a Cardiorespiratory Endurance Exercise Program   95
    Components of a Cardiorespiratory Exercise Prescription   96
        Modality   *96*
        Frequency   *96*
        Intensity   *97*
            Heart Rate Methods   *98*
                Maximal Heart Rate   *99*
                Heart Rate Reserve   *100*
                Rate of Perceived Exertion   *100*
                Percent of VO_2 Maximum   *102*
        Duration   *102*
        Progression   *103*
            Initial Conditioning Stage   *103*
            Improvement Stage   *103*
            Maintenance Stage   *104*
    Determination of Heart Rate   *105*
        Procedures for Determining Heart Rate Electronically   *105*
        Procedures for Palpating Pulse   *105*
    Components of the Daily Cardiorespiratory Exercise Session   *105*
        Warm-Up   *106*
        Conditioning   *106*
        Cool-Down   *106*
    Exercise Prescriptions and Weight Loss   *107*
    Cardiorespiratory Endurance Training Risk   *107*
    Detraining: The Effect of Exercise Training Reduction or Stoppage on Cardiorespiratory
       Endurance   *109*

Chapter 6: Principles of Muscular Strength and Endurance   121

    Introduction   *123*
    What Is the Difference Between Muscular Strength and Muscular Endurance   *123*
    Benefits of Resistive Training   *123*
    Principle of Overload—Resistive Training   *124*
    Principle of Specificity of Exercise—Resistive Training   *124*
    Detraining: The Effects of Resistive Exercise Training Reduction or Stoppage on Skeletal
       Muscle Tissue   *125*
    Types of Skeletal Muscular Contraction   *125*
        Isometric (Static) Contractions   *126*
        Concentric Contractions   *126*
        Eccentric Contractions   *126*
    Skeletal Muscle Actions   *126*
    Types of Skeletal Muscle Fibers   *126*
        Slow Twitch (Type I)   *127*
        Fast Twitch (Type IIa and Type IIb)   *128*
    Factors Affecting Muscular Strength and Endurance Training   *128*
        Muscle Size   *128*
        Gender   *128*
        Age   *128*
    Muscle Soreness   *129*

Basic Techniques of Resistance Training   *129*
    Isometric Training   *129*
    Isotonic (Progressive Resistive Exercise) Training   *129*
    Isokinetic Training   *130*
Principles of Training   *130*
    Introduction   *130*
        Time Course of Cellular Adaptation and Increased Strength   *130*
    Isometric Training Principles   *131*
    Isotonic Training Principles   *131*
        Training for Muscular Strength   *132*
        Training for Muscular Endurance   *132*
        Training for Muscular Power   *132*
        Training for Hypertrophy   *133*
        Inter-Set and Inter-Session Rest Periods   *133*
        Practical Guidelines for Isotonic Training   *133*
    Isokinetic Training Principles   *134*
Additional Resistance Activities   *134*
    Circuit Training   *134*
    Plyometrics   *134*
    Calisthenics   *135*
    Body Building   *135*
Additional Considerations for Resistive Training Programs   *135*

Chapter 7: Resistive Training Activities   *149*

General Considerations When Performing Resistance Training Exercises   *151*
    Breath Control (Breathing) During Resistive Training   *151*
        Valsava Maneuver   *151*
    Weight Belts   *152*
    Knee Wraps   *152*
    Hand Grips and Placement   *152*
    Body Positioning   *153*
    Spotting   *153*
Machines vs. Free Weights   *154*
    Advantages/Disadvantages of Variable Resistance Machines   *154*
    Advantages/Disadvantages of Free Weights   *155*
Progressive, Variable, and Cable Resistance Machine Exercises   *156*
Free Weight Barbell Exercises   *170*
Free Weight Dumbbell Exercises   *178*
Resistance Training Without Free Weights or Resistance Machines   *189*

Chapter 8: Principles of Flexibility   *195*

What Is Flexibility?   *197*
    Active Flexibility   *197*
    Passive Flexibility   *197*
Benefits of Flexibility   *197*
Factors That Influence Flexibility   *197*
    Muscle Spindles   *198*
    Golgi Tendon Organs   *198*
    Joint Structure   *198*
    Soft Body Tissue   *198*
    Age   *198*
    Gender   *199*

Muscle Temperature *199*
Pregnancy *199*
Principles and Procedures of Flexibility Training or Stretching *199*
How Can Range of Motion Be Improved? *199*
Static Stretching *200*
Dynamic or Ballistic Stretching *200*
Proprioceptive Neuromuscular Facilitation (PNF) *201*

Chapter 9: Flexibility Activities *221*

Stretching Protocols: General Guidelines *223*
Static Stretching Activities *223*
Contraindicated Static Stretching Activities *224*
Plough *224*
Hurdler's Stretch *224*
Full or Deep Knee Squats or Lunges *224*
Standing Straight Legged Toe Touch *225*
Standing Straight Legged Straddle Toe Touch *225*
Full Neck Rolls *225*
Waist Circles *226*
Back Bends (Bridges) *226*
Recommended Static Stretching Activities *226*
Feet *226*
Lower Legs *227*
Upper Legs *229*
Adductors *230*
Hips *230*
Back and Trunk *230*
Neck *232*
Chest *233*
Shoulders *233*
Arms *234*
Ballistic Stretching Activities *235*
Proprioceptive Neuromuscular Facilitation Stretching Activities *235*
Upper Leg *236*
Lower Back *237*
Chest *237*
Shoulders *238*
Adductors *238*

Chapter 10: Principles of Nutrition *239*

Nutrition *241*
High Nutrient Density *241*
Exploring the Essential Nutrients *241*
Carbohydrates *241*
Simple Carbohydrates *242*
Complex Carbohydrates *242*
Fiber *243*
Soluble Fiber *243*
Insoluble Fiber *243*
Fats *243*
Saturated Fat *244*
Hydrogenation and Trans Fatty Acids *244*

Unsaturated Fat *245*
  Monounsaturated Fat *245*
  Polyunsaturated Fat *246*
  Olestra (Olean) *246*
 Proteins *246*
  Amino Acid Supplementation *247*
   Creatine *248*
 Vitamins *248*
  Fat Soluble Vitamins *248*
  Water Soluble Vitamins *248*
  Antioxidant Vitamins *248*
 Minerals *249*
  Sodium and Potassium *249*
  Iron *249*
  Calcium *249*
 Water *249*
Nutrient Recommendation *250*
Understanding the MyPyramid Food System *250*
Supplements *253*
Herbal Supplements *255*
Food for Performance *255*
 How Soon Can I Exercise after I Eat? *255*
 Dietary Needs for the Physically Active *256*
  Carbohydrate Intake *256*
  Carbohydrate Loading *256*
  Fat Intake *257*
  Protein Intake *257*
  Sodium Replacement *257*
  Fluid Replacement *258*
  Vitamin and Mineral Supplementation *258*
Caffeine *259*
Understanding the New Food Label *259*
 % Daily Values *259*
 Health Claims *260*
 Nutrient Content Descriptors *261*

Chapter 11: Principles of Weight Management *267*

Introduction *269*
Understanding Body Fat *269*
Understanding Obesity *270*
Regional Body Fat Storage *270*
Understanding Energy Balance *271*
Understanding Energy Balance and Weight Loss *273*
Causes of Obesity *273*
 Labor-Saving Devices/Technology *273*
 Genetics *273*
 Family Lifestyle *274*
 Childhood Fatness *274*
 Set Point Theory *274*
Understanding the Role of Exercise in Weight Control *275*
Spot Reduction *276*
Behavior Modification and Successful Weight Management *276*
Eating Disorders *281*
 Anorexia Nervosa *281*

Bulimia *282*
Practical Guidelines for Gaining Weight *283*

Chapter 12: Low Back: Health and Fitness Management *311*

Introduction *313*
The Lower Back: An Anatomical Review *313*
    Components of the Vertebral Column *313*
    Curvatures of the Vertebral Column *314*
    Structure and Function of the Vertebral Column *314*
Causes, Prevention, and Treatment of Low Back Pain *315*
    Causes of Low Back Pain *315*
    Prevention of Low Back Pain *316*
        Lifting/Weight Belts *316*
        Postural and Fitness Considerations *317*
        General Guidelines *317*
    Treatment of Low Back Pain *318*
        Body Composition *318*
        Cardiorespiratory Fitness *318*
        Muscular Strength and Endurance *319*
        Flexibility *319*
Recommended Exercises for the Lower Back *319*
    Low Back Exercises *319*
        Prone Single Arm Lift *319*
        Prone Double Arm Lift *320*
        Prone Single Leg Lift (Extension) *320*
        Kneeling Arm and Leg Extension *320*
        Pelvic Tilt *321*
        Curl-ups *321*
        Bridging *322*
    Additional Low Back Flexibility Exercises *322*
    Contraindicated Low Back Exercises *322*
        Curl-ups—Grasping behind the Head *322*
        Double Leg Lifts *323*
        Prone Double Leg Raise *323*
        Simultaneous Arm and Leg Lifts *323*
        Straight Leg Sit-ups *324*

Chapter 13: Prevention and Treatment of Common Fitness Injuries *331*

Heat-Related Illness *333*
    Heat Cramps *333*
    Heat Exhaustion *333*
    Heat Stroke *331*
Prevention and Treatment of Heat-Related Illness *333*
    Prevention *333*
    Treatment *334*
Prevention of Hypothermia: Exercising in Cold Weather *334*
Prevention and Treatment of Common Fitness Injuries *334*
    Shinsplints *335*
    Muscle Cramps or Spasms *335*
    Side Stitch *335*
    Sprains *335*
    Strains *335*
    Contusion *335*

Tendonitis and Bursitis *336*
Muscle Soreness *336*
Skeletal Fractures *336*
 Stress Fractures *336*
 Simple Fracture *336*
 Compound Fracture *336*
Skin Wounds *337*
 Open Wounds *337*
 Closed Wounds *337*
Treatment and Management of Injuries Using RICE *337*
Treatment and Management of Injuries Using Heat *337*

References *339*

Brief Contents

Chapter 1: Concepts of Health and Wellness 1

Chapter 2: Understanding and Changing Human Behavior 35

Chapter 3: Beginning a Health-Related Fitness Program 53

Chapter 4: Understanding the Cardiovascular System 75

Chapter 5: Principles of Cardiorespiratory Endurance 93

Chapter 6: Principles of Muscular Strength and Endurance 121

Chapter 7: Resistive Training Activities 149

Chapter 8: Principles of Flexibility 195

Chapter 9: Flexibility Activities 221

Chapter 10: Principles of Nutrition 239

Chapter 11: Principles of Weight Management 267

Chapter 12: Low Back: Health and Fitness Management 311

Chapter 13: Prevention and Treatment of Common Fitness Injuries 331

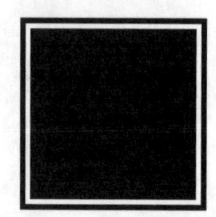

List of Laboratories

Laboratory 1-A:	Statement of Informed Consent: Participation in Physical Activities	*15*
Laboratory 1-B:	Statement of Informed Consent: Participation in Fitness Evaluations	*17*
Laboratory 1-C:	Lifestyle Self-Assessment	*19*
Laboratory 1-D:	Pre-Exercise Self-Assessment	*25*
Laboratory 1-E:	Medical/Health Questionnaire	*29*
Laboratory 2-A:	Implementing Behavior Change	*49*
Laboratory 2-B:	Readiness for Behavioral Change	*51*
Laboratory 3-A:	Personal Exercise Prescription	*63*
Laboratory 4-A:	Blood Pressure Measurement	*87*
Laboratory 4-B:	Coronary Heart Disease Risk Appraisal	*91*
Laboratory 5-A:	Cardiorespiratory (VO_2Max): Rockport Walking Test	*113*
Laboratory 5-B:	Cardiorespiratory (VO_2Max): 1.5-Mile Run Test	*117*
Laboratory 5-C:	3-Mile Walk/Run Test	*119*
Laboratory 6-A:	Muscle Endurance: One-Minute Bent Knee Sit-up Test	*139*
Laboratory 6-B:	Muscle Strength: Upper Leg Press	*141*
Laboratory 6-C:	Muscular Strength: Bench Press	*143*
Laboratory 6-D:	Muscular Endurance: Push-Ups	*145*
Laboratory 6-E:	Muscular Endurance: Curl-Up (Crunch) Test	*147*
Laboratory 8-A:	Flexibility: Shoulder and Wrist Elevation	*205*
Laboratory 8-B:	Flexibility: Trunk and Neck Extension	*207*
Laboratory 8-C:	Flexibility: Ankle Plantar Flexion	*209*
Laboratory 8-D:	Flexibility: Ankle Dorsi Flexion	*211*
Laboratory 8-E:	Flexibility: Modified (Accuflex) Sit and Reach	*213*
Laboratory 8-F:	Flexibility: Long Axis Body Rotation	*217*
Laboratory 8-G:	Flexibility: Sit and Reach	*219*
Laboratory 10-A:	Food Labeling	*265*
Laboratory 11-A:	Body Composition Assessment: Procedural Instructions	*287*
Laboratory 11-B:	Body Composition Assessment: Three Site Skinfold—Female	*291*
Laboratory 11-C:	Body Composition Assessment: Three Site Skinfold—Male	*295*
Laboratory 11-D:	Body Composition Assessment: Seven Site Skinfold—Male and Female	*299*
Laboratory 11-E:	Body Composition Assessment: Body Mass Index (BMI)	*301*
Laboratory 11-F:	Regional Fat Distribution: Waist-to-Hip Ratio	*303*
Laboratory 11-G:	Determining Basal Metabolic Rate	*305*
Laboratory 11-H:	Determining Estimated Daily Caloric Needs	*307*
Laboratory 11-I:	Food Log	*309*
Laboratory 12-A:	Low Back: Back-Extension	*327*
Laboratory 12-B:	Low Back: Hip and Lumbar Flexibility	*329*

List of Tables

Table 1-1: Estimated Contribution of Four Factors to the Ten Leading Causes of Death before Age Seventy-Five 9
Table 1-2: "LifeScore" Life Expectancy 19
Table 1-3: Ideal Weights Based on Height and Body Build 23
Table 1-4: Estimated Frame Size by Elbow Breadth 23
Table 1-5: Social Readjustment Rating Scale 24
Table 1-6: Classification of Individual Health Status Prior to Exercise Testing or Participation 26
Table 1-7: Coronary Artery Disease Risk Factor Thresholds 27
Table 1-8: ACSM Recommendations for (A) Current Medical Examination and Exercise Testing Prior to Participation and (B) Physician Supervision of Exercise Tests 27
Table 2-1: Routine Health Screening: Recommendations for Disease Prevention 39
Table 2-2: Stages of the Transtheoretical Model 41
Table 2-3: Stages and Descriptive Timeframes of the Transtheoretical Model 52
Table 3-1: Normative Values for Determining Fitness Classifications by Percentile Score 65
Table 4-1: Coronary Artery Disease Risk Factors 79
Table 4-2: Normative Values for Classifying Blood Pressure in Adults Age 18 and Older 80
Table 4-3: Classification of Risk on Total, HDL, and LDL Cholesterol (mg/dl) 81
Table 4-4: Normative Values for Classifying Blood Pressure in Adults Age 18 and Older 88
Table 4-5: Relative Risk Categories: Risko 91
Table 5-1: Recommended Exercising Intensity for Developing Health-Related and Fitness-Related Benefits 95
Table 5-2: Recommended Exercise Frequency Based on Fitness Level 97
Table 5-3: Recommended Exercise Percent HHR Based on Initial Fitness Levels 100
Table 5-4: Rate of Perceived Exertion Scale 101
Table 5-5: Classification of Intensity of Exercise Based on 20–60 Minutes of Endurance Training 102
Table 5-6: Relationship of Percent of Maximum Heart Rate, Heart Rate Reserve, and Maximal Oxygen Uptake 102
Table 5-7: Recommended Exercise Duration Based on Fitness Level 103
Table 5-8: Example Exercise Progression for an Apparently Healthy 20-Year-Old Student 104
Table 5-9: The Relationship of Exercise Frequency, Intensity, Duration and Energy Expenditure 108
Table 5-10: Normative Values by Age and Gender for VO_{2max} (ml/kg/min) 114
Table 6-1: Recommended Isotonic Training Guidelines Based on Type of Resistive Training 132
Table 6-2: Normative Values by Age and Gender for 1-Minute Sit-up Muscular Strength and Endurance Test 140
Table 6-3: Normative Values by Age and Gender for 1 RM Absolute Upper Leg Strength Normalized by Body Weight 142

Table 6-4:	Normative Values by Age and Gender for 1 RM Absolute Bench Press Strength Normalized by Body Weight *144*
Table 6-5:	Normative Values by Age and Gender for Push-up Muscular Endurance *146*
Table 6-6:	Normative Values by Age and Gender for Curl-ups (Crunches) *148*
Table 7-1:	Advantages and Disadvantages of Variable Resistance Weight Machines *155*
Table 7-2:	Advantages and Disadvantages of Free Weights *156*
Table 8-1:	Recommended Guidelines for Static, PNF, and Ballistic Flexibility Training *200*
Table 8-2:	Normative Values by Gender for Shoulder and Wrist Elevation *206*
Table 8-3:	Normative Values by Gender for Trunk and Neck Extension *208*
Table 8-4:	Normative Values by Gender for Ankle Plantar Flexion *210*
Table 8-5:	Normative Values by Gender for Ankle Dorsi Flexion *212*
Table 8-6:	Normative Values by Age and Gender for Sit and Reach Box (Inches) *214*
Table 8-7:	Normative Values by Age and Gender for Sit and Reach Box (cm) *215*
Table 8-8:	Normative Values by Age and Gender for Long Axis Body Rotation *218*
Table 8-9:	Normative Values by Age and Gender for Wooden Sit and Reach Box (cm) *220*
Table 9-1:	Sequence of Action for Static Stretching Activities *223*
Table 9-2:	Sequence of Action for Proprioceptive Neuromuscular Facilitation Stretching Activities *236*
Table 10-1:	Recommended Daily Intake for Fat, Protein, and Carbohydrate Based on Low, Average, and High Levels of Caloric Intake *242*
Table 10-2:	Recommended Methods to Lower Total Fat, Saturated Fat, and Cholesterol Intake *245*
Table 10-3:	MyPyramid Food Intake Pattern Calorie Levels *252*
Table 10-4:	What Counts? *253*
Table 10-5:	Recommended Daily Food Intake For Each Food Group By Calorie Level *254*
Table 10-6:	Descriptive Phases of the Carbohydrate Loading Procedure *257*
Table 10-7:	Examples of Low Nutrient Content Descriptors *261*
Table 11-1:	Classification of Body Fatness by Gender *270*
Table 11-2:	Comparison of a Traditional Daily Diet and a Healthy Choice Daily Diet *279*
Table 11-3:	Understanding Food Serving or Portion Sizes *280*
Table 11-4:	Percent Body Fat Classification for Women *292*
Table 11-5:	Percent Body Fat Values for Women Based on the Sum of Three Skinfolds (Triceps, Hip, and Thigh) and Age *293*
Table 11-6:	Percent Body Fat Classifications for Men *296*
Table 11-7:	Percent Body Fat Values for Men Based on the Sum of Three Skinfolds (Chest, Abdomen, and Thigh) and Age *297*
Table 11-8:	Normative Values for Classifying Disease Risk Based on Body Mass Index (BMI) and Waist Circumference *302*
Table 11-9:	Risk Classification by Gender and Waist-to-Hip Ratio (WHR) *303*
Table 12-1:	Normative Values for Back-Extension *328*
Table 12-2:	Normative Values for Hip and Low Back Flexibility *330*

List of Figures

Figure 1.1: Elbow Breadth Determination *24*
Figure 4.1: Blood Pressure Determination *87*
Figure 5.1: Pulse Palpation: Carotid *115*
Figure 5.2: Pulse Palpation: Radial *115*
Figure 6.1: One-Minute Bent Knee Sit-up *140*
Figure 6.2: Leg Press *142*
Figure 6.3: Bench Press *144*
Figure 6.4: Push-up *146*
Figure 6.5: Bent Knee Push-Up *146*
Figure 6.6: Curl-up *148*
Figure 7.1: Machine - Bench Press *157*
Figure 7.2: Machine - Vertical Chest Press *157*
Figure 7.3: Machine - Vertical Pec *158*
Figure 7.4: Machine - Fly *158*
Figure 7.5: Machine - Assisted Dips *159*
Figure 7.6: Machine - Seated Arm Curls *159*
Figure 7.7: Machine - Standing Cable Arm Curls *160*
Figure 7.8: Machine - Seated Triceps Extension *160*
Figure 7.9: Machine - Standing Triceps Extension *161*
Figure 7.10: Machine - Overhead Press *161*
Figure 7.11: Machine - Standing Upright Cable Row *162*
Figure 7.12: Machine - Seated Lateral Raise (Abduction) *162*
Figure 7.13: Machine - Seated Posterior Deltoid *163*
Figure 7.14: Machine - Lat Pull Down *163*
Figure 7.15: Machine - Seated Rowing *164*
Figure 7.16: Machine - Back Extension *165*
Figure 7.17: Machine - Abdominals *165*
Figure 7.18: Machine - Hip Sled *166*
Figure 7.19: Machine - Leg Abduction *166*
Figure 7.20: Machine - Seated Leg Press *167*
Figure 7.21: Machine - Seated Leg Extension *167*
Figure 7.22: Machine - Prone Leg Curl *168*
Figure 7.23: Machine - Seated Leg Curl *168*
Figure 7.24: Machine - Leg Adduction *169*
Figure 7.25: Machine - Foot Plantar Flexion *169*
Figure 7.26: Free Weight Barbell - Barbell Bench (Chest) Press *170*
Figure 7.27: Free Weight Barbell - Barbell Incline Bench (Chest) Press *171*

Figure 7.28: Free Weight Barbell - Standing Barbell Curl   *171*
Figure 7.29: Free Weight Barbell - Seated Barbell Curl Using Curling Bench   *172*
Figure 7.30: Free Weight Barbell - Lying Barbell Triceps Extension   *173*
Figure 7.31: Free Weight Barbell - Sitting Triceps Extension   *173*
Figure 7.32: Free Weight Barbell - Lying Closed Grip Bench Press   *174*
Figure 7.33: Free Weight Barbell - Barbell Wrist Curl   *174*
Figure 7.34: Free Weight Barbell - Barbell Wrist Extensions   *175*
Figure 7.35: Free Weight Barbell - Overhead Barbell Press   *175*
Figure 7.36: Free Weight Barbell - Barbell Inclined Overhead Press   *176*
Figure 7.37: Free Weight Barbell - Standing Barbell Upright Row   *177*
Figure 7.38: Free Weight Barbell - Barbell Bent Over Row   *177*
Figure 7.39: Free Weight Barbell - Barbell Pull-over   *178*
Figure 7.40: Free Weight Barbell - Standing Barbell Heel Raise   *178*
Figure 7.41: Free Weight Dumbbell - Dumbbell Fly, Chest Adduction, Bench (Chest) Press   *179*
Figure 7.42: Free Weight Dumbbell - Dumbbell Incline Bench (Chest) Press   *180*
Figure 7.43: Free Weight Dumbbell - Standing Dumbbell Curl   *181*
Figure 7.44: Free Weight Dumbbell - Standing Hammer Curl   *181*
Figure 7.45: Free Weight Dumbbell - Seated Dumbbell Curl   *182*
Figure 7.46: Free Weight Dumbbell - Seated Thigh Dumbbell Curl   *183*
Figure 7.47: Free Weight Dumbbell - Seated Dumbbell Curl Using Curling Bench   *183*
Figure 7.48: Free Weight Dumbbell - Lying Dumbbell Triceps Extension   *184*
Figure 7.49: Free Weight Dumbbell - Sitting Triceps Extension   *184*
Figure 7.50: Free Weight Dumbbell - Dumbbell Wrist Curl   *185*
Figure 7.51: Free Weight Dumbbell - Dumbbell Wrist Extensions   *185*
Figure 7.52: Free Weight Dumbbell - Seated Overhead Dumbbell Press   *186*
Figure 7.53: Free Weight Dumbbell - Standing Dumbbell Lateral Row   *186*
Figure 7.54: Free Weight Dumbbell - Standing Dumbbell Upright Row   *187*
Figure 7.55: Free Weight Dumbbell - Dumbbell Bent over Row   *188*
Figure 7.56: Free Weight Dumbbell - Dumbbell Pull-over   *188*
Figure 7.57: Free Weight Dumbbell - Standing Dumbbell Heel Raise   *189*
Figure 7.58: Resistance Training - Reversed, Closed Grip Pull-up   *189*
Figure 7.59: Resistance Training - Dips   *190*
Figure 7.60: Resistance Training - Chair Dips   *190*
Figure 7.61: Resistance Training - Push-up   *191*
Figure 7.62: Resistance Training - Closed Hand Push-up   *191*
Figure 7.63: Resistance Training - Pull-up   *192*
Figure 7.64: Resistance Training - Crunches (Curl-ups)   *192*
Figure 7.65: Resistance Training - Inclined Bent Knee Sit-ups   *193*
Figure 8.1: PNF - Initial Position   *201*
Figure 8.2: PNF - Isometric Contraction   *201*
Figure 8.3: PNF - Passive Stretch Following Contraction   *202*
Figure 8.4: Shoulder and Wrist Elevation   *206*
Figure 8.5: Trunk and Neck Extension   *208*
Figure 8.6: Ankle Plantar Flexion   *210*
Figure 8.7: Ankle Dorsi Flexion   *212*
Figure 8.8: Modified (Accuflex) Sit and Reach   *215*
Figure 8.9: Long Axis Body Rotation   *218*
Figure 8.10: Sit and Reach   *220*

Figure 9.1:	Plough	*224*
Figure 9.2:	Hurdler's Stretch	*224*
Figure 9.3:	Full or Deep Knee Squats or Lunges	*225*
Figure 9.4:	Standing Straight Legged Toe Touch	*225*
Figure 9.5:	Standing Straight Legged Straddle Toe Touch	*225*
Figure 9.6:	Full Neck Rolls	*226*
Figure 9.7:	Waist Circles	*226*
Figure 9.8:	Back Bends (Bridges)	*226*
Figure 9.9:	Plantar Arch Stretch	*227*
Figure 9.10:	Anterior Foot and Toes Stretch	*227*
Figure 9.11:	Anterior Lower Leg Stretch Procedure #1	*228*
Figure 9.12:	Anterior Lower Leg Stretch Procedure #2	*228*
Figure 9.13:	Lateral Lower Leg Stretch	*228*
Figure 9.14:	Posterior Lower Leg Stretch	*229*
Figure 9.15:	Anterior Upper Leg Stretch	*229*
Figure 9.16:	Posterior Upper Leg Stretch	*229*
Figure 9.17:	Adductor Stretch	*230*
Figure 9.18:	Hip Stretch	*230*
Figure 9.19:	Supine Single Leg Trunk Rotation	*230*
Figure 9.20:	Supine Double Leg Hip Rotation	*231*
Figure 9.21:	Cat Stretch	*231*
Figure 9.22:	Double Leg Hip Flexion	*231*
Figure 9.23:	Single Leg Hip Flexion	*232*
Figure 9.24:	Anterior Neck Stretch	*232*
Figure 9.25:	Lateral Neck Stretch	*232*
Figure 9.26:	Posterior Neck Stretch	*233*
Figure 9.27:	Chest Stretch	*233*
Figure 9.28:	Anterior Shoulder Stretch	*233*
Figure 9.29:	Posterior Shoulder Stretch	*234*
Figure 9.30:	Anterior Upper Arm (Biceps) Stretch	*234*
Figure 9.31:	Posterior Upper Arm (Triceps) Stretch	*234*
Figure 9.32:	Sequence of Action PNF Stretching - Step 1	*235*
Figure 9.33:	Sequence of Action PNF Stretching - Steps 2 and 3	*235*
Figure 9.34:	Sequence of Action PNF Stretching - Steps 4–6	*235*
Figure 9.35:	PNF Anterior Upper Leg Stretch	*236*
Figure 9.36:	PNF Posterior Upper Leg Stretch	*237*
Figure 9.37:	PNF Low Back and Hamstring Stretch	*237*
Figure 9.38:	PNF Chest Stretch	*237*
Figure 9.39:	PNF Anterior Shoulder Stretch	*238*
Figure 9.40:	PNF Adductor Stretch	*238*
Figure 10.1:	The MyPyramid Symbol	*251*
Figure 11.1:	Ectomorph Somatotype	*269*
Figure 11.2:	Mesomorph Somatotype	*269*
Figure 11.3:	Endomorph Somatotype	*269*
Figure 11.4:	Android Obesity	*271*
Figure 11.5:	Gynoid Obesity	*271*
Figure 11.6:	Energy Balance	*272*
Figure 11.7:	Chest Skinfold	*288*

Figure 11.8: Triceps Skinfold *288*
Figure 11.9: Axilla Skinfold *289*
Figure 11.10: Subscapular Skinfold *289*
Figure 11.11: Abdominal Skinfold *289*
Figure 11.12: Suprailium Skinfold *289*
Figure 11.13: Thigh Skinfold *289*
Figure 11.14: Waist Measurement *304*
Figure 11.15: Hip Measurement *304*
Figure 12.1: Components and Curvature of the Vertebral Column *314*
Figure 12.2: Lordosis/Pelvic Tilt *317*
Figure 12.3: Proper Pelvic Position *317*
Figure 12.4: Prone Single Arm Lift *320*
Figure 12.5: Prone Double Arm Lift *320*
Figure 12.6: Prone Single Leg Lift *320*
Figure 12.7: Kneeling Arm and Leg Extension *321*
Figure 12.8: Pelvic Tilt *321*
Figure 12.9: Curl-ups *321*
Figure 12.10: Bridging *322*
Figure 12.11: Curl-ups - Grasping Behind the Head *322*
Figure 12.12: Double Leg Lifts *323*
Figure 12.13: Prone Double Leg Raise *323*
Figure 12.14: Simultaneous Arm and Leg Lifts *324*
Figure 12.15: Straight Leg Sit-ups *324*
Figure 12.16: Low Back: Back-Extension *328*
Figure 12.17: Low Back: Hip and Lumbar Flexibility Lab - Initial Position *330*
Figure 12.18: Low Back: Hip and Lumbar Flexibility Lab - Final Position *330*

Acknowledgments

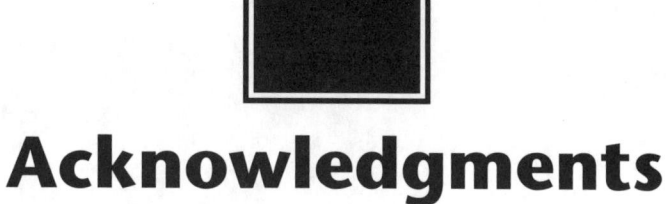

I would like to thank my colleagues for their support during the development and writing of this manuscript. Additionally, I would like to thank those in University administration for their support in providing some of the time needed to prepare the document.

Finally, a special and deep felt thanks to my loving wife, Harriette. Your patience, love, and support mean everything to me. I know the sacrifices you made to allow me the time to complete this work. Your direct assistance played a critical role in defining this product. I thank you and I love you.

1

Concepts of Health and Wellness

Those who do not find time for exercise will have to find time for illness.
Anonymous

■ Chapter Outline ■

Introduction: 24-7
The Power of Choice
    Causes of Death
    Cardiovascular Disease
    Smoking
    Obesity
    Diabetes
    Physical Inactivity/Sedentary Lifestyle
    Serum Cholesterol
    Hypertension
Exercise Is Power
What Is Health?
Components of Health
    Physical Health
    Mental Health
    Social Health
    Intellectual Health
    Spiritual Health
What Is Wellness?
    Differences between Health and Wellness
    The Health Field Concept
Why Physical Fitness?
U.S. Surgeon General's Report
Physical Fitness, Physical Exercise, and Physical Activity
Benefits of Being Physically Fit
Economic Benefits of Being Physically Fit

■ Learning Objectives ■

The student should be able to:

- Discuss the role of lifestyle choices as they relate to health and wellness.
- Define health and wellness.
- Describe the components of health.
- Differentiate between health and wellness.
- Explain the Health Field Concept.
- Discuss the determinants of behavior.
- Describe the three levels of prevention.
- List and explain the six stages of change.
- Define physical fitness.
- Define physical activity.
- Identify the health-related and skill-related components of fitness.
- Identify physical and economic benefits of being physically fit.

Keywords

- Cardiovascular disease
- Coronary artery disease
- Diabetes
- Health
- Health field concept
- Health-related components of fitness
- Hypertension
- Hypokinetic diseases
- Intellectual health
- Lifestyle choices
- Mental health
- Physical activity
- Physical exercise
- Physical fitness
- Physical health
- Sedentary lifestyle
- Skill-related components of fitness
- Social health
- Spiritual health
- Wellness

Introduction: 24 - 7

Are you frustrated with your body weight or level of fitness? Do you want to lose weight but don't know how? Perhaps you have tried dieting and still have an unwanted level of fatness? Would you like to "firm-up" musculature while at the same time lose a couple extra pounds?

So many people have tried to lose weight and failed. Are you one of them? Have you struggled through a diet, lost weight, only to watch yourself gain back the unwanted weight? You may have even found, after all your struggles and efforts, you added additional weight.

Do you know how to select and prepare foods that will lead to a healthier lifestyle? Do you know how to modify your diet to lower serum cholesterol levels? Is it safe to eat oysters and salt? What does it mean when a food label indicates lean, or low fat?

Are there foods that, if eaten, can raise or lower serum cholesterol levels? Are there foods that have special body fat burning properties? Is cancer related to dietary intake?

Maybe you are concerned about your current fitness level. How fit are you? Have you tried to get involved in an exercise program? Perhaps you have even gone to the expense to join a health/fitness club only to find that your attempts to improve your fitness levels left you sore and unable or uninterested in continuing your conditioning program. Do you find fitness activities boring? Do you find fitness equipment intimidating? Do you know how to use the various pieces of equipment? Do you know how to properly train and condition? Do you fear injury or life threatening events if you engage in activity?

Do you have pre-existing conditions, such as illness or physical limitations, which you believe will prevent you from participating in regular physical activity? Is it safe for a hypertensive individual to exercise? Should pregnant women exercise or will it harm the unborn child? What effect does aging have on individual fitness levels?

Do you know how to prevent and/or treat fitness related injuries? What affects do environmental conditions such as temperature have on an individual wanting to exercise? Can it be too hot or too cold to exercise? Can breathing cold air during exercise freeze your lungs?

Are you constantly plagued with low back pain? Are there activities that you can engage in to help prevent or treat your problem?

In simple, there are many questions associated with implementing a healthy lifestyle. The answers to these questions and the choices we make directly impact our health and our quality of life. What can be done? How can we take control over our lives? What steps will allow each and every one of us to live fully and completely? Are you living life to the fullest, or is your life being controlled by your current health and fitness status?

Isn't it sad to think that daily living activities, family vacations, and other aspects of our lives are planned based on our health and fitness levels? Have you ever wanted to participate in an activity but chose not to for fear that you didn't have the physical capability? Are you one of the many forced to drive around parking lots looking for a parking space just a little closer to the mall or in front of a particular store because you get tired walking? Are you a sports spectator and not a sports participant because you do not have the physical ability to play?

No one has to be a couch potato. Each of us has the power to change our lives. We have the power to take control of our health and our fitness levels. We have the power to control our future.

If you are reading this, you have taken the first step to changing your life. The purpose of this text is to provide you with: (1) answers to many of your health and fitness related questions and (2) the information you will need to help you change your life. It is important, however, that you accept that you are changing your life. The information contained **does not** provide a quick fix or immediate remedy. This cannot be emphasized enough. There is no easy way. You must be motivated and willing to make long-term alterations in your current lifestyle. Face it, how you currently live, what you eat, and what levels of exercise you are participating in may have left you unsatisfied, frustrated and wanting change. Accept this. If you do, it will be easier for you to move forward with your behavior modifications. **Don't try to hang on to a bad past, but rather create a positive, meaningful future.**

Accept the fact that many of the behaviors you may want to change have been developed over a lifetime. Unfortunately, many may reflect a lifetime of body neglect and bad choice. Do not expect to erase your past quickly, without effort, and without long-term change. Brief periods of diet and exercise will not allow for long-term gains in health and fitness. In fact, neither will allow for safe, effective short-term changes. It is extremely important that you recognize and accept the changes you make; **you are making for a lifetime.** You must change 24 – 7. From here out, 24 hours a day, 7 days a week, for the rest of your life, you will lead a new life.

Fortunately, the body will respond to your efforts. You should also be advised or, maybe more appropriately, warned, that the body will respond to either good or bad behavior. If you choose to live wisely, you will benefit from a healthy, fit life. If you make poor choices, you will suffer the immediate and long-term consequences of those bad choices. Illness, excessive body weight, poor physical fitness, poor psychological well-being and self-esteem potentially represent your future.

Positive living is one of life's great blessings. Health and fitness are to be enjoyed. Take pleasure in knowing, through proper intervention, you can change and improve the quality of your life. You can reap the benefits of healthy living.

This text will help guide you as you choose to move toward a more active lifestyle. Laboratory activities will help you assess your current health or fitness status. Text information can be used to help you establish your own health/fitness program designed to meet individual needs. Fundamental information is provided to assist you in making informed, positive lifestyle choices. Guidelines are provided to help you establish safe, individualized, intervention programs that can address your immediate and long-term needs and objectives.

The Power of Choice

Do the choices we make regarding fitness activities and dietary intake really impact our health and fitness? Are disease states or illnesses related to lifestyle choices? These are important questions. Let us look at the facts as reported by the American Heart Association (www.americanheart.org) and the National Center for Chronic Disease Prevention and Health Promotion (www.cdc.gov). Discussed below are statistical findings related to disease states or illnesses associated with poor or improper lifestyle choices. Subheaders have been used for reader ease.

Causes of Death

More than half of today's health problems are **lifestyle related** and **preventable.** That's right! Fifty-one (51) percent of the health problems we experience as a population, we **choose to experience.** Moreover, nine out of the ten underlying causes of death in the United States are related to our **lifestyle.** What are the most prevalent health problems in our nation? Currently, the three leading causes of death are: cardiovascular disease, cancer and stroke. All three are lifestyle related. Fortunately, 80% of the negative, troubling aspects associated with these health problems can be **prevented or delayed** by living a positive, physically active, healthy life. This may seem surprising to some. Many perceive that death due to childhood diseases, aging, sexually related diseases, and accidents are the primary culprits to mortality. This assumption is simply wrong. *On average, physically active individuals outlive sedentary individuals.* In addition, physically active people lead a more functionally independent, and fuller life than inactive individuals.

Cardiovascular Disease

Cardiovascular disease (CHD) alone accounts for more than 40% of all deaths. It is the leading cause of death among women. No one is immune. Cardiovascular disease affects both men and women of all races and ethnic groups. More money is spent treating heart disease than any other illness. In 1997, 274 billion dollars were spent on the treatment of CHD. Fifty-eight million Americans currently suffer from one or more forms of cardiovascular disease. In order to put this number in perspective, this represents almost ¼ of the nation's population. Most of these individuals can positively change this state of health by actively engaging in a positive, healthy lifestyle. People who live a sedentary life double their risk of heart disease by choosing to remain inactive. Proper exercise and dietary intervention can have a significant impact on this negative disease.

Smoking

There are other negative influences on our health that result from our choice of sedentary living, poor diet and other harmful lifestyle choices. For example, the use of cigarettes and other tobacco products is considered the leading preventable cause of death in the United States and is the primary cause of lung cancer. A smoker presents twice the risk of heart attack compared to non-smokers. One in every five deaths associated with cardiovascular disease can be attributed or linked to smoking. Additionally, smoking is directly linked to coronary artery disease by speeding up the atherosclerosis process. Statistically, 430,000 deaths annually are directly related to tobacco use and between 37,000 to 40,000 deaths annually are related to secondary smoke. Medical care costs related to tobacco use exceed 50 billion dollars annually.

What is the impact of stopping smoking? Will I benefit from smoking cessation, or is the damage permanent? How will I benefit if I choose to quit smoking? The evidence shows the power of positive health-related interventions. Statistically, one year after smoking cessation, the risk of coronary heart disease is lowered by 50%. Fifteen years after stopping, the risk of coronary heart disease for an ex-smoker is close to that of a non-smoker.

Obesity

Obesity is the second most preventable cause of death in the United States. Sixty-one percent of adults and more than 25% of children are overweight. The percentage of overweight children and adolescents has more than doubled in the last 30 years. Obesity is related to a number of illnesses, including, but not limited to, increased risk of coronary artery disease, arthritis, renal disease, and pulmonary disease. Proper exercise and dietary intervention can assist in eliminating excessive weight and maintaining normal body weight.

Diabetes

Diabetes is strongly related to obesity and sedentary lifestyles. In fact, obesity is the number one link to adult onset diabetes. A 20% increase in body weight has been shown to double the risk of developing diabetes. Diabetes affects almost nine million Americans and is responsible for more than 60,000 deaths annually. Almost 800,000 cases of Type 2 (non-insulin dependent) diabetes are diagnosed every year. Individuals presenting diabetes have 2–4 times greater risk of heart disease or stroke than those who are disease free. Proper exercise and dietary intervention can assist in preventing or controlling diabetes.

Physical Inactivity/Sedentary Lifestyle

Sadly, and unfortunately, 24% of adults lead *completely sedentary lives*. Nearly 50% of American youth between the ages of 12–21 do not participate in regular vigorous activity. Twenty-eight percent of Americans ages 18 or older have reported no physical activity in the last 30 days. Only 15% of American adults participate in regular physical activity for five or more days per week for 30 minutes or longer each activity session.

Serum Cholesterol

Sedentary living and poor dietary choices are also related to high cholesterol, hypertension, obesity, and diabetes. Fifty-one percent of American adults have serum cholesterol levels greater than 200 mg/dl. A level considered high and related to coronary artery disease. Twenty percent have levels greater than 240 mg/dl which is considered extremely high and dangerous to individual health. These dangerously high levels are not restricted to adults. Thirty-six percent of American youth age 19 or under have serum cholesterol levels of 170 mg/dl or higher. These levels are comparable to a level of 200 mg/dl in adults. Ten percent have levels exceeding 200 mg/dl, which represents an extremely high serum cholesterol level. Proper exercise and dietary intervention can assist in lowering and controlling serum cholesterol levels.

Hypertension

Hypertension, or high blood pressure, affects 50 million adults aged 6 or older. This represents 1 out of every 5 Americans and, more specifically, 1 out of every 4 adults. Sadly, almost 32 percent of these individuals are unaware of their status. Forty-one percent are not on any form of therapy or intervention, or they are on medication but do not have their hypertension under control. In fact, only 27 percent of hypertensive individuals are on medications and are properly managing and controlling their blood pressure. As a result, during the ten-year period between 1988 and 1998, the mortality rate associated with hypertension increased 16 percent, while the actual number of deaths rose to slightly over 40 percent. In general, sedentary individuals present a 30–50% greater risk of developing hypertension. As you may expect, proper exercise and dietary intervention can assist in lowering and controlling blood pressure.

Exercise Is Power

The findings above are staggering. It appears we are choosing to be a **health care society** rather than a **health prevention society**. What can we do to change? How can exercise influence the damaging affects of poor lifestyle choices?

The power of modern medicine is remarkable. New technologies in such areas as medications and surgical procedures have assisted many individuals in leading more advanced, productive lives. Yet, to date *there is no single drug that can positively affect the human body and its health status the way regular exercise can.*

As mentioned above, regular exercise has been shown to prevent premature death, reduce the risk of heart disease, and reduce the risk of developing diabetes and hypertension. Additionally, it is related to weight reduction and maintenance, psychological well-being, and reduction in depression and anxiety. Specific physiological benefits of exercise are itemized later in this chapter (see Benefits of Being Physically Fit).

Exercise is power. It is the power to control our futures. It gives us the power we need to control our lives. There is no greater way to influence our health and fitness status than exercise.

What Is Health?

A universally accepted definition of health is difficult to develop because health is a personal value, not a scientific absolute. In other words, there is no formula that will guarantee an individual will be free from disease and injury.

Health long ago was considered freedom from disease. Probably the most widely accepted definition of health comes from the World Health Organization (1947), which declared, "health is a state of complete physical, emotional and social health, not merely the freedom from disease and illness." That statement still has meaning today, although a "state of complete health" in reality seems impossible to attain and therefore makes the definition inappropriate.

In more recent years the concept of longevity has been attached to life, as if to suggest long life equals health. While longevity certainly is a reflection of health, a more contemporary definition typically has elements of vitality or vigor and a positive approach to all life has to offer. Health can be described as a temporary state resulting from the ability of an individual to balance physical, mental, intellectual, social and spiritual dimensions in a way that makes him/her happy, satisfied and productive. The important ingredients in the definition are happy, satisfied, and productive. These elements reflect the personal values an individual attaches to health.

Health status reflects a measurement of the various dimensions of our well-being. Height, weight, body composition, blood pressure, cholesterol, intelligence tests, and personality indexes would represent some of the measures that would be taken to determine a person's health status. Using this data would result in an overall health score much like those estimated from currently available health risk appraisals. The score would represent some type of status ranging from excellent to poor health. This information could be used to initiate behavior change if so desired by the individual completing the health inventory. The Lifestyle Self-Assessment (Laboratory 1-C) from the Center for Corporate Health Promotion presented at the end of this chapter can give you an indication of your current health status.

Components of Health

Physical Health

Physical health is based on the biological integrity of the human organism. The level of susceptibility to disease, body weight, visual acuity, strength, coordination, level of endurance, and powers of recuperation are physiological and structural characteristics that enable people to participate in daily activities. In a healthy person, the cells, tissues, organs and systems of the body function properly and the individual feels well. If the body is compromised in some way, the individual will exhibit measurable or observable *signs* of disease such as fever or changes in white blood cell count. The person may also have complaints such as fatigue or body aches. These subjective reports are described as *symptoms* of a disease or illness.

Mental Health

Mentally healthy people are able to deal positively with life's challenges. They are able to cope with stress, remain flexible and compromise to resolve conflict. They are able to realistically evaluate situations that may occur over a lifespan and limit the negative impacts of events such as divorce and death. To be mentally healthy requires an ability to identify barriers to mental well-being and create solutions that will allow mental health to be maintained or improved. The establishment of mental health also requires an exploration of personal thoughts and feelings. This can lead to the development of self-esteem, self-acceptance, self-confidence, self-control and self-actualization. The development of these qualities can also have a positive impact on social health.

Social Health

Satisfying interpersonal relationships are essential to social well-being and overall health. In order to achieve interpersonal well-being, we must be able to learn communication skills, acquire the capacity for intimacy, and develop a network of caring people. Social health is all about the formation of warm, loving relationships with family members and friends, as well as belonging to organizations such as civic clubs and churches.

Intellectual Health

Intellectual health is characterized by an ability to absorb, understand, and utilize information in a variety of forms. It requires the capacity to view situations critically and select or create solutions that benefit the individual as well as society. Problem-solving, decision-making, and critical thinking are all components of intellectual health. The end result of effective intellectual skills is that individuals should feel more in control of their lives.

Spiritual Health

Spiritual health can be described as a belief in a higher power. It is a sense of being part of the universe and connected to other living things. Spiritual health may be cultivated through organized religion, but may also be developed through involvement in the arts, communing with nature or providing service to others. The result is a set of values and beliefs that give life meaning and purpose. For those whose lives have meaning and purpose there is typically a sense of inner peace and harmony.

What Is Wellness?

Wellness is a concept that has often been used interchangeably with health. Halbert Dunn has been given credit for coining the term wellness, which according to Dunn (1961) is a process involving a zest for living. Don Ardell (1982) describes it as a self-designed style of living that allows you to live your life to the fullest. Wellness is a dynamic process that allows individuals to function at an optimal level and adapt to a wide variety of environmental situations. Wellness behaviors include: physical activity, appropriate nutrition, maintaining appropriate body weight, stress management, wise use of all drugs, and protection from disease and injury.

Differences between Health and Wellness

Simply stated, *health is a status, while wellness is a process*. Health is the end result of personal behaviors combined with an individual's genetics and environmental surroundings, and also the appropriate utilization of available health care. Wellness, on the other hand, is the *process* of choosing health-enhancing behaviors. It is the daily conscious efforts of an individual to choose behaviors that have been identified as having a positive influence on health status. So, while health is an end result and can be measured, wellness behaviors are those observable activities an individual participates in that result in some state of health.

The Health Field Concept

The Health Field Concept (Laframboise, 1973) was developed as a result of the need to develop a framework to investigate all matters that affect health. The four components in the Health Field Concept are lifestyle, heredity, environment, and health care. According to LaLonde (1974), these four elements were identified through an examination of the causes and underlying factors of sickness and death within a population. With the development of this concept, a number of studies have been completed which provide a better understanding of the contributors to morbidity and mortality in a society and also what health professionals and individuals can do to improve health. See Table 1-1 for the results of one study using the Health Field Concept.

Lifestyle choices have the greatest impact on an individual's health in the United States. The use of tobacco, dietary excess or inadequacies, and sedentary living are the three main lifestyle contributors or risk factors associated with the leading causes of disease and death in this country.

The physical, emotional, and social environments play a significant role in the health of an individual. Environmental toxins, violence, abuse and isolation can be major contributors to the disease process and impact the decisions people make about personal behaviors.

Both the genetic disposition of an individual and the aging process play an important role in the development of disease or the maintenance of a healthy organism. Numerous studies have been done that reflect a genetic predisposition for a variety of diseases such as heart disease and cancer.

The component of the Health Field Concept that has the least impact on an individual's health is health care. However, because of the success of the medical profession in restoring

Table 1-1 ■ Estimated Contribution of Four Factors to the Ten Leading Causes of Death Before Age Seventy-Five

Cause of Death	Lifestyle (%)	Environment (%)	Biology/Heredity (%)	Inadequate Health Care (%)
Heart disease	54	9.0	25	12
Cancer	37	24	29	10
Motor vehicle Accidents	69	18	1	12
Other Accidents	51	31	4	13
Stroke	50	22	21	7
Homicide	63	35	2	0.0
Suicide	60	35	2	3
Cirrhosis	70	9	18	3
Influenza/pneumonia	23	20	39	18
Diabetes	34	0.0	60	6
All ten causes together	51.5	20.1	19.8	10

Source: From J.R. Terborg, "Health Promotion at the Worksite" in K. H. Rowland & G. R. Ferris (Eds.) *Research in Personnel and Human Resource Management,* Volume 4, Greenwich, CT: JAI Press, 1986.

our health, it is often times given credit for protecting and maintaining our health. Actually it is helping us recover from disease, illness or injury. Most people follow the philosophy, "if it ain't broke don't fix it," when it comes to their health. As a result they wait until some component of their overall health is manifesting overt signs and symptoms of some disease or illness before they go for help. The problem frequently is diagnosable and remedied through drugs or surgery. Therefore it is called "health care," when in actuality it is illness care. In recent years, health care organizations have begun to practice preventive medicine by providing health education and screening for various diseases. These activities are more consistent with the true meaning of health care.

Why Physical Fitness?

Widespread interest in health and preventative medicine has led to an increase in the number of people participating in physical fitness programs. Do not, however, be misled. The numerical values related to this statement leave much to be desired. Approximately 60% of adults in the United States exercise regularly, and 55% or more of Americans are (97 million) overweight. Unfortunately, 27% (24% adults) of Americans do not exercise at all. They choose to live a totally sedentary lifestyle.

As a result of these lifestyles, we are a more overweight and unfit nation than ever before. Our sedentary (sit-around) lifestyle has developed into a society that is experiencing an ever-increasing number of hypokinetic diseases. Hypokinetic diseases pose a real threat to the health of our nation. Improper lifestyle choices account for 51% of the deaths in the U. S. These diseases include, but are not limited to, coronary artery disease, hypertension, obesity, osteoporosis, maturity onset diabetes, ulcers, stress, and low back pain.

These disease states are costing our health care systems billions of dollars. More money is spent annually treating heart disease than any other illness. In 1997, health costs related to heart disease were approximately 275 billion dollars (AMA, 1998). Hypokinetic diseases also take a toll on the quality of life that individuals may anticipate. These diseases, for the most part, are preventable, or at least, positively influenced, through proper dietary intervention, and the implementation and adherence to a regular exercise program. Appropriate levels of fitness will not only prevent diseases and improve quality of life, but will extend longevity.

U. S. Surgeon General's Report

Every ten years the Department of Health and Human Services releases objectives for disease prevention and health promotion for our nation. In July of 1996, *Healthy People 2000* was released. It stated: "regular moderate physical activity provides substantial benefits in health and well-being for the vast majority; preventing premature death, unnecessary illness, and disability. Lack of regular physical activity is a serious threat to the health of our nation." In January 2000, *Healthy People 2010* was released. Of particular interest, **physical activity** was identified as one of the Ten Leading Health Indicators.

In consideration of these facts, the focus of this text is on the *Health-Related Components of Fitness.* These include: Cardiovascular Endurance, Muscular Strength and Endurance, Flexibility, and Body Composition. These components are concerned with, and result in, efficient bodily functioning. The focus of physical activity will be those activities an individual can be involved with for a lifetime and will have a direct, positive impact on individual health status and fitness.

Traditionally, courses of this nature have centered on the **Skill-Related Components of Fitness:** Agility, Balance, Coordination, Reaction Time, Speed, and Power. Success in sport has been tied specifically to the development of these components. These components of fitness are important and should not to be undervalued. They are not, however, related to health risk and are therefore not fully addressed in this text.

Physical Fitness, Physical Exercise, and Physical Activity

Physical fitness may be defined as the general capacity to adapt and respond favorably to physical effort. An individual is considered physically fit when systems of his/her body (i.e., cardiovascular, respiratory, muscular) are healthy and functioning efficiently. A fit person should be able to engage in daily living activities without undue fatigue. To attain or maintain a proper level of physical fitness, regular physical activity must become a part of an individual's lifestyle.

Physical activity may include everyday tasks such as walking to the store, washing the car by hand, gardening, and taking the stairs or exercise related activities such as jogging, swimming, or cycling. No matter the nature of activity, to be beneficial it must involve enough body movement and energy expenditure to reduce health risk.

Benefits of Being Physically Fit

- Lowers risk for chronic diseases and illness (CAD, cancer, strokes)
- Decreases mortality rate from chronic diseases
- Improves *quality* of life
- Improves appearance and posture
- Regulates and improves all body functions
- Increases size, strength, and power of muscles
- Develops greater lean body mass
- Increases size and strength of heart
- Increases size of the vascular system
- Increases blood volume
- Lowers resting heart rate
- Lowers blood pressure
- Helps prevent type II diabetes
- Helps sleeping patterns

- Prevents chronic back pain
- Reduces anxiety/stress
- Extends longevity
- Motivates one toward positive lifestyle changes
- Helps maintain proper weight

Economic Benefits of Being Physically Fit

Corporations implement fitness programs because participation in fitness programs leads to:

- Lower medical costs
- Fewer insurance claims
- Fewer expenses to keep workers healthy than to treat for illnesses
- Increased job productivity
- Decreased employee absenteeism
- Less depression
- Prevention of premature death
- Prevention of disability
- Reduced job turnover rate

Laboratory Activities

CHAPTER 1

For women only: If you smoke at all and take birth control pills
 −4

5. Alcohol

Figure the amount of alcoholic beverages you drink each day. One drink equals 1½ ounces of liquor or 8 ounces of beer or 6 ounces of wine. If your drinks are larger, multiply accordingly.

If your average daily number of mixed drinks, beers, or glasses of wine totals

0	0
1–2	+1
3–4	−4
5–6	−12
7–9	−20
10 or more	−30

6. Car Accidents

Most people think they wear seatbelts more than they actually wear them. Take a minute to honestly figure out how much of the time you wear seatbelts.

If the time you wear seatbelts is

Less than 25%	0
About 25%	+2
About 50%	+4
About 75%	+6
About 100%	+8

7. Stress

One way of measuring the stress in your life is to look at the changes in your life. The Holmes Scale (see Table 1-5) is designed to do this. Look at the table and add up the points for all the events on the scale that have happened to you in the past year, plus the points for all the events you expect in the near future.

If your Holmes score is

Less than 150	0
150–250	−4
251–300	−7
Over 300	−10

8. Personal History Factors

If you have been in close contact for a year or more with someone with tuberculosis
 −4

If you have had radiation (x-ray) treatment of tonsils, adenoids, acne, or ringworm of the scalp
 −6

If you have had substantial exposure to asbestos and do not smoke
 −2

If you have had substantial exposure to asbestos and do smoke
 −10

If you have had substantial exposure to vinyl chloride
 −4

9. Family History Factors

If a parent, brother, or sister had a heart attack before age 40
   −4

If a grandparent, uncle, or aunt had a heart attack before age 40
   −1

If a parent, brother, or sister has high blood pressure requiring treatment
   −2

If a grandparent, uncle, or aunt has high blood pressure requiring treatment
   −1

If a parent, brother, or sister developed diabetes **before** age 25
   −6

If a grandparent, uncle, or aunt developed diabetes **before** age 25
   −2

If a parent, brother, or sister developed diabetes **after** age 25
   −2

If a grandparent, uncle, or aunt developed diabetes **after** age 25
   −1

If you have a parent, grandparent, brother, sister, uncle, or aunt with glaucoma
   −2

If you have a parent, grandparent, brother, sister, uncle, or aunt with gout
   −1

For women, if your mother or a sister has had cancer of the breast
   −1

10. Medical Care

If you have had the following procedures regularly, score the points indicated.

Blood pressure check every year
   +4

Self-examination of breasts monthly plus examination by physician every year or two
   +2

Pap smear every year or two
   +2

Tuberculosis skin test every 5 to 10 years
   +1

Glaucoma test every 4 years after age 40
   +1

Test for hidden blood in stool every two years after age 40, every year after age 50
   +1

Proctosigmoidscopy once after age 50
   +1

11. Medical Problems

Please indicate if you have any of the following medical problems:

Arthritis	yes	no
Asthma	yes	no
Cancer	yes	no
Diabetes	yes	no
Emphysema	yes	no
Heart Problem	yes	no
High Blood Pressure	yes	no
Stroke	yes	no

Table 1-3 ■ Ideal Weights Based on Height and Body Build

\multicolumn{4}{c	}{Women}	\multicolumn{4}{c}{Men}
Height Feet	Inches	Small Frame	Medium Frame	Large Frame	Height Feet	Inches	Small Frame	Medium Frame	Large Frame

Height Feet	Inches	Small Frame	Medium Frame	Large Frame	Height Feet	Inches	Small Frame	Medium Frame	Large Frame
4	10	102–111	109–121	118–131	5	2	128–134	131–141	138–150
4	11	103–113	111–123	120–134	5	3	130–136	133–143	140–153
5	0	104–115	113–126	122–137	5	4	132–138	135–145	142–156
5	1	106–118	115–129	125–140	5	5	134–140	137–148	144–160
5	2	108–121	118–132	128–143	5	6	136–142	139–151	146–164
5	3	111–124	121–135	131–147	5	7	138–145	142–154	149–168
5	4	114–127	124–138	134–151	5	8	140–148	145–157	152–172
5	5	117–130	127–141	137–155	5	9	142–151	148–160	155–176
5	6	120–133	130–144	140–159	5	10	144–154	151–163	158–180
5	7	123–136	133–147	143–163	5	11	146–157	154–166	161–184
5	8	126–139	136–150	146–167	6	0	149–160	157–170	164–188
5	9	129–142	139–153	149–170	6	1	152–164	160–174	168–192
5	10	132–145	142–156	152–173	6	2	155–168	164–178	172–197
5	11	135–148	145–159	155–176	6	3	158–172	167–182	176–202
6	0	138–151	148–162	158–179	6	4	162–176	171–187	181–207

Source: Metropolitan Life Insurance Company.

Table 1-4 ■ Estimated Frame Size by Elbow Breadth*

Height — **Elbow Breadth***

Men	Small Frame	Medium Frame	Large Frame
< 5'4"	< 2½	2½–2⅞	> 2⅞
5'4"–5'7"	< 2⅝	2⅝–2⅞	> 2⅞
5'8"–5'11"	< 2¾	2¾–3	> 3
6'0"–6'3"	< 2¾	2¾–3⅛	> 3⅛
> 6'3"	< 2⅞	2⅞–3¼	> 3¼

Women	Small Frame	Medium Frame	Large Frame
< 5'0"	< 2¼	2¼–2½	> 2½
5'0"–5'3"	< 2¼	2¼–2½	> 2½
5'4"–5'7"	< 2⅜	2⅜–2⅝	> 2⅝
5'8"–5'11"	< 2⅜	2⅜–2⅝	> 2⅝
> 5'11"	< 2½	2½–2¾	> 2¾

*Elbow breadth measured by determining the distance between the medial and lateral epicondyles of the elbow (see Figure 1.1).

Source: Metropolitan Life Insurance Company.

Table 1-5 ■ Social Readjustment Rating Scale

Rank	Life Event	Life Change Units
1	Death of spouse	100
2	Divorce	73
3	Marital separation	65
4	Jail term	63
5	Death of close family member	63
6	Personal injury or illness	53
7	Marriage	50
8	Fired at work	47
9	Marital réconciliation	45
10	Retirement	45
11	Change in health of family member	44
12	Pregnancy	40
13	Sex difficulties	39
14	Gain of new family member	39
15	Business readjustment	39
16	Change in financial state	38
17	Death of close friend	37
18	Change to different line of work	36
19	Change in number of arguments with spouse	35
20	Large mortgage (i.e., house)	31
21	Foreclosure of mortgage or loan	30
22	Change in responsibilities at work	29
23	Son or daughter leaving home	29
24	Trouble with in-laws	29
25	Outstanding personal achievement	28
26	Wife begins or stops work	26
27	Begin or end school	26
28	Change in living conditions	25
29	Revision of personal habits	24
30	Trouble with boss	23
31	Change in work hours or conditions	20
32	Change in residence	20
33	Change in school	20
34	Change in recreation	19
35	Change in church activities	16
36	Change in social activities	18
37	Smaller mortgage or loan (i.e., car, stereo)	17
38	Change in sleeping habits	16
39	Change in number of family get-togethers	15
40	Change in eating habits	15
41	Vacation	14
42	Christmas	13
43	Minor violations of the law	11

Source: Modified from Holmes, T. and Rahe, R. (1967). The social readjustments rating scale, *Journal of Psychosomatic Research*, *11*: 213.

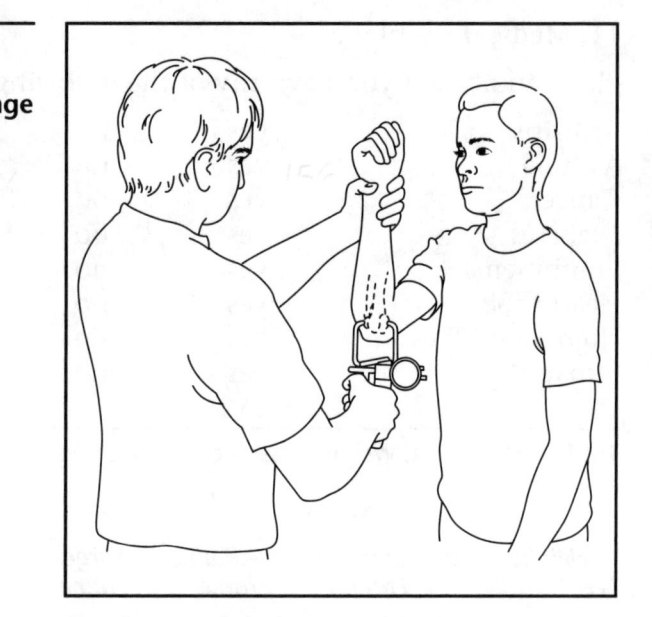

Figure 1.1 ■ Elbow Breadth Determination

Concepts of Health and Wellness ■ 27

Table 1-7 ■ Coronary Artery Disease Risk Factor Thresholds

Positive Risk Factors	Defining Criteria
Family History	MI or sudden death before age 55 in father or other male first-degree relative (i.e., brother or son), or before 65 years of age in mother or other female first-degree relative (i.e., sister or daughter)
Cigarette smoking	Current cigarette smoker or those who quit within the previous 6 months
Hypertension	Systolic blood pressure => 140 mm Hg or diastolic blood pressure => 90 mm Hg, confirmed by measurements METs on at least two separate occasions; or on anti-hypertensive medication (see Lab 4-A)
Hypercholesterolemia	Total serum cholesterol > 200 mg/dL (5.2 mmol/L) or high-density lipoprotein cholesterol of < 40 mg/dL (0.9 mmol/L), or on lipid-lowering medication. If low-density lipoprotein cholesterol is available use > 130 mg/dL (3.4 mmol/L) rather than total cholesterol of > 200 mg/dL
Impaired fasting glucose	Fasting blood glucose => 100 mg/dL (6.1 mmol/L) confirmed by measurements on at least 2 separate occasions
Obesity	Body Mass Index of => 30 kg/m^2 or waist girth of > 102 cm for men and > 88 cm for women or waist/hip ratio: = or > 0.95 for men and = or > 0.86 for women
Sedentary lifestyle	Persons not participating in a regular exercise program or meeting the minimal physical activity recommendations (accumulating 30 min. or more of moderate physical activity on most days of the week) from the U.S. Surgeon General's report

Negative Risk Factor	Defining Criteria
High serum HDL cholesterol	> 60 mg/dL (1.6 mmol/dL)

Notes: (1) It is common to sum risk factors in making clinical judgments. If HDL is high, subtract one risk factor from the sum of positive risk factors because high HDL decreases CAD risk; (2) Professional opinions vary regarding the most appropriate markers and thresholds for obesity.

Source: American College of Sports Medicine. *ACSM's Guidelines for Exercise Testing and Prescription* (7th ed.). Baltimore: Lippincott Williams & Wilkins, 2006.

Table 1-8 ■ ACSM Recommendations for (A) Current Medical Examination and Exercise Testing Prior to Participation and (B) Physician Supervision of Exercise Tests

	Low Risk	Moderate Risk	High Risk
Current Medical Examination (< one year)			
Moderate exercise*	Not Necessary***	Not Necessary	Recommended
Vigorous exercise**	Not Necessary	Recommended	Recommended
Physician Supervision of Exercise Tests			
Submaximal Test	Not Necessary	Not Necessary	Recommended
Maximal Test	Not Necessary	Recommended****	Recommended

* Absolute moderate exercise is defined as activities that approximate 3–6 METs, or the equivalent of brisk walking at 3 to 4 mph for most healthy adults. Nevertheless, a pace of 3 to 4 mph might be considered "hard" to "very hard" by some sedentary, older persons. Moderate exercise may alternatively be defined as an intensity well within the individual's capacity, one which can be comfortably sustained for a prolonged period of time (appr. 45 min.), which has a gradual initiation and progression, and is generally noncompetitive. If an individual's exercise capacity is known, relative moderate exercise may be defined by the range of 40–60% maximal oxygen uptake.

** Vigorous exercise is defined as activities of > 6 METs. Vigorous exercise may alternatively be defined as exercise intense enough to represent substantial cardiorespiratory challenge. If an individual's exercise capacity is known, vigorous exercise may be defined as an intensity of > 60% maximal oxygen uptake.

*** The designation of "Not Necessary" reflects the notion that a medical examination, exercise test, and physician supervision of exercise testing would not be essential in the preparticipation screening; however, they should not be viewed as inappropriate.

**** When physician supervision of exercise testing is "Recommended," the physician should be in close proximity and readily available should there be an emergent need.

Source: American College of Sports Medicine. *ACSM's Guidelines for Exercise Testing and Prescription* (6th ed.). Baltimore: Lippincott Williams & Wilkins, 2000.

Name: _____ Class Time/Day: _____ Score: _____

LABORATORY 1-E

Medical/Health Questionnaire

■ **Test Purpose:** This laboratory will help to determine pretest and preparticipation medical history.

■ **Precautions:** None

■ **Equipment:** Health/Medical Questionnaire (Source: Nieman, D. (1999)). *Exercise Testing and Prescription: A Health Related Approach* (4th ed.), Mountain View, CA: Mayfield.)

■ **Procedure:** Complete the questionnaire as accurately as possible.

■ **Scoring:** None

■ **Data/Calculations:**

Name: Date: / /

Gender: Age: Height: Weight:

Medical/Health Questionnaire

Personal Information

Please print your name _____

Signature _____

Age _____   Sex ___ Male ___ Female

What is your marital status? ___ Single; ___ Married; ___ Widowed; ___ Divorced/Separated

Race or ethnic background:

    ___ White, not of Hispanic origin   ___ American Indian/Alaskan native   ___ Asian

    ___ Black, not of Hispanic origin   ___ Pacific Islander   ___ Hispanic

Symptoms or Signs Suggestive of Disease

Yes   No

_____ _____ Have you experienced unusual fatigue or shortness of breath at rest, during usual activities, or during mild-to-moderate exercise (e.g., climbing stairs, carrying groceries, brisk walking, cycling)?

_____ _____ Have you had any problems with dizziness or fainting?

_____ _____ When you stand up, or sometimes during the night while you are sleeping, do you have difficulty breathing?

_____ _____ Do you suffer from swelling of the ankles (ankle edema)?

_____ _____ Have you experienced an unusual and rapid throbbing or fluttering of the heart?

_____ _____ Have you experienced severe pain in your leg muscles during walking?

_____ _____ Has a doctor told you that you have a murmur?

Chronic Disease Risk Factors

Yes   No

_____ _____ Are you a male over age 45 years, or a female over age 55 years, or a female who has experienced premature menopause and is not on estrogen replacement therapy?

_____ _____ Has your father or brother had a heart attack or died suddenly of heart disease before age 55 years; has your mother or sister experienced these heart problems before age 65 years?

_____ _____ Are you a current cigarette smoker? If yes, how many per day (on average)? _____

_____ _____ Has your doctor told you that you have high blood pressure (more than 140/90 mm Hg), or are you on medication to control your blood pressure?

_____ _____ Is your total serum cholesterol greater than 240 mg/dl, or has a doctor told you that your cholesterol is at a high-risk level?

_____ _____ Do you have diabetes mellitus?

_____ _____ Are you physically inactive and sedentary (little physical activity on the job or during leisure time)?

_____ _____ During the past year, would you say that you experienced enough stress, strain, and pressure to have a significant effect on your health?

_____ _____ Do you eat foods nearly every day that are high in fat and cholesterol, such as fatty meats, cheese, fried foods, butter, whole milk, or eggs?

_____ _____ Do you tend to avoid foods that are high in fiber such as whole-grain breads and cereals, fresh fruits or vegetables?

_____ _____ Do you weigh 30 or more pounds than you should?

_____ _____ Do you average more than two alcoholic drinks each day?

Medical History

Please check which of the following conditions you have had or now have. Also check medical conditions in your family (father, mother, brother(s), or sister(s)). Check as many as apply.

Personal	Family	Medical Condition
_____	_____	Coronary heart disease, heart attack, coronary artery surgery
_____	_____	Angina
_____	_____	High blood pressure
_____	_____	Peripheral vascular disease
_____	_____	Phlebitis or emboli
_____	_____	Other heart problems (specify: _____)
_____	_____	Lung cancer
_____	_____	Breast cancer
_____	_____	Prostate cancer
_____	_____	Colorectal cancer (bowel cancer)
_____	_____	Skin cancer
_____	_____	Other cancer (specify: _____)
_____	_____	Stroke
_____	_____	Chronic obstructive pulmonary disease (emphysema)
_____	_____	Pneumonia
_____	_____	Asthma
_____	_____	Bronchitis
_____	_____	Diabetes mellitus
_____	_____	Thyroid problems
_____	_____	Kidney disease
_____	_____	Liver disease (cirrhosis of the liver)
_____	_____	Hepatitis
_____	_____	Gallstones/gallbladder disease
_____	_____	Osteoporosis
_____	_____	Arthritis
_____	_____	Gout
_____	_____	Anemia (low iron)
_____	_____	Bone fracture
_____	_____	Major injury to foot, leg, knee, hip, or shoulder
_____	_____	Major injury to back or neck
_____	_____	Stomach/duodenal ulcer
_____	_____	Rectal growth or bleeding
_____	_____	Cataracts

		Glaucoma
____	____	Hearing loss
____	____	Depression
____	____	High anxiety, phobias
____	____	Substance abuse problems (alcohol, other drugs, etc.)
____	____	Eating disorders (anorexia, bulimia)
____	____	Problems with menstruation
____	____	Hysterectomy
____	____	Sleeping problems
____	____	Allergies
____	____	Any other health problems (specify and include information on any recent illnesses, hospitalizations, or surgical procedures):

_____

_____

Please check any of the following medications you currently take regularly. Also give the name of the medication

Medication	Name of Medication
____ Heart medicine	_____
____ Blood pressure medicine	_____
____ Blood cholesterol medicine	_____
____ Hormones	_____
____ Birth control pills	_____
____ Medicine for breathing/lungs	_____
____ Insulin	_____
____ Other medicine for diabetes	_____
____ Arthritis medicine	_____
____ Medicine for depression	_____
____ Medicine for anxiety	_____
____ Thyroid medicine	_____
____ Medicine for ulcers	_____
____ Painkiller medicine	_____
____ Allergy medicine	_____
____ Other (please specify)	_____

Physical Fitness, Physical Activity/Exercise

In general, compared to other persons your age, rate how physically fit you are:

1 __ 2 __ 3 __ 4 __ 5 __ 6 __ 7 __ 8 __ 9 __ 10 __

Not at all   Somewhat   Extremely
physically fit   physically fit   physically fit

Outside of your normal work or daily responsibilities, how often do you engage in exercise that at least moderately increases your breathing and heart rate and makes you sweat for at least 20 minutes (such as brisk walking, cycling, swimming, jogging, aerobic dance, stair climbing, rowing, basketball, racquetball, vigorous yard work)?

 __ 5 or more times per week __ 3–4 times per week __ 1–2 times per week

 __ less than 1 time per week __ seldom or never

How much hard physical work is required on your job?

 __ a great deal __ a moderate amount __ a little __ none

How long have you exercised or played sports regularly?

 __ I do not exercise regularly __ less than 1 year __ 1–2 years

 __ 2–5 years __ 5–10 years __ more than 10 years

Diet

On average, how many servings of fruit do you eat per day? (One serving = 1 medium apple, banana, orange, etc.; ½ cup of chopped, cooked, or canned fruit; ¾ cup of fruit juice.)

 __ none __ 1 __ 2 __ 3 __ 4 or more

On average, how many servings of vegetables do you eat per day? (One serving = ½ cup cooked or chopped raw, 1 cup raw leafy, ¾ cup of vegetable juice.)

 __ none __ 1–2 __ 3 __ 4 __ 5 of more

On average, how many servings of bread, cereal, rice, or pasta do you eat per day? (One serving = 1 slice of bread, 1 ounce of ready-to-eat cereal, ½ cup of cooked cereal, rice, or pasta.)

 __ none __ 1–3 __ 4–6 __ 7–9 __ 10 or more

When you use grain and cereal products, which do you emphasize

 __ whole grain, high fiber __ mixture of whole grain and refined __ refined, low fiber

On average, how many servings of red meat (not lean) do you eat per day? (One serving = 2–3 ounces of steak, roast beef, lamb, pork chops, hamburgers, etc.)

 __ none __ 1 __ 2 __ 3 __ 4 or more

On average, how many servings of fish, poultry, lean meat, cooked dry beans, peanut butter, or nuts do you eat per day? (One serving = 2–3 ounces of meat, ½ cup of cooked dry beans, two tablespoons of peanut butter, or ⅓ cup of nuts.)

 __ none __ 1 __ 2 __ 3 __ 4 or more

On average, how many servings of dairy products do you eat per day? (One serving = 1 cup of milk or yogurt, 1.5 ounces of natural cheese, 2 ounces of processed cheese.)

___ none ___ 1 ___ 2 ___ 3 ___ 4 or more

When you use dairy products, which do you emphasize?

___ regular ___ low fat ___ nonfat

How would you characterize your intake of fats and oils (e.g., regular salad dressings, butter or margarine, mayonnaise, vegetable oils)?

___ high ___ moderate ___ low

Body Weight

How tall are you (without shoes)? _____ feet _____ inches

How much do you weigh (minimal clothing and without shoes)? _____ pounds

What is the most you have ever weighed? _____ pounds

Are you *now* trying to:

___ lose weight ___ gain weight ___ stay about the same ___ not do anything

Psychological Health

How have you been feeling in general during the past month?

___ in excellent spirits ___ in good spirits mostly ___ in low spirits mostly
___ in very good spirits ___ up and down in spirits a lot ___ in very low spirits

During the past month, would you say that you experienced _____ stress?

___ a lot of ___ moderate ___ relatively little ___ almost no

In the past year, how much effect has stress had on your health?

___ a lot ___ some ___ hardly any or none

On average, how many hours of sleep do you get in a 24-hour period?

___ less than 5 ___ 5–6.9 ___ 7–9 ___ more than 9

Substance Use

Have you smoked at least 100 cigarettes in your entire life? ___ yes ___ no

How would you describe your cigarette smoking habits?

___ never smoked ___ used to smoke

How many years has it been since you smoked? _____ years ___ still smoke

How many cigarettes a day do you smoke on average? _____ cigarettes / day

How many alcoholic drinks do you consume? (A "drink" is a glass of wine, a wine cooler, a bottle / can of beer, a shot glass of liquor, or a mixed drink).

___ never use alcohol ___ less than 1 per week ___ 1–6 per week
___ 1 per day ___ 2–3 per day ___ more than 3 per day

Source: Nieman, D. (1999). *Exercise Testing and Prescription: A Health Related Approach* (4th ed.), Mountain View, CA: Mayfield.

2

Understanding and Changing Human Behavior

'Tis easier to prevent bad habits than to break them.
Ben Franklin

■ Chapter Outline ■

Understanding Our Behaviors
Determinants of Behavior
    Predisposing Factors
    Reinforcing Factors
    Enabling Factors
    Levels of Prevention
Developing a Behavior Change Plan
    Locus of Control
    Transtheoretical Model
    Six Stages of Change
        Precontemplation
        Contemplation
        Preparation
        Action
        Maintenance
        Termination
Making the Change
    Step 1: Choose a Problem Behavior
    Step 2: Learn Your Actions and Behaviors
    Step 3: Establish Personal Goals and Objectives
    Step 4: Prepare a Plan of Action
    Step 5: Implement Your Plan
    Step 6: Revaluate and Modify Your Plan

■ Learning Objectives ■

The student should be able to:

- Discuss the determinants of behavior, including but not limited to, predisposing factors, reinforcing factors, and enabling factors.
- Describe the three levels of prevention and the role prevention plays in living a positive, healthy lifestyle.
- Define and discuss the role of internal locus of control in influencing our behaviors.
- Define and discuss the role of external locus of control in influencing our behaviors.
- List and explain the six stages of change as described in the Transtheoretical Model.
- Identify and discuss steps or courses of action taken when attempting to modify behavior.

Keywords

- Action stage
- Barriers
- Contemplation stage
- Efficacy
- Enabling factors
- External locus of control
- Internal locus of control
- Maintenance stage
- Negative reinforcement
- Positive reinforcement
- Precontemplation stage
- Predisposing factors
- Preparation stage
- Primary prevention
- Reinforcing factors
- Secondary prevention
- Sedentary lifestyle
- Termination stage
- Tertiary prevention
- Transtheoretical model

Understanding Our Behaviors

Why do we act the way we do? Why do we make the choices we make? What behavioral choices are we making that directly influence our health-related fitness? The answers to these and other related questions are important.

Most of us have tried to make a long-term change in our lifestyles. For example, we may have tried to lose a couple of extra pounds by altering our diet and beginning a regular walking program. Yet, over time we found ourselves noncompliant and returned back to our old, bad habits and ways. Unfortunately, as a result of this process, we quickly learn, behavior change is not easy and it doesn't simply happen because we want it to.

Why does this occur? Why do some people find success in managing and/or changing their lifestyle and behavior, while others only struggle and fail?

In many cases, personal history and previous attitudes and knowledge may play critical and important roles in our behavior. For example, our past history with physical activity may have been negative. We may have been picked last for a team when we were young and remember the sting of rejection. We may have improperly tried to implement a regular fitness program into our lifestyle only to find our inappropriate approach left us sore and unwilling to continue.

To begin to understand our behavior, let's look to see what factors may influence or alter our behaviors. These are discussed under the subheader *Determinants of Behavior* below. Then we will review three levels of prevention that may help us to develop a better understanding of activities that may restrict or prevent a behavior from occurring. Finally, we will look at how to change our behavior. By developing an understanding of the behavioral-change process, we are better prepared to successfully implement a positive, long-term lifestyle change.

Determinants of Behavior

Predisposing Factors

Predisposing factors are described as what an individual knows, feels or believes about a certain behavior or situation. Predisposing factors can influence our behaviors and make it difficult for us to be willing to change our current behavior. For example, knowledge of nutrition may *predispose* some individuals to make proper food choices that enable them to meet nutritional guidelines. In contrast, how individuals feel about a particular food may result in a failure to apply what he/she knows about nutrition. For example, some may know that eating excessive amounts of cheese in their diet would mean they are consuming a diet high in fat. Yet, because they enjoy the taste of cheese they continue to eat large quantities. This example demonstrates one common finding regarding predisposing factors. Just because a person may know the right health related behavior, doesn't mean he/she will practice it. *There is little evidence to support that raising an individual's knowledge, in and of itself, will result in behavioral change.*

Another interesting finding regarding predisposing factors is that our beliefs are more powerful than our knowledge and attitudes in terms of influencing our health-related fitness behaviors. Hales (2002) has suggested that individuals are more likely to change their behavior if they have three beliefs. These include:

- They believe they are *susceptible or at risk* because of their current behavior.
- They believe the price they will pay for their behavior is too *severe.*
- They believe they will *benefit* by changing their behavior to a more appropriate behavior.

Other predisposing factors may influence our health-related fitness. Unfortunately, we may not be able to positively change these factors. For example, some of us are genetically linked to families with health histories of elevated cholesterol levels, heart disease, or diabetes. Alternatively, we may have grown up in a family that had a history of poor diet and sedentary living. While we cannot change our parents, we can take positive action to recognize these factors and try to positively address them in our lifestyles. We do not have to choose to live a sedentary lifestyle and eat a poor diet.

Reinforcing Factors

Reinforcing factors are identified as the social support people have for participating or not participating in a particular behavior. If one member of a family chooses to begin an exercise program and others within the family encourage and assist that person, it would be seen as **positive reinforcement**.

If, on the other hand, a family member or somebody working within an office environment attempts to quit smoking and those around that person do not respect that choice and continue to smoke and ridicule the person's attempts to quit, this lack of support would be seen as **negative reinforcement** and would make it difficult to change that behavior.

It is important to recognize the value of reinforcing factors. Praise and rewards have an extremely positive role in behavioral management. This is particularly true when new behaviors are being acquired. Over time, however, the commitment to change must come from within the individual.

For example, consider the individual mentioned above who has chosen to begin an exercise program. There is little doubt that being praised, respected, and maybe even admired by family and friends for his/her efforts will help to continue in the program objective. In time, however, this individual will have to rely on his/her own internal motivation, commitment, and sense of accomplishment if he/she hopes to be successful and enjoy the health and fitness related benefits of maintaining a long-term program.

Enabling Factors

Enabling factors are environmental and organizational barriers or facilitators to behaviors. An example of an enabling factor that facilitates wellness behavior would be the development of bike paths, routes or trails around a community. The bike paths, in and of themselves, provide the individual the opportunity to bike without fear of being on an open highway and exposed to the risks of riding in traffic.

In contrast, **barriers** work in opposition to enabling factors. For example, a barrier to a proper diet or appropriate food consumption might be the constant exposure to the plethora of franchise food establishments and vending machines. The ease of access and convenience of these establishments have the potential to negatively influence us to choose a fast food meal instead of taking the time to properly prepare healthier meals containing the whole grains, fresh fruits and vegetables, lean meats, and low-fat dairy products that we should be consuming.

Levels of Prevention

In most cases, people choose to worry about their health and health-related fitness levels after they have lost them. Few have the foresight and wisdom, 1) to understand the value of preventing bad health habits from developing, and 2) to take appropriate steps to lead active lives. One of the most obvious and often neglected steps a person can take to assist in health-related lifestyle management is prevention.

The power of prevention cannot go unstated. For example, eighty percent (80%) of the deaths associated with cardiovascular diseases could be avoided, or at a minimum delayed, by preventative measures. Hales (2002) indicates that 2 out of 3 deaths, and 1 out of 3 hospitalizations, could be prevented by altering our lifestyles.

How then can individuals live a preventative lifestyle? What aspects of their lives should they be concerned? What steps can they take to prevent a health/fitness related problem from presenting itself in their lives? These are important questions. The value of proper prevention and the negative costs, both financial and physical, of not taking proper preventive measures has been clearly established.

The health care profession has begun to recognize the value of prevention and is beginning to practice more preventive medicine. Although most of us have a simple definition of prevention (activities that don't allow something to occur), prevention actually occurs on three levels. These are delineated as primary, secondary, and tertiary prevention.

Primary prevention reflects what most of us believe prevention is all about such as activities that prevent an illness, disease or injury from ever occurring. Examples of these activities include health education and immunizations.

Secondary prevention activities involve early detection and treatment of a disease in order to limit the duration and severity of the disease. Examples of secondary prevention activities include screenings for blood pressure, cholesterol and skin cancer. There are a number of routine exams that health consumers should participate in. These can be found in Table 2-1.

Table 2-1 ■ Routine Health Screening: Recommendations for Disease Prevention

Medical Test/Measurement	Recommended Frequency
Blood Pressure	Every medical visit; at least once every 2 years
Height/Weight (by health care practitioner)	Every 1 to 3 years
Cholesterol	Every 5 years after 18 years of age
Glucose (diabetes screening)	Every year after 50 years of age
Dental	Every 6 to 12 months
Glaucoma	Annually after age 65 years of age
Prostate (PSA)	Annually after 50 years of age
Breast Examination (by health care practitioner)	Annually after 40 years of age
Breast Examination (by women)	Annually after 20 years of age
Mammograms	Baseline by age 40; every 1 to 2 years between 40 and 49; annually after 50 years
Pap test for cervical cancer	Every 1 to 3 years after first sexual intercourse; if previous screenings have been normal, no testing is needed after 65 years of age
Flu Vaccination	Annually for people 65 years of age and older

Source: Adapted from Sox, H.C. 1994. Preventive Health Services in Adults. *Journal of the American Medical Association, 330,* 1589–1595.

The third level of prevention is called **tertiary prevention.** Activities at this level focus on rehabilitation. They may involve cardiac rehabilitation for an individual who had a cardiac event, or physical therapy for someone who had an orthopedic problem (Cottrell, Girvan, and McKenzie, 1999).

No matter what level of prevention considered, preventive efforts have proven to be positive. In terms of the four health-related fitness areas, increased physical activity and weight management have been positively effected by preventive measures.

Developing a Behavior Change Plan

When attempting to achieve a positive lifestyle and optimal health and fitness, all of us will have to fight unique personal battles. It would be nice if everyone practiced primary prevention and avoided all illness, disease and injury. That, however, is simply not the case. Ultimately, many of us choose to use tobacco, pay little or no attention to dietary needs, fail to remain active throughout life, engage in risky sexual behavior, inappropriately use alcohol and illicit drugs, and drive our vehicles in an unsafe fashion.

The good news is that we can change. Change must come from within. The state of readiness required to initiate a behavior change can be developed by reading books, attending classes, or from life's experiences. Motivation for change in the American culture most likely involves short-term personal goals such as looking better, being more popular, or improving at a sport, rather than being concerned about what is going to happen when we get older.

Increasing our awareness of the risks associated with behaviors may heighten motivation. Increased motivation may also come from external forces such as the social pressure to stop smoking. The most common behaviors people want to change are: use of tobacco, alcohol consumption, caffeine consumption, sleeping patterns, stress management, dietary habits, and *physical activity*. Some goals related to these behaviors include losing weight, developing more friendships, and becoming more spiritually-centered.

Locus of Control

What external events occur in our lives? What internal forces stimulate us or motivate us to change? Internal and external forces are important for us to recognize as we attempt to identify sources of responsibility for the events that occur in our lives. Some of us believe we are in control of our lives and its course of action. Others of us believe that external events control our destiny.

People who believe they have control over their lives are said to have an **internal locus of control.** These individuals believe that they can make a difference and control or positively influence their state of health and fitness.

Individuals who believe factors beyond their control are impacting and controlling their lives are said to have an **external locus of control.** These individuals believe factors such as heredity, family histories, and their environment have more control over their lives than they do. As a result, they place little value in preventative health care and will take few steps to manage their state of health and fitness.

Efficacy is the belief that one is capable of changing a behavior. If you believe you can make a change, you most likely will succeed. If you believe it is unlikely that you can succeed in your efforts to change, you most likely will fail.

Those with an internal locus of control possess an extremely important quality and are more likely to be successful in managing their lifestyle and controlling their health and fitness related behaviors. Since these individuals believe they can make a difference, they are more motivated and optimistic about achieving a positive outcome. Individuals who present a high external locus of control are more likely to fail in their attempts at behavioral management.

There is no precise formula for change that is 100% successful, but there are models for change that set the stage for individuals to make health-enhancing alterations in their lifestyle. Essentially, behavior change involves *self-assessment, self-management and reassessment*.

Transtheoretical Model

Behavioral change is a processs, not an event. As a result, various models have been developed to help explain human behavior, as well as assist in the process of changing human behavior. The diet we choose to eat and the level of physical activity we regularly participate in are direct expressions of our behaviour. One of the most effective models in helping individuals change, their health-fitness related behaviors over time, is the **Transtheoretical Model** (Prochaska, 1979). This model has been used to assist in changing a variety of health and fitness related behaviors, including but not limited to, weight management (Prochaska, Norcross, Fowler, Follick, & Abrams, 1992; Prochaska & DiClemente, 1985) and physical inactivity.

In his model, Prochoska and his colleagues (1994) describe six stages of change individuals may pass through on their way to healthy behavior. These stages are: precontemplation, contemplation, preparation, action, maintenance, and termination. They are discussed under separate headers below and summarized in Table 2-2. The use of the model seems warranted in the health related areas of weight management, smoking cessation, substance abuse, and correcting for a sedentary or inactive lifestyle. For purposes of illustration, throughout the description of the six stages of change we will hypothetically consider the example of a sedentary individual going through the process of changing lifestyle and becoming more active.

Table 2-2 ■ Stages of the Transtheoretical Model

Stage	Description and Timeframe
Precontemplation	Resistant and unwilling to change behavior within the next 6 months
Contemplation	Considering change in the future (< 6 months)
Preparation	Gathering information and getting ready to change in the immediate future (< 1 month)
Action	Actively attempting to change
Maintenance	Actively living the changed behavior (< 5 years)
Termination	Maintained the changed behavior of over 5 years

Six Stages of Change

Precontemplation

Precontemplation is characterized by an individual who has no intention of changing a behavior, at least not within the next 6 months, or is giving no thought to the behavior. It does not matter that those around him may recognize the potential harm associated with the behavior. An individual in the precontemplation stage makes no attempt to recognize the problem, or if he does recognize it, he denies it. He will avoid or resist any attempts to help in changing the behavior.

Individuals who are in this stage have little chance of successfully altering their behavior over the long-term. In fact, few will even initiate a change in behavior unless pressured externally by family or friends. Normally, some event or series of events must occur before this individual is willing to move to the next stage. During the precontemplation stage, raising an individuals level of awareness and knowledge about negative lifestyle behaviors may help him to move forward toward the stage of contemplation.

Consider our hypothetical example of the sedentary individual. In the precontemplation stage, this individual places no value on regular physical activity and may openly avoid any form of physical activity. Helping this individual understand the positive health-related benefits of regular physical activity might help him to move forward into the second stage.

Contemplation

The second stage in the transtheoretical model is the contemplation stage. **Contemplation** begins when a person acknowledges that his/her behavior is a problem and may negatively impact his/her life. During this stage, the person is willing to investigate the underlying causes and possible solutions to the problem or behavior. This may involve reading information about the behavior and its effects or listening to others who have dealt with a similar situation. *It does not mean that the individual is ready to make a commitment and begin to take action to change his/her behavior.* Individuals may remain in this stage for long periods of time, even though they may believe they are intending to take action in the next couple of months.

Consider again our hypothetical example of the sedentary individual. In the contemplation stage, this individual is now willing to openly discuss and consider the positive benefits of regular physical activity and is able to admit that current behavior of a sedentary lifestyle is or will negatively impact his/her life. During the stage of contemplation, this individual is carefully considering and weighing out the pros and cons of beginning a regular physical activity program. In truth, the more knowledge and facts about the benefits of regular physical activity he can gain, the more likely he will be to move forward and begin an exercising program. External support from family and friends, and any information he can gain about the benefits of regular activity will help in moving forward to the next stage, the stage of preparation.

Preparation

The third stage of the transtheoretical model is referred to as the preparation stage. **Preparation** involves the final adaptations required before actually beginning a behavior change. During this stage, the individual presents both intention and behavioral change criteria. For example, he/she may establish intent to quit smoking by identifying a quit date. He/she may present behavioral change criteria by starting to cut back on the number of cigarettes they are smoking in preparation for the quit date.

Another way to get prepared for a change is to establish some baseline data about the behavior. This may come in the form of recording food intake or recording information about smoking in a journal. After summarizing the data, some specific goals can be established. It may be a good idea to *enter into a personal contract* that indicates starting and beginning dates for the behavior change process and the amount of time and personal resources that will be required.

Consider again our hypothetical example of the sedentary individual. In the contemplation stage, this individual may begin investigating the services provided by local fitness clubs. He might purchase clothes and shoes that he believes he will need for exercising. This individual may begin to establish personal goals and program objectives he hopes to achieve after beginning the fitness program. He might seek active membership in a fitness club to coincide with their predetermined start date.

Action

The fourth stage of the transtheoretical model is the action stage. **Action** is the most obvious of the stages and the one that requires the most time and energy. The person engaging in the behavior change is now applying what was learned during the contemplation stage and visualized during the preparation stage. As he begins to exhibit a new behavior, whether it is diet modification or smoking cessation or whatever, this is the stage where he will receive attention from those around him. Positive reinforcement is crucial and family, friends, and co-workers should be encouraged to aid in this process.

In addition, the action phase should include a diary or journal to keep track of progress toward desired goals. If the action phase is continued, then the individual will be able to move forward into the next stage, the stage of maintenance.

Consider again our hypothetical example. During this stage, our sedentary individual will actively begin to participate in a program of regular fitness activities. This individual may demonstrate his actions by walking, jogging, cycling, or resistive training. The specific actions presented will be consistent with predetermined goals and objectives formulated during the earlier stages and potentially detailed in the behavioral management contract. In addition to increasing his aerobic activity, this individual may begin to change other health and fitness related behaviors, such as altering his diet by eating less calories or reducing fat intake.

It is important that during the action stage the participant gains self-confidence and participates in activities he enjoys. In this stage, it would also be appropriate for this individual to develop a reward structure that positively reinforces him when he accomplishes established goals.

Maintenance

The last stage of the transtheoretical model is the maintenance stage. The **maintenance** stage requires the individual to take steps to sustain the change and resist temptation to relapse. Basically, he is fine-tuning and adapting to the new lifestyle. This is the time to utilize the information gathered during the contemplation and preparation stages about the obstacles and the temporary setbacks that may occur during the change process. The person must continue to monitor the behavior and follow through with the system of rewards that have been predetermined and are typically identified in the behavior contract.

According to Prochaska, Norcross, Fowler, Follick, & Abrams (1992), for addictive behaviors, the maintenance stage begins about six months after the overt action to change begins. The initiation of this stage has not been defined for many other non-addictive behaviors.

In our hypothetical example, the maintenance stage is nothing more than a continuation of the fitness program and all the positive behaviors that have been developed. At this point, our previously sedentary individual is working to keep the gains he has made as a result of the new behavior. He is working to avoid relapsing back into old habits and behaviors. The object of the maintenance stage for this individual is to maintain the new active, healthy lifestyle for a lifetime.

Termination

The **termination** of the behavior change process occurs when the new behavior becomes fully integrated into the individual's lifestyle. For example, ex-smokers may continue to have memories of cigarettes, but the urge to smoke is under control. The same goes for those who have begun exercise programs or have modified their diets. Their new way of life becomes a "mostly permanent" way of life. "Mostly permanent" because as with any behavior, the threat of relapse is constant. At the termination stage, however, conscious efforts are not directed at changing behavior. Instead, the individual is simply living his/her life.

Remember that you did not develop any particular behavior overnight, so do not expect change to occur rapidly. In a similar vein, an acquired behavior is not lost with a single relapse. *Lifestyle behavioral management is an ongoing, process.* It should be viewed positively and as a means of helping to assist individuals in establishing and living full and optimal lives.

Making the Change

Once individuals understand the consequences of their behaviors and recognize a need to change those behaviors, what can they do to begin to alter their behaviors? What are the steps that people can make that will help them succeed in changing a bad behavior into a good behavior? Below is a common course of action that, when followed, may assist in helping a person to establish behavioral change. The steps include:

1. Choose a Problem Behavior
2. Learn your Actions and Behaviors
3. Establish Personal Goals and Objectives
4. Prepare a Plan of Action
5. Implement Your Plan
6. Revaluate and Modify Your Plan

Step 1: Choose a Problem Behavior

The first step in making a change is to identify the behavior you wish to alter. Be selective. The chance of successfully altering one behavior is far greater than trying to alter many. *Don't try and change all your negative behaviors at once.* It is highly unlikely that you can lose weight, increase your physical activity levels, lower your alcohol consumption, and stop smoking all at one time. For purposes of illustration, a hypothetical example of an overweight individual wanting to reduce his body fatness will be provided.

Step 2: Learn Your Actions and Behaviors

Once you have targeted a behavior you would like to change, examine your actions and how they are linked to the targeted behavior. Using a journal or log may prove helpful. Using the hypothetical example proposed above, our overweight individual may want to begin to record the types of foods he/she is eating and their quantity of intake. He also needs to determine other factors such as, time of day, his moods, where he was located, and how hungry he was when he ate. It is not uncommon to find patterns of behavior or stimuli that are related to overeating. Certain foods may be identified as being abused. Mood swings or job situations may be linked to excessive eating. Many people find they eat when they are not really hungry, but rather when they have the time. Some may find they have developed relationships between their eating behaviors and other activities such as watching television. Others may find they eat when they are lonely or depressed.

It may also be helpful to gain as much knowledge about the benefits of your proposed behavioral change. Understanding the risks of being overweight or living a sedentary life may help in developing a better understanding of why an individual may want to change a behavior. *Knowledge is power*. In this situation, that power can be used to motivate and encourage an individual to remain steadfast in his/her desire to change a negative behavior.

Step 3: Establish Personal Goals and Objectives

Establishing realistic and achievable goals is critical in being able to successfully change a behavior. Establish goals that can be measured in both the short-term and the long-term. Avoid the use of long-term goals only. Be specific when establishing goals. Avoid vague goals. Successful accomplishment of any goal must be clearly established. Adherence to any behavioral change typically results from finding small successes that can be built upon.

Establish a **personal contract** regarding the behavior change. This will help establish personal commitment and responsibility. This should be a written agreement. Use your personal goals and objectives to guide you. Evaluate and update this contract regularly. The contract should be flexible.

Contracts need to provide opportunities for success, but must not be so easy that they have limited meaning. Slightly challenging contractual agreements offer the opportunity to build success and provide opportunities to build confidence. In contrast, if the contract establishes unrealistic goals and objectives, it will ensure failure and frustration. Unrealistic goals and objectives in personal contracts should be avoided.

Consider again our hypothetical example. It is unrealistic for our overweight individual to set a goal of losing 30 pounds in 30 days. Not only is this goal unrealistic, it would also be an unhealthy approach to accomplishing his/her objective. A better goal would be to lose 2 pounds per week.

Goals that are more specific could also be established. For example, a number of easily identifiable and short-term goals could include cutting out snacks, eating only at meal times, eliminating all candy bars from the diet and replacing them with a piece of fruit. Accomplishing these short-term goals will help to establish confidence and lead to long-term success.

Step 4: Prepare a Plan of Action

After specific goals and objectives have been established it is important to develop an appropriate plan or course of action that will lead to a successful change in the desired behavior. Establish or determine specific techniques or strategies that will lead to proper change. These strategies may include modifications in personal lifestyle, changes in the current environment, developing a support system with friends and family, and identifying specific rewards when goals have been accomplished.

Identify known or suspected barriers that will hinder successful change. Develop alternative courses of action to help remove these barriers. Remember, no barrier is so large that it will prevent a successful change in behavior unless you allow it. All barriers can be moved, by passed, or walked over. The key to success is determining how what works.

Continuing our hypothetical example, our overweight individual may include in his plan, a dietary intake log and an activity log designed to monitor caloric intake and exercise related behavior. This individual may establish or prepare weekly meal plans that are designed to meet predetermined caloric intake goals. He may establish a calendar that identifies specific dates when he will measure his body fatness to assess his progress and achievements. He may develop a strategy to alter his normal diet to adjust for unusual situations such as a wedding reception, travel, illness, or holidays. He may develop specific grocery lists that prevent the purchase of unnecessary snack items or tempting foods.

He may advise his friends and family of his intentions and ask for their support. He may even prepare a list of "do's and don'ts" designed to reinforce his desired behavior change objective. For example, he may specifically ask family members to not prepare for his consumption selected foods such as cakes or pies. He may ask for support during meals by requesting family members or friends to not tempt or encouraged him to eat more than his plan has established. Statements like "Go ahead, one little helping isn't going to hurt you," should be discouraged.

The plan of action may include specific rewards. For example, our overweight individual may establish specific body weight objectives so that when he achieves these new lower levels he will reward himself with the purchase of a new clothing item.

Step 5: Implement Your Plan

After the plan of action has been developed, the next step toward behavioral change is to implement the plan. Be firm. Avoid the temptation of complacency and procrastination. Now is the time to begin. Focus on why you want to make the change. Remember that you are in charge of your future. Do not allow external factors to change your course of action. Keep your motivation up and enjoy the positive benefits that your plan will provide.

Self-management is critical to success. While it is important to take advantage of the social support offered by friends, coworkers, and family, do not rely on them. Praise from others, while important, will not in and of itself guarantee success. Trust yourself and your actions.

Use your predetermined strategies and techniques to keep you focused. Honestly determine your successes and failures. Evaluate why you failed and develop strategies to avoid these pitfalls in the future. Do not be afraid to revise your plan of action. Remember, changing behavior is an ongoing process. It is not the action of a single event.

Refer back to our hypothetical example. What can our overweight individual expect? What temptations will he face? What can he do to stay the course? First, it is important for this individual to recognize that he developed his negative behavior and their excessive levels of body fatness over the course of his life. He must recognize that his plan is not going to bring an instant change. He must recognize that while there are safe and reliable methods for successfully losing body fat, none provide quick results.

We live in a fast-paced world. We have grown to expect everything in our lives to occur rapidly. Behavioral change does not happen rapidly. Like our hypothetical individual, all of us must learn to accept this and be patient. *Change can and will occur over time.* Do not forget, there is a future for all of us. Time will pass. The question is, "What will the future for our hypothetical candidate hold?" Will he find success or failure one year from now? One thing is certain; one year from now will present itself no matter what he does or what course of action he takes. This finding will be the same for you. Where will you be one year from now? What changes will have occurred in your life?

In our example, our overweight subject must also recognize that changing his behavior is not a short-term fix to a bad problem in his life. His plan is designed to alter the way he lives. He must be willing and motivated to make this lifetime alteration and commitment. He must look positively to the gains he expects from the success of the plan. He must not view the new behavior as a negative aspect in his life that is forcing him to make a change and/or forcing him to sacrifice or give up something he is not willing and ready to let go.

This individual must also accept the change he is making in his life will not come easily. He will fail at times and relapse back into old bad habits. He must be prepared for these occurrences. He must implement preprepared action plans to address failure. He cannot and should not dwell on the failure, but should analyze it and determine why he failed.

This individual must learn to use his dietary log and exercise journal. He needs to vigilantly record his actions and behaviors. By studying this record, he will be able to identify triggers to success and triggers to failure. He will be able to develop strategies to avoid the negative triggers.

Step 6: Revaluate and Modify Your Plan

It is extremely important to periodically revaluate and modify your plan. No one develops the perfect model. Change will be necessary and should be expected. Do not view this as negative. Look to find ways to better assist you in achieving your goals and objectives. Look for areas of weakness and refine your plan to address them. Don't be afraid to take new approaches that meet current needs. Monitor your level of enjoyment and boredom.

Continuing with our example, our hypothetical candidate should carefully monitor his food intake and exercise habits. He/she should be willing to explore different positive and healthy approaches to his/her diet or activity habits. By varying diet and exercise history, he/she can prevent the risk of boredom and the potential for relapse.

Laboratory Activities

CHAPTER 2

Name: _____ Class Time/Day: _____ Score: _____

LABORATORY 2-A

Implementing Behavior Change

■ **Purpose:** To identify a health-related fitness behavior you would like to change by either increasing or decreasing.

■ **Precautions:** None

■ **Equipment:** Note pad and pencil.

■ **Procedure:**

Step 1: Choose a Problem Behavior:

a. Identify a health-related fitness behavior you would like to change.

Step 2: Learn Your Actions and Behaviors:

a. Examine your actions and behaviors related to the chosen behavior for one week. Record this information in a log.

b. Develop an itemized list of the health-related benefits of changing your chosen behavior.

1.

2.

3.

c. Develop an itemized list of health-related *risks* associated with **not** changing your chosen behavior.

1.

2.

3.

Step 3: Establish Personal Goals and Objectives:

a. Establish realistic short-term and long-term goals related to your behavior change objective. Be specific.

Short-Term

1.

2.

3.

Long-Term

1.

2.

3.

    b. Use your itemized short-term and long-term goals to establish a personal contract.

Step 4: Prepare a Plan of Action

    a. Prepare and itemize specific strategies you plan to use to help in changing your behavior.

        1.

        2.

        3.

    b. Identify suspected or known barriers that will hinder your success in changing your behavior.

        1.

        2.

        3.

    c. Identify specific actions to help remove known or suspected barriers to successful change of your behavior.

        1.

        2.

        3.

    d. Identify specific rewards you plan to enjoy when stated short-term and long-term objectives are achieved.

        1.

        2.

        3.

Step 5: Implement Your Plan

Step 6: Revaluate and Modify Your Plan

■ **Scoring:** None

■ **Data/Calculations:** None

Name: _____ Class Time/Day: _____ Score: _____

LABORATORY 2-B

Readiness for Behavioral Change

■ **Purpose:** To identify behaviors that inhibit your health-related fitness and to determine your willingness to change those behaviors by matching them to the stages of the Transtheoretical Model.

■ **Precautions:** None

■ **Equipment:** Note pad and pencil.

■ **Procedure:** Identify and itemize behaviors that inhibit your health-related fitness. Determine your willingness to change each behavior by matching your current thinking with the descriptions and timeframes presented in Table 2-3. Enter the appropriate stage in the space provided.

Health-Inhibiting Behavior	Stage
1.	
2.	
3.	
4.	
5.	
6.	
7.	
8.	
9.	
10.	

■ Scoring:

Table 2-3 ■ Stages and Descriptive Timeframes of the Transtheoretical Model

Stage	Description and Timeframe
Precontemplation	Resistant and unwilling to change behavior within the next 6 months
Contemplation	Considering change in the future (< 6 months)
Preparation	Gathering information and getting ready to change in the immediate future (< 1 month)
Action	Actively attempting to change
Maintenance	Actively living the changed behavior (< 5 years)
Termination	Maintained the changed behavior of over 5 years

■ Data/Calculations: None

Name: Date: /   /

Gender: Age: Height: Weight:

Which behaviors are you most likely ready to change?

1.

2.

3.

4.

5.

3

Beginning a Health-Related Fitness Program

*Begin where you are. But don't stay where you are.
Improvement begins with "I."*
Unknown

■ Chapter Outline ■

Basic Considerations When Beginning a Fitness Program
Beginning a Fitness Program: Basic Training Principles
    Principle of Adaptation
    Principle of Overload
    Principle of Progressive Overload
    Principle of Reversibility (Disuse)
    Principle of Consistency
    Principle of Specificity
    Principle of Individuality
    Principle of Hard and Easy
    Principle of Safety
Three Basic Elements of a Daily Exercise Session
    Warm-up
    Conditioning (Workout)
    Cool-Down
Exercise Precautions
    Overtraining

■ Learning Objectives ■

The student should be able to:

- Define and discuss basic principles of training and conditioning, including but not limited to, the principle of adaptation, the principle of overload, the principle of progressive overload, the principle of reversibility, the principle of consistency, the principle of specificity, the principle of individuality, the principle of hard and easy, and the principle of safety.
- Identify and discuss the three basic elements of a daily exercise session, including but not limited to warm-up, conditioning (workout) and cool-down.
- Identify and discuss signs and symptoms associated with overtraining.

Keywords

- Adaptation
- Chronic physiological adaptation
- Cool-down
- Conditioning
- Consistency
- Disuse
- Individuality
- Overload
- Overtraining
- Progressive overload
- Progression
- Reversibility
- Safety
- Specificity
- Warm-up

Basic Considerations When Beginning a Fitness Program

When beginning a fitness program, there are several issues that should be examined to insure success. Initially, it is important to determine current fitness status. Physical assessments will help to identify individual strengths and weaknesses.

Secondly, specific fitness goals should be identified. These goals should address individual desires and the identified weakness. When establishing goals, **be realistic.** It takes time for the body to physiologically adjust to regular activity. Unrealistic expectations will lead to unrealized objectives, frustration, and ultimately, to exercise program attrition. While it is exciting to take control of your life and positively address fitness objectives, realize these are lifelong changes that are being made. Give your body time to adjust. You will have a lifetime to enjoy the change.

Finally, physical activities should be selected that will allow specific goals to be accomplished. For example, a student may set a goal of losing ten pounds. To accomplish this goal he/she may choose weight training as the mode of activity. Is this an appropriate choice? Clearly, weight training is important and should be considered an integral part of any exercise prescription. It has been established to build lean muscle mass and increase the basal metabolic rate. It is not, however, the best mode of activity to meet this objective. This student would be better served if he/she developed an exercise program that primarily emphasized aerobic activities and secondarily emphasized weight training.

An exercise prescription is an individualized logical "plan" for physical activity, which is based on one's objectives, needs, functional capacity, and interests. Precaution should be taken to carefully prepare this plan. It will serve as your guide. If properly developed, the exercise prescription should address your initial fitness programming needs. Additionally, the exercise prescription should be a flexible plan. It should be easy to alter or adapt the plan depending on new needs that will arise as your body physiologically adapts to a healthier, more active lifestyle. Additional instructions on how to write an exercise prescription dealing with cardiovascular endurance, muscular strength and endurance, flexibility, and body composition can be found in the chapters of this text that relate specifically to these topics.

Beginning a Fitness Program: Basic Training Principles

Before beginning a fitness program, it is important to understand how the body will respond to increases or decreases in physical conditioning and training. The following are scientifically proven training principles that are known to influence human response to changes in physical activity levels.

It is extremely important to recognize these principles are absolute. They apply to everyone. They are not influenced by differences in race, gender, fitness levels, and health status. *These are the rules of the body and there are no exceptions.* Collectively, they describe how the body will respond. While the exact physiologic change that occurs will differ between systems of the body (i.e., cardiovascular, muscular), the fact that a change will occur is consistent to all systems.

These changes are referred to as chronic physiological adaptations. They occur *over time* and are a direct result of the stress placed on the body by repeated exposure to specific levels of activity. Reoccurring bouts of increased activity will result in positive adaptations. Chronic exposure to low levels of activity will result in negative physiological adaptations.

Principle of Adaptation

The principle of adaptation states, "if a specific physiological capacity is taxed by a physical training stimulus within a certain range and on a regular basis, this physiological capacity usually expands" (Holly & Shaffrath, 2001). The underlying premise of adaptation stems back to the early work of Dr. Hans Selye (1956). His work suggested the body responds and specifically adapts to physical stress over time. He referred to this phenomenon as the General Adaptation Syndrome.

For example, in the case of physical training, consider a sedentary individual who possesses poor cardiac and respiratory function. He/she can improve these functions by repeatedly stressing his/her cardiorespiratory system by gradually and carefully implementing increased levels of physical activity into his/her daily lifestyle. Over time, his/her heart and lungs will adjust to the new and higher levels of demand by becoming stronger and functioning more efficiently. Without the increased training stimulus, none of these positive changes could or would occur. *The body cannot improve function without being repeatedly physically stressed at a higher level than it currently has adapted to.*

Principle of Overload

The **principle of overload** involves a gradual increase in the frequency (how often), duration (how long) or intensity (how hard) of the activity. This principle is based on the principle of adaptation. As previously stated, the underlying premise of *adaptation* is the body's ability to change its structure and/or function to better adjust to a new environment. In other words, overloading entails exerting beyond the "comfort zone," yet not to the point of pain or injury, on a regular basis and allowing the body to develop physiologically to meet the needs or demands placed on it. It is best to "overload" initially, with frequency or duration (or a combination of both) rather than intensity.

From an applied, practical standpoint, consider the following example. A poorly conditioned individual wants to improve his or her fitness level by jogging. He or she should begin his/her training by participating in a low-level walking program. This will introduce the body physiologically to increased activity and metabolism. Over time, the body will adjust and adapt. As the individual gradually increases his or her frequency and duration, higher levels of fitness will be attained.

After these initial physical adaptations have occurred, it would be appropriate to increase intensity. The individual may then incorporate some jogging or participate in some run-walk type activities. This additional intensity will "overload" the body. The body will then, over time, adapt to this new level of demand and allow for even higher levels of fitness to be achieved. At this time, it would be appropriate for this individual to participate in more challenging and physically demanding training activities (i.e., fark-lets, hill repeats, and interval training.)

The process of overloading and allowing the body to adapt to the new level of demand can be continued until the desired level of physical fitness has been reached. At this point, the individual can maintain his/her fitness level by continuing to participate in activities with similar levels of intensity. Precaution should be taken, however, to not lower exercise frequency, intensity, or duration when fitness levels or exercising goals are met. If this happens, unfortunately the body will physiological adapt to the new lower demand, thus causing the person to lose physical fitness (see Principle of Reversibility). Maintenance of any fitness level can occur only when the body is similarly stressed.

Principle of Progressive Overload

The **principle of progressive overload** states that in order for an individual to continually benefit or improve his/her fitness level, the training intensity must be **progressively** increased, as the body adapts to the current level of conditioning or training. The rate of progression is highly individualized. Factors such as initial fitness levels, age, and the nature of training activities will influence the actual rate of progression. It should be emphasized that unless a progressive increase in training intensity occurs, the body cannot continue to improve and will actually lose fitness should lower levels of training occur. Like the principle of overload, the principle of progressive overload requires a careful manipulation of training frequency, duration, and intensity in conjunction with chronic changes in training adaptation.

Principle of Reversibility (Disuse)

The **principle of reversibility** is also referred to as the *principle of disuse*. It states that when physical training is stopped or reduced, the body will adjust to the new and diminished level of physiological stress. The specific level of adaptation will be in accordance to the new level of activity. In common parlance, it is often summarily stated by the cliché "Use it or lose it." The principle of reversibility can and should be considered the opposite of the principle of overload. This principle is particularly important when considering health-related fitness in that it directly applies to the health-fitness levels of the skeletal, cardiorespiratory, and muscular systems.

From a practical standpoint, the principle suggests that *the body cannot store fitness levels* or any gains in fitness for any appreciable amount of time. Once a person gains a particular level of fitness, he/she must continue to train or he/she will lose any gains he/she experienced. These loses present themselves in the forms of lower levels of muscular strength and endurance, and decreased cardiorespiratory fitness levels. When and how much loss occurs varies. Factors such as 1) the level of fitness, 2) the length of time a person has been trained, and 3) the system involved (i.e., cardiovascular, muscular), all play important roles.

The health/fitness levels of the human body must be considered on a continuum where optimal health/fitness is at one end and death is at the other. Where a person lies on that continuum is directly related to how he/she chooses to live. Positive lifestyle choices will result in positive gains. Negative lifestyle choices will result in lost gains. A highly trained individual, like anyone else, will lose his/her fitness if he/she makes negative choices and reduce his/her levels of activity.

The effects of decreased physical activity usually present themselves after only 1 or 2 weeks of reduced activity. The specific nature and magnitude of loss is dependent on the type and level of reduced activity. Dudley and Ploutz-Snyder (2001) suggest reduced muscle activity can occur from detraining, bed rest, casting, use of crutches, paralysis, aging, and weightlessness occurring in space flight.

For example, compare the magnitude of fitness loss for an individual presented with two similar and yet different situations. The situations are similar in that in both cases, the individual is unable to participate in resistive training for a period of two weeks. The difference is only in the causative nature as to why he/she was unable to participate. In the first scenario, consider a situation where the individual is restricted to a bed, for two weeks, as a result of illness. In the second scenario, this same individual misses two weeks of resistive training as a result of being on a vacation and having no access to any resistive training equipment. The magnitude of loss in muscular fitness would be far greater in the first situation than the second.

Principle of Consistency

The **principle of consistency** would indicate, for most non-symptomatic individuals, exercise sessions should be scheduled a minimum of 3 to 5 times weekly. Alternating days of activity with rest is recommended. This allows the body adequate time to recover and adapt to training. "Weekend Warriors," or those who try to exercise on a Friday, Saturday, Sunday approach, find little carry-over of gains, and have an increased potential of exercise induced injury. The practice of training like a "Weekend Warrior" should be discouraged.

Principle of Specificity

The **principle of specificity** states that the body will adapt very specifically to the type and nature of training. The principle of specificity applies to all types of training (i.e., weight training, cardiorespiratory training, flexibility).

For example, muscle adaptations are influenced by specific speed of contraction, the type of muscular contraction, the muscle groups involved and the energy source utilized. From a practical standpoint, you must train as similar to the activity and type of performance as you can.

Consider the practical example of long distance running. This type of training will not make you a better cyclist or swimmer even though each activity requires a high level of cardiovascular endurance. Long distance running will not make you run faster even though you are performing virtually the same leg movements. Long distance running will only make you a better long distance runner.

To improve cycling or swimming performance, an individual would have to specifically train by participating in cycling and swimming activities. To develop running speed, an individual would have to mimic similar speeds of muscle contraction in training. Simply stated, he/she has to train by running fast.

Principle of Individuality

The **principle of individuality** is two-fold. First, it is conceived based on the idea that each individual has his/her own fitness level, fitness objectives, and levels of enjoyment. In simple, individual participation in physical activity is highly individualized and stems from a variety of influencing factors.

For example, traditionally, women have been encouraged to participate in less vigorous, less contact oriented activities than men. It has been only in recent history that a women marathon (26.2 miles) has been added to the Olympic games. It is still extremely rare to have a woman participate in the sport of football.

Both genders tend to associate lower levels of activity with aging. Past experiences in activities stemming from school or other social situations may also influence a person's desire to participate. Individual levels of confidence may encourage or discourage participation. Access to facilities, time, and other related issues influence participation.

The desire to participate in activity is related to our abilities to understand short and long-term benefits. Individuals who clearly understand the personal health and fitness benefits tend to be more physically active. Without question, perceived and realized levels of enjoyment and satisfaction are highly related to participation and adherence to any exercise program.

This issue is extremely important. *Exercise program attrition is high.* Approximately 50% of those who begin a program will drop out within 3–6 months. Each individual should find an activity that is readily available, personally enjoyable, and able to meet his/her fitness goals and objectives. If he/she does, he/she will significantly increase his/her chances of developing a new, positive, healthy, lifestyle that includes regular participation in physical activity.

The second tenet of individuality stems from a physiological perspective. With the exception of identical twins, no two people are alike. As a result, physiologic adaptations to exercise will vary from person to person. This variance stems from such factors as cellular growth rate, metabolism, and neural and endocrine regulation. In simple, two people participating in the same activity or exercise program may respond to that activity completely different.

In closing, the principle of individuality must be considered when developing and implementing exercise programs. The specific fitness objectives, goals, fitness levels, and individual rates of physiological adaptation must be considered to ensure maximal exercise program effectiveness.

Principle of Hard and Easy

The **principle of hard and easy** states that an easier day of training should follow after one to two days of hard training. This easy day allows the body to physically recover from hard training while still remaining active. Hard training may be either high intensity work or long duration activities. Failure to follow the principle of hard and easy will likely lead to activity or training induced physical injury.

Principle of Safety

The **principle of safety** stresses the importance of making the workout as safe as possible. Walkers, joggers, and bikers should choose safe routes and wear a reflective vest before sunrise and after sunset. Walkers and joggers should proceed against the flow of the traffic, while bikers (wearing helmets, of course) should ride with the traffic flow.

Three Basic Elements of a Daily Exercise Session

Warm-Up

The purpose of the warm-up is to: gradually stimulate the cardiorespiratory system, increase muscle temperature, stretch tendons and muscles, increase flexibility, and prevent injury and muscle soreness. The warm-up phase of a daily exercise session should last between 10–15 minutes. A warm-up should consist of two parts:

1. A general whole body low intensity warm-up activity that elevates the heart rate.
2. A period of light stretching, calisthenics, and low level participation in an activity specifically related to a chosen sport or the chosen conditioning activity.

Conditioning (Workout)

In a total exercise program, cardiovascular endurance, muscular strength and endurance, and joint range of motion should be considered. Normally, stretching activities designed to improve range of motion are included in the warm-up and cool-down components of the daily exercise session. Changes in cardiovascular endurance and muscular strength and endurance must stem from specific conditioning activities.

To establish these changes and ultimately improve physical fitness, the conditioning or workout phase should last approximately 20 to 30 minutes. This is considered a minimum recommendation. Specific guidelines for establishing either cardiovascular fitness or muscular strength and endurance are discussed in Chapters 5 and 6, respectively. In either situation, the conditioning phase does not include time spent in warm-up and cool-down activities.

Longer conditioning phases are appropriate and may be considered by individuals who are more physically fit. The participant should be cautioned. There is a positive and exponential relationship between exercise duration and increased risk of injury. This relationship can be simply stated: "as the time of conditioning increases, the risk of musculoskeletal injury increases." These "workout" related injuries can be avoided if the participant does not extensively overtrain and allows the body time to properly adapt to the longer training or conditioning sessions.

Cool-Down

Cool-down is a critical and often neglected component of the daily work out session. It should last approximately 5–10 minutes. During this time, the intensity of the activity should be gradually reduced to allow the participant's heart rate and blood pressure to return gradually back to normal. Abrupt exercise stoppage should be avoided.

If a cool-down is not incorporated into the overall exercise plan, blood pooling will occur. This may lead to dizziness, faintness, cardiac abnormalities and muscle tissue damage and soreness. In some cases, though rare, catecholamine levels will remain elevated and may contribute to serious and potentially fatal heart arrhythmias. After normal heart rate and blood pressure have returned, it is advisable to incorporate stretching exercises into the cool-down (see Chapters 8 and 9).

Exercise Precautions

Overtraining

How much training is enough? Is it possible to train so intensely or at such a high level or volume that the body will negatively respond to the training effect? The answer to these types of questions is yes. Overtraining can lead to a variety of emotional and physiological responses. By definition, overtraining occurs whenever overload training is so great that the body is unable to adapt or properly recover. Overtraining leads to decreased exercise performance. To prevent injury, training overload and volume need to be immediately reduced when signs and symptoms of overtraining are present. The following are suggested signs and symptoms of overtraining (Robergs and Roberts, 1997):

- An increase in resting heart rate
- Loss of body weight
- Decrease in appetite
- Long-term muscle soreness (greater than 24 hours)
- Greater susceptibility to illness
- Constipation or diarrhea
- Decreased performance
- Decrease in desire to train or compete

What are the risks of overtraining? The answer is that the risks vary. The level of overtraining appears to be the most significant influencing factor. For example, in summarizing a series of studies on 2,500 male and female runners conducted by the Center of Disease Control and Prevention, Robergs and Roberts (1997) offer the following:

- One year injury incidence rate is about 2.5 to 12 injuries per 1000 hours of running
- 37% developed orthopedic injuries serious enough to reduce weekly training
- Risk of injury increase with increase running
- 60% of all injuries involved the knee or foot
- Average runner has a 1 in 3 chance of being injured within a year
- Average runner has a 1 in 10 chance of an injury that will require medical attention
- A runner averaging 15 miles a week can expect 1 injury every 2 years

Laboratory Activities

CHAPTER 3

Name: _____ Class Time/Day: _____ Score: _____

LABORATORY 3-A

Personal Exercise Prescription

- **Purpose:** This lab will help: 1) To identify your health-related fitness levels, 2) to identify health-related behaviors you would like to change by either increasing or decreasing, and 3) to establish a personal health-related fitness program.

- **Precautions:** Students are cautioned to follow the guidelines as describe in this book when establishing their personal health-related fitness program. *This laboratory experience should be completed after full study of the contents of this book.*

- **Equipment:** Selected lab activity results, note pad, and pencil.

- **Procedure:** Complete Laboratory 3-A Form A, Form B, Form C, Form D, and Form E.

- **Scoring:** Form A requires a total fitness profile score to be computed and fitted to the normative data provided.

- **Data/Calculations:** With the exception of the total fitness profile score, all measures should be calculated as described by the identified health-related fitness lab.

Name: _____ Class Time/Day: _____ Score: _____

FORM A

Total Health-Fitness Profile

- **Purpose:** This lab component will assist in determining your total fitness profile as measured by selected health-related fitness examinations.

- **Precautions:** None

- **Equipment:** Selected completed health-related fitness labs, note pad and pencil.

- **Procedure:** Determine your health-related fitness classification and percentile scores from each of the identified labs. Multiply the percentile score by the correction factor provided. Determine your total fitness profile score by summing the computed scores.

- **Scoring:** After the total fitness profile score has been computed, determine your total health fitness classification by using Table 3-1.

Table 3-1 ■ Normative Values for Determining Fitness Classification by Percentile Score

Total Health Fitness Classification	Total Percentile Score
Excellent	90
	80
Above Average	70
	60
Average	50
	40
Below Average	30
	20
Poor	10

Data/Calculations:

Laboratory Activity	Classification	Percentile Score x Correction Factor	Score
Cardiorespiratory Fitness			
Rockport Walk: Lab 5-A		× .35	
Muscular Strength			
Upper Leg Press: Lab 6-B		× .0625	
Bench Press: Lab 6-C		× .0625	
Muscular Endurance			
Push-Ups: Lab 6-D		× .0625	
Curl-Ups: Lab 6-E		× .0625	
Flexibility			
Sit and Reach: Lab 8-E or 8-G		× .15	
Body Composition			
3-Site Skinfold: Lab 11-B or 11-C		× .25	

Sum Total = _____

Total Health Fitness Percentile: _____

Total Health Fitness Classification: _____

Name: _____ Class Time/Day: _____ Score: _____

FORM B

Cardiorespiratory Fitness Program

■ **Purpose:** This lab component will assist in identifying behaviors related to your cardiorespiratory fitness you would like to change and help you to establish a cardiorespiratory fitness program.

■ **Precautions:** Precaution should be taken to follow the guidelines suggested in this text when establishing the cardiorespiratory training program.

■ **Equipment:** Selected completed health-related fitness labs, calculator, note pad, and pencil.

■ **Procedure:**

Step 1: Review your cardiorespiratory lab results and establish your current aerobic fitness level.

Step 2: Learn Actions and Behaviors: Examine your actions and identify behaviors and determine how they are linked to your cardiovascular fitness.

1.
2.
3.

Step 3: Establish Your Goals and Objectives:

Short-Term

1.
2.

Long-Term

1.
2.

Step 4: Prepare a Plan of Action: Use the cardiorespiratory fitness program form below to develop your personalized cardiorespiratory fitness training program. Carefully consider your current fitness levels when establishing exercise frequency, intensity, and duration.

Cardiorespiratory Fitness Program

Name:

Age:

Body Weight:

Resting Heart Rate:

Estimated MHR:

Determined VO_{2max}:

	Week	Frequency	%VO2max Min.	Target	Max.	Recommended Heart Rates Heart Rate Reserve Min.	Target	Max.	Ex. Time	Sets	Duration
Initial Stage	1										
	2										
	3										
	4										
	5										
	6										
Improvement Stage	7										
	8										
	9										
	10										
	11										
	12										
	13										
	14										
	15										
	16										
	17										
	18										
	19										
	20										
	21										
	22										
	23										
	24										
	25										
	26										
	27										
Maintenance Stage	28										

Name: _____ Class Time/Day: _____ Score: _____

FORM C

Muscular Strength and Endurance: Fitness Program

- **Purpose:** This lab component will help you to: 1) identify behaviors related to your muscular strength and endurance you would like to change, and 2) help you establish a muscular strength and endurance training program.

- **Precautions:** Precaution should be taken to follow the guidelines suggested in this text when establishing the muscular strength and endurance training program.

- **Equipment:** Selected completed health-related fitness labs, calculator, note pad, and pencil.

- **Procedure:**

Step 1: Review your muscular strength and endurance lab results and determine areas of strength and weakness.

Step 2: Learn Actions and Behaviors: Examine your actions and identify behaviors and determine how they are linked to your muscular strength and endurance.

　　1.
　　2.
　　3.

Step 3: Establish Your Goals and Objectives:

Short-Term
　　1.
　　2.

Long-Term
　　1.
　　2.

Step 4: Prepare a Plan: Complete the form below by selecting appropriate resistive training activities. Choose activities based on your personal muscular strength and endurance goals and objectives and current fitness levels. Carefully consider your current fitness levels when establishing exercise intensity, sets, and repetitions.

Activity by Region	Intensity (Load)	Sets	Repetitions
Chest			
1.			
2.			
3.			
Shoulders			
1.			
2.			
3.			
Upper Arm (Anterior)			
1.			
2.			
3.			
Upper Arm (Posterior)			
1.			
2.			
3.			
Back			
1.			
2.			
3.			
Abdominal			
1.			
2.			
3.			
Upper Leg (Anterior)			
1.			
2.			
3.			
Upper Leg (Posterior)			
1.			
2.			
3.			
Lower Leg (Anterior)			
1			
2.			
3.			
Lower Leg (Posterior)			
1.			
2.			
3.			

Name: _____ Class Time/Day: _____ Score: _____

FORM D

Flexibility: Fitness Program

- **Purpose:** This lab component will assist you identifying behaviors related to your total body flexibility you would like to change, and help you to establish a flexibility training program.

- **Precautions:** Precaution should be taken to follow the guidelines suggested in this text when establishing the flexibility training program.

- **Equipment:** Selected completed health-related fitness labs, calculator, note pad, and pencil.

- **Procedure:**

Step 1: Review your flexibility lab results and determine areas of strengths and weaknesses.

Step 2: Learn Actions and Behaviors: Examine your actions and identify behaviors and determine how they are linked to your flexibility levels.

    1.

    2.

    3.

Step 3: Establish Your Goals and Objectives:

Short-Term

    1.

    2.

Long-Term

    1.

    2.

Step 4: Prepare a Plan: Complete the form below by selecting appropriate flexibility activities. Choose activities based on your personal flexibility goals and objectives and current levels of joint range of motion. Carefully consider your current flexibility levels when establishing exercise activities, sets, and repetitions.

Activity by Region	Sets	Repetitions
Chest		
1.		
2.		
3.		
Shoulders		
1.		
2.		
3.		
Upper Arm (Anterior)		
1.		
2.		
3.		
Upper Arm (Posterior)		
1.		
2.		
3.		
Back		
1.		
2.		
3.		
Abdominal		
1.		
2.		
3.		
Upper Leg (Anterior)		
1.		
2.		
3.		
Upper Leg (Posterior)		
1.		
2.		
3.		
Lower Leg (Anterior)		
1.		
2.		
3.		
Lower Leg (Posterior)		
1.		
2.		
3.		

Name: _____ Class Time/Day: _____ Score: _____

FORM E

Body Composition: Fitness Program

■ **Purpose:** This lab component will assist you in identifying behaviors related to your body composition you would like to change, and help you to establish a dietary management program.

■ **Precautions:** Precaution should be taken to follow the guidelines suggested in this text when establishing the dietary management program.

■ **Equipment:** Selected completed health-related fitness labs, calculator, note pad, and pencil.

■ **Procedure:**

Step 1: Review your body composition lab results and determine your needs.

Step 2: Learn Actions and Behaviors: Examine your actions and identify behaviors and determine how they are linked to your body composition and dietary intake.

1.
2.
3.

Step 3: Establish Your Goals and Objectives:

Short-Term

1.
2.

Long-Term

1.
2.

Step 4: Prepare a Plan: Are there particular foods you tend to abuse that you should avoid? Are there particular emotional states that stimulate you to eat that you need to pay particular attention? Do you have a tendency to eat more alone or when eating with others? Are there particular behaviors you associate with eating such as watching television? Are you planning on keeping a dietary log and recording it in nutritional software packages to determine nutritional information regarding your diet?

4

Understanding the Cardiovascular System

Fifty-eight million Americans have one or more forms of cardiovascular disease.
Center for Disease Control and Prevention

More money is spent treating heart disease than any other illness.
Center for Disease Control and Prevention

■ Chapter Outline ■

Cardiorespiratory System: Function
Anatomical Considerations of the
  Cardiovascular System
Exercise and Cardiovascular Disease
Understanding Cardiovascular Risk: Coronary
  Risk Factors
    Smoking
    Blood Pressure and Hypertension
    Measurement of Blood Pressure

Hypercholesterolemia/Hyperlipidemia
Physical Inactivity
Diabetes Mellitus and Glucose Intolerance
Obesity
Stress
Age
Family History
Gender
Physical Activity and Coronary Risk

■ Learning Objectives ■

The student should be able to:

- Identify and discuss the impact of cardiovascular disease on the population of the United States.
- Discuss the anatomical structure and function of the cardiovascular system.
- Identify the primary and secondary coronary risk factors.

- Discuss the relationship of cigarette smoking and coronary artery disease risk.
- Discuss the relationship of blood pressure and coronary artery disease risk.
- Discuss the relationship of hypercholesterolemia and hyperlipidemia and coronary artery disease risk.
- Discuss the relationship of physical inactivity and coronary artery disease risk.

- Discuss the relationship of diabetes mellitus, glucose intolerance and coronary artery disease risk.
- Discuss the relationship of obesity and coronary artery disease risk.
- Discuss the relationship of unmanaged stress and coronary artery disease risk.
- Discuss the relationship of advancing age and coronary artery disease risk.
- Discuss the relationship of family history of coronary artery disease and coronary artery disease risk.
- Discuss the relationship of gender and coronary artery disease risk.
- Discuss the relationship of regular physical activity and the reduction of coronary artery disease risk.

■ Keywords ■

Android obesity
Atria
Atrioventricular valves
Cigarette smoking
Coronary artery disease
Diabetes mellitus
Diastolic blood pressure
Family history
Glucose intolerance

Gynoid obesity
HDL cholesterol
Hypercholesterolemia
Hyperlipidemia
Hypertension
LDL cholesterol
Obesity
Physical inactivity
Pulmonary system

Pulse pressure
Sedentary lifestyle
Semilunar valves
Smoking
Stress
Systemic system
Systolic blood pressure
Total cholesterol
Ventricle

Cardiorespiratory System: Function

The cardiorespiratory system is composed of the heart, blood, blood vessels, and lungs. These components make up the cardiovascular and respiratory systems. The cardiorespiratory system is a cooperative system combining the efforts of the cardiovascular system and the respiratory system. One of the primary functions of the cardiorespiratory system is to transport gases to and from the lungs and body tissues.

The respiratory system serves to bridge the gap between atmospheric air and the body. Oxygen (O_2) in the inhaled air is able to pass from the lungs into the blood. The heart then serves to pump the oxygenated blood to the working muscles and other body tissues. Carbon dioxide (CO_2), a by-product of metabolism, is picked up at the tissue level and transported, in blood, back to the heart and lungs. At the lungs, CO_2 leaves the blood and is exhaled into the atmosphere.

In addition to the function of gas transport, the cardiovascular system functions to deliver nutrients to, and remove waste products from, the cells of the body. It helps to deliver hormones, assist in body temperature regulation, and balance body fluid levels to prevent dehydration during activity. In simple, most body functions and body tissues rely on the cardiovascular system.

Anatomical Considerations of the Cardiovascular System

The heart is a muscular pump about the size of a grown adult's fist. It is located in the mediastium of the chest cavity, just under, and slightly off center (toward the left), of the sternum or breastbone. It functions to contract and propel blood throughout the pulmonary and systemic systems.

The heart is a four chambered structure. It is divided into right and left sides by muscular tissue known as the septum. The upper chambers are known as atria and the lower chambers are referred to as ventricles. By being divided into left and right sides, the heart is able to serve two different systems. These are the pulmonary system and the systemic system. The right side of the heart functions to serve the pulmonary system by returning deoxygenated blood from the body tissues to the lungs. At the lungs, gas exchange occurs and CO_2 is removed from the blood by the lungs and is exhaled into the atmosphere. At the same time, O_2 is picked up from the lungs by the blood. The blood returns from the lungs to the left side of the heart. The left side serves the systemic system or the body tissues. The oxygenated blood is pumped from the left ventricle to the body tissues. At the tissue level, O_2 is removed from the blood and CO_2 is picked up. As the oxygen-poor blood leaves the tissues it returns to the right side of the heart where it will be pumped to the lungs for reoxygenation.

To help in directing blood flow through the heart there are one-way valves. These include the atrioventricular valves and the semilunar valves. The right and left atrioventricular valves are located between the atria and ventricles. Because of the number of cusps that make up the valves, they are also referred to as tricuspid and bicuspid (mitral) valves, respectively. The semilunar valves are three cusps valves and include the pulmonary and aortic valves. The right and left atrioventricular valves are located between the atria and ventricles. The pulmonary valve lies between the right ventricle and the pulmonary artery. The aortic valve lies between the aorta and the left ventricle.

Exercise and Cardiovascular Disease

Cardiovascular disease is the number one cause of death in the United States. In 1993, the American Heart Association (AMA) reported that cardiovascular diseases annually (Wilmore & Costill, 1999):

- Affects more than 60 million Americans.
- Result in nearly 1 million deaths.
- Cost individuals, government, and private industry nearly $275 billion.

Additionally, the AMA estimates that annually:

- More than 1.5 million heart attacks occur.
- About 500,000 Americans die from heart attacks.
- More than one out of every five Americans suffers some form of cardiovascular disease.

Lastly, Wilmore and Costill (1999) indicate that in 1995, there were more than:

- 573,000 coronary artery bypass surgeries.
- 419,000 coronary angioplasties.
- 2,345 heart transplants.

As staggering as these findings may seem, they are far more positive than those previously reported. Beginning in the late 1960's, the deaths related to cardiovascular disease began to decline. Between 1980 and 1990 alone, the mortality rates declined by 26.7% and by more than 50% from the peak rates of the mid 1960's.

Cardiovascular disease presents itself in a variety of forms. These include, but are not limited to:

- Angina pectoris
- Cerebral vascular accidents (strokes)
- Congenital heart disease
- Congestive heart failure
- Coronary artery disease
- Hypertension
- Peripheral vascular disease
- Rheumatic heart disease
- Valvular heart disease

The majority of reported deaths are related to coronary artery disease. Coronary artery disease and other selected cardiovascular diseases are described under separate headers. It must be emphasized that *cardiovascular disease is not an infectious disease, but is often preventable and lifestyle related.*

Understanding Cardiovascular Risk: Coronary Risk Factors

Research has attempted to identify personal behaviors and characteristics, lifestyle behaviors, disease status, environmental factors, and inherited characteristics that are related to the development of coronary artery disease (CAD). Identified factors are grouped as either primary or secondary. Primary risk factors are those that have been definitively associated with, or directly cause coronary artery disease. These include cigarette smoking, hyperlipidemia, inactivity, hypertension, obesity, and diabetes. Secondary factors are believed to contribute to or advance the severity of atherosclerosis and CAD. These include gender, family history of CAD, unmanaged stress, and age. Primary and secondary factors are often grouped as to whether they can be altered or controlled by lifestyle, or whether they are unalterable. Table 4-1 presents a summary of these factors and groupings.

The impact of disease risk associated with one or more risk factors is significant and exponential. For example, an individual with one risk factor will have twice the risk of CAD as an individual with no risk factors. A person with two risk factors will have three times the risk, and a person with three risk factors will have ten times the risk of CAD.

Table 4-1 ■ Coronary Artery Disease Risk Factors

Primary Risk Factors (Lifestyle Related)	**Secondary Risk Factors (Lifestyle Related)**
Diabetes mellitus	Unmanaged Stress
Hypertension	
Hypercholesterolemia	**Secondary Risk Factors (Uncontrollable)**
Obesity	Age (Advancing)
Physical inactivity	Gender (Male)
Smoking	Heredity (Family history of CAD)

Smoking

Cigarette smoking and passive smoke inhalation are highly related to CAD. In fact, it has been reported that smokers have a 70% greater level of coronary risk than nonsmokers (ACSM, 1998). Marks (2001) cites that approximately 90% of lung cancers, 80% of emphysema, 75% of bronchitis, and 30% coronary heart disease is accredited to smoking. The magnitude of risk is related to the number of cigarettes smoked daily. Cigarette smoking acts on the body by:

- Injuring the inner lining of the artery
- Increasing the risk of blood clotting
- Increasing the risk of myocardial infarction
- Lowering levels of HDL cholesterol

Fortunately, these negative effects are reversible upon smoking cessation. Mangan and Golding (1984) suggest that after 15 years of complete smoking cessation the mortality ratio between smokers and ex-smokers is similar.

Blood Pressure and Hypertension

Blood pressure is the driving force that moves blood throughout the body. It is directly related to heart contraction and relaxation. When the ventricles of the heart contract, blood is driven to the lungs (**pulmonary system**) and to the body tissues (**systemic system**). **Systolic blood pressure** is a measure of the highest pressure in the arterial vessels and occurs when the heart is contracting and ejecting blood from its ventricles. This phase of the cardiac cycle is known as systole. **Diastolic blood pressure** is a measure of the lowest pressure in the arterial vessels and occurs during heart diastole. During diastole the heart is resting and refilling with blood. Normative values for resting systolic and diastolic blood pressure for adults are presented in Table 4-2. These values are normally recorded with systolic pressure first (i.e. 120/80).

Blood pressure varies between individuals. In addition to hypertensive medication, extraneous factors such as time of day, full bladder content, body posture, recent intake of caffeine, nicotine, alcohol, and recent strenuous activity, can influence blood pressure.

Pressure varies within the blood vessels as the heart contracts and relaxes and is referred to as pulse pressure. **Pulse pressure** is the difference between the systolic and diastolic pressures.

Hypertension or chronically elevated blood pressure is strongly related to coronary heart disease. The American Heart Association (1993) and National Institute of Health (1992) report more than 25% or 50 million Americans are hypertensive. Most (67%) are not being treated and almost one-half are unaware of the complication. Contributing factors include age, race (particularly African-American), sodium sensitivity, chronic alcohol abuse, the use of oral contraceptives, and sedentary living. Additionally, hypertension is related to other coronary risk factors such as elevated serum cholesterol and/or lipids, obesity, diabetes mellitus, and cigarette smoking.

Hypertension causes the cardiac muscle or heart to overwork. There is direct relationship between vascular injury and excessive pressure on the vascular wall. Additionally, negative

Table 4-2 ■ Normative Values for Classifying Blood Pressure in Adults Age 18 and Older

Classification	Systolic (mm Hg)		Diastolic (mm Hg)
Normal	< 120	and	< 80
Prehypertension	120–139	or	80–89
Stage 1 Hypertension	140–159	or	90–99
Stage 2 Hypertension	=> 160	or	=> 100

Source: *Seventh Report of the Joint National Committee on Prevention, Detection, Evaluation and Treatment of High Blood Pressure (JNC 7) Express.* National Heart, Lung, and Blood Institute. Bethesda, MD. 2003. JAMA 2003; 289:2560-2571.

effects on the heart or myocardium resulting from increases muscular stress and myocardial oxygen demands are apparent. These conditions lead to arterial damage and ultimately, if left untreated, heart failure and stroke.

Fortunately, there are a number of lifestyle related, non-pharmacological interventions that can facilitate the lowering of high blood pressure and/or assist in the maintenance of normal blood pressure. Included are weight reduction and/or maintenance of normal body weight, smoking cessation, and regular physical activity. Appropriate physical activities should emphasize continuous, rhythmical, large muscle group activities such as walking, jogging, swimming, and cycling. Other therapeutic approaches include dietary interventions that emphasize the reduction of fat consumption and dietary cholesterol.

Measurement of Blood Pressure

Blood pressure can be measured directly or indirectly. Direct measurement is an invasive procedure requiring the insertion of a needle into a blood vessel. Because of the inherent risks and the impractical aspects associated with this action, the direct measurement of blood pressure is rarely used.

Indirect measurement of blood pressure is less accurate, but is a relatively routine procedure. Indirect measurement requires the use of a sphygmomanometer and a stethoscope (see Figure 4.1). The sphygmomanometer consists of an adjustable cloth cuff that includes an inflatable bladder, an inflation-deflation pump with a release valve, and a manometer that can measure the pressure in the bladder. Specific procedures for measurement are described in Laboratory 4-A. It should be noted that posture directly influences blood pressure. The procedures described in Laboratory 4-A determine seated resting blood pressure.

Typically, blood pressures should rise slightly as one moves from a supine, to a sitting, to a standing position. Individuals experiencing light-headedness or fainting during standing may be presenting postural hypotension. To determine postural hypotension, pressure should be measured immediately and 1 to 5 minutes after standing (American Society of Hypertention, 1992).

Hypercholesterolemia/Hyperlipidemia

Elevated serum cholesterol levels (**hypercholesterolemia**) and elevated lipid or fat levels (**hyperlipidemia**) in the blood are strongly related to CAD. To consider total cholesterol (TC) only is not adequate when determining coronary risk. As a result, separating total cholesterol into fractions is warranted. Lipids are insoluble in blood and therefore bind to protein when transported in the body. This combination is referred to as a lipoprotein. There are several lipoproteins that are related to CAD. High-density lipoproteins (HDL) offer a protective effect against CAD. Increasing HDL level is desirable and will contribute to lowering coronary disease risk. Low-density lipoproteins (LDL) and very-low-density lipoproteins (VLDL) are considered undesirable and are associated with increase CAD risk. Low-density lipoproteins are considered one of the leading carriers of cholesterol in the body.

Because of the difference in coronary risk associated with HDL and LDL cholesterol fractions, one of the best methods of determining CAD risk is to determine the ratio of total cholesterol to high-density lipoproteins. This may be determined using the following formula: TC/HDL. Values equal to or greater than 5.0 for men and 4.5 for women are associated with greater risk. Table 4-3 summarizes a classification of risk based on total, HDL, and LDL cholesterol levels.

Table 4-3 ■ Classification of Risk Based on Total, HDL, and LDL Cholesterol (mg/dl)

Total Cholesterol	
Desirable cholesterol	< 200
Borderline-high cholesterol	200–239
High cholesterol	> 240
HDL Cholesterol	
Desirable HDL cholesterol	=> 35
Low HDL cholesterol	< 35
LDL Cholesterol	
Optimal LDL cholesterol	< 100
Desirable LDL cholesterol	< 130
Borderline-high LDL cholesterol	130–159
High LDL cholesterol	> 159

Source: American Heart Association (1993). *Journal of American Medical Association, 269*: 3015–3023 and Robergs, R. and Roberts, S. (1997). *Exercise Physiology: Exercise, Performance, and Clinical Applications*. St. Louis, MO.: Mosby.

Physical Inactivity

Physical activity levels and CAD are strongly *inversely related*. In other words, as physical activity levels go down, the risk of CAD goes up, and visa versa. Morris and colleagues (1973, 1980) report that sedentary individuals have a two to three times greater risk of CAD than physically active individuals. Additionally, Powell and his colleagues (1987) at the Center for Disease Control indicate *individuals living a sedentary lifestyle double their risk of having a fatal heart attack*. The level of risk appears to be similar to that of cigarette smoking, hypertension, and elevated serum cholesterol levels. Yet, because of the positive effects of regular physical activity, the reduction or elimination of a sedentary lifestyle may arguably be the single best method of controlling or reducing CAD.

There are a number of interrelated explanations as to why increasing physical activity levels help in reducing the risk of CAD. These seem to stem from the positive effects of regular physical activity on other coronary risk factors. For example, physical activity helps to establish and maintain normal blood pressure. It helps to control obesity, glucose intolerance, and other factors which contribute to diabetes mellitus. Physical activity has an extremely positive effect in controlling hypercholesterolemia and hyperlipidemia. It assists in raising HDL levels, while lowering LDL, triglyceride, and total cholesterol levels. Finally, physical activity may assist in controlling or managing an individual's stress levels.

Diabetes Mellitus and Glucose Intolerance

Glucose intolerance and diabetes mellitus are directly related to obesity. Diabetes mellitus, especially type II or adult onset, is strongly related to hypercholestrolemia, hypertension, elevated LDL and total cholesterol levels, and lower HDL levels. As previously indicated, all of these lead to an increased risk of CAD. A diabetic male has twice the risk of CAD, while a diabetic female has three times the risk of CAD compared to nondiabetic same gender individuals.

Obesity

Obesity is directly related to many of the other identified coronary risk factors. For example, glucose intolerance, diabetes, and sedentary or physically inactive lifestyles all contribute to obesity. As a result, obesity is related to CAD and is now considered a primary risk factor by some organizations.

Interestingly, the pattern of fat distribution is important and related to the level of CAD risk. Individuals who carry excessive levels of fat on their trunks are at greater risk of CAD than those who carry excessive fat lower in their bodies (i.e., hips and legs). The term **android obesity** (see Chapter 11 - Figure 11.4) is used to describe higher or upper body fat distribution, while **gynoid obesity** (see Chapter 11 - Figure 11.5) is used to describe lower body fat distribution.

Stress

Unmanaged stress is related to CAD. This is especially true for individuals that present type A personalities. These individuals are extremely driven to succeed and are extremely competitive. Other related characteristics include a sense of time urgency. The relationship between stress and CAD appears stronger in white middle-aged men than in women, Blacks, Hispanics, and younger adults.

Age

Men over the age of 45 and women over the age of 55 appear to have greater risk of CAD. CAD is related to women who present premature menopause and do not undertake estrogen replacement therapy.

Family History

Individuals with a family history of CAD are at greater risk than those whose families are clinically free of CAD. The risk is greater when the father or other first-degree relative has experienced a myocardial infarction (heart attack) or sudden death before the age of 55. The same is true when the mother or another first-degree female family member before the age of 65 presents the same conditions. Individuals with family histories of diabetes, hypertension, and hyperlipidemia are at greater risk.

Gender

Statistically, men have a greater history of presenting CAD earlier in life than women. As a result, many falsely believe that CAD is a male-oriented disease. As earlier indicated, men are at greater risk beginning around 45 years of age, while women appear to be at higher risk after the age of 55. Yet, as both genders share more common lifestyles in terms of work place, occupational and psychosocial stress levels, dietary behaviors, physical activity levels, etc., these differences have become smaller. CAD is not a gender selective disease. Both males and females who practice bad lifestyle behaviors, such as cigarette smoking, improper diet, and inadequate physical activity levels, are at risk.

Physical Activity and Coronary Risk

Regular, proper, and adequate physical activity or exercise is one of the best, if not the best, method known to assist in controlling coronary artery disease risk. Exercise has been shown to strengthen the myocardium or heart muscle. It has been established that regular physical activity helps increase coronary artery circulation, decrease resting heart rate, and increase resting and exercising stroke volume. These factors, and others, help to establish and maintain normal systolic and diastolic blood pressures. Additionally, individuals who exercise regularly are less likely to develop hypertension.

Since physical activity is associated with increased caloric or energy expenditure, it helps to reduce body weight and control obesity. Physical activity has been shown to assist in limiting glucose intolerance complications. Specifically, it acts to lower blood glucose levels. Both are related to diabetes mellitus. As a result, physical activity can reduce the risk of developing adult onset diabetes, as well as help to control the complications of both type I and type II diabetes.

One of the more positive effects of physical activity is its action on blood profiles. Exercise has been shown to assist in normalizing blood lipid and cholesterol profiles. Regular aerobic activity has been shown to raise HDL levels, while lowering LDL, triglyceride, and total cholesterol levels. Finally, physical activity has proven beneficial in assisting individuals with Type A personalities to control and manage their stress levels.

Clearly, regular physical activity can reduce CAD risk. When coupled with other risk factor reductions, such as improved diet, smoking cessation, weight management, etc., will significantly improve an individual's health status.

Laboratory Activities

CHAPTER 4

Name: _____ Class Time/Day: _____ Score: _____

LABORATORY 4-B

Coronary Heart Disease Risk Appraisal

- **Purpose:** This lab will estimate your coronary heart disease risk.

- **Precautions:** None

- **Equipment:** Risko Coronary Heart Disease Risk Appraisal Survey

- **Procedure:** Each subject should complete the survey as accurately as possible. For each variable, identify the descriptor that most fits you. The value in paraphrases represents your score for that variable. Variable explanations are as follows:
  - **Age:** Your chronological age in years.
  - **Hereditary:** Parents, or immediate family (i.e. brothers and sisters) who have a history of heart attack or stroke.
  - **Weight:** Your body weight measured in pounds compared to standard recommended weights for individuals of your age and gender.
  - **Tobacco Smoking:** Your current smoking status. If you smoke and inhale deeply and/or smoke a cigarette completely, **add** one point to the provided score. **Do not** correct by subtracting a point if you smoke partial cigarettes or do not inhale.
  - **Exercise:** Your current exercising status. If you exercise consistently and frequently with moderate intensity, **subtract** one point from your score.
  - **Cholesterol or Fat % in Diet:** Recent, determined serum cholesterol level. If cholesterol levels are not available, estimate as accurately as possible the amount of saturated (solid) fat that you eat.
  - **Blood Pressure:** Recent, determined resting blood pressure.
  - **Gender:** Your gender.

- **Scoring:** Table 4-5 should be used to determine relative coronary heart disease risk.

Table 4-5 ■ Relative Risk Categories: Risko

Score	Relative Risk Category
6–11	Risk well below average
12–17	Risk below average
18–24	Average risk
25–31	Moderate risk
32–40	High risk
41–62	Very high risk

Risko: Coronary Heart Disease Risk Appraisal Survey

	(1)	(2)	(3)	(4)	(6)	(8)
Age	10 to 20 years	21 to 30 years	31 to 40 years	41 to 50 years	51 to 60 years	61 and over

	(1)	(2)	(3)	(4)	(6)	(7)
Heredity	No known history of heart disease	1 relative with heart disease over 60	2 relatives with heart disease over 60	1 relative with heart disease under age 60	2 relatives with heart disease under age 60	3 relatives with heart disease under age 60

	(0)	(1)	(2)	(3)	(5)	(6)
Weight	More than 5 lbs. below standard weight	−5 to +5 lbs. standard weight	6–20 lbs. overweight	21–35 lbs. overweight	36–50 lbs. overweight	51–65 lbs. overweight

	(0)	(1)	(2)	(4)	(6)	(10)
Tobacco Smoking	Nonsmoker	Cigar and/or pipe; live or work with someone who smokes	10 cigarettes or less per day	11–20 cigarettes per day	21–30 cigarettes per day	40 or more cigarettes per day

	(1) Intensive occupational and recreational exertion	(2) Moderate occupational and recreational exertion	(3) Sedentary work and intense recreational exertion	(5) Sedentary occupational and moderate recreational exertion	(6) Sedentary work and light recreational exertion	(8) Complete lack of all exercise
Exercise						

	(1)	(2)	(3)	(4)	(5)	(7)
Cholesterol or Fat % in diet	Cholesterol below 180 mg/dl; Diet contains no animal or solid fats	Cholesterol 181–205 mg/dl; Diet contains 1–10% animal or solid fats	Cholesterol 206–230 mg/dl; Diet contains 11–20% animal or solid fats	Cholesterol 231–255 mg/dl; Diet contains 21–30% animal or solid fats	Cholesterol 256–280 mg/dl; Diet contains 31–40% animal or solid fats	Cholesterol 281–300 mg/dl; Diet contains 50% animal or solid fats

	(1)	(2)	(3)	(4)	(5)	(7)
Blood Pressure	100–119 systolic	120–139 systolic	140–159 systolic	160–179 systolic	180–199 systolic	200 or over systolic

	(1)	(2)	(3)	(4)	(6)	(7)
Gender	Female under age 40	Female aged 40–50	Female over age 50	Male	Stocky Male	Bald stocky male

Source: Modified from: McArdle, W., Katch, F., & Katch, V. (1996). *Exercise Physiology: Energy, Nutrition, and Human Performance.* Philadelphia, PA: Williams & Wilkins.

■ Data/Calculations:

Subject: _____ Date: _____

Gender: _____ Age: _____ Height: _____ Weight: _____

Cumulative Score: _____

Relative Risk Category: _____

5

Principles of Cardiorespiratory Endurance

Half of American adults do not achieve the recommended level of physical activity, and more than one-fourth report no leisure-time physical activity.
Center for Disease Control and Prevention

■ Chapter Outline ■

Purpose of the Cardiorespiratory Endurance Exercise Program
Health vs. Fitness: Program Considerations
Benefits of a Cardiorespiratory Endurance Exercise Program
Components of a Cardiorespiratory Exercise Prescription
    Modality
    Frequency
    Intensity
        Heart Rate Methods
            Maximal Heart Rate
            Heart Rate Reserve
        Rate of Perceived Exertion
        Percent of VO_2 Maximum
    Duration
    Progression
    Initial Conditioning Stage
    Improvement Stage
    Maintenance Stage
Determination of Heart Rate
    Procedures for Determining Heart Rate Electronically
    Procedures for Palpating Pulse
Components of the Daily Cardiorespiratory Exercise Session
    Warm-up
    Conditioning
    Cool-Down
Exercise Prescriptions and Weight Loss
Cardiorespiratory Endurance Training Risk
Detraining: The Effect of Exercise Training Reduction or Stoppage on Cardiorespiratory Endurance

■ Learning Objectives ■

The student should be able to:

- Identify the benefits and importance of good cardiorespiratory fitness.
- Identify the differences between health-related and fitness-related benefits of exercise.
- Develop a cardiorespiratory exercise prescription following recommended criteria for modality, frequency, intensity, duration, and progression.
- Demonstrate the ability to establish appropriate exercise intensities using the

following procedures: Percentage of Maximum Heart Rate, Percentage of Heart Rate Reserve, Percentage of Maximum Oxygen Consumption (VO_{2max}), and Rate of Perceived Exertion.
- Demonstrate the ability to determine resting and exercise heart rates through pulse palpation.
- Demonstrate the ability to develop a daily exercise session, including warm-up, conditioning, and cool-down phases.
- Demonstrate the ability to tailor an exercise prescription to meet specific caloric expenditure needs.
- Identify the risks of regular and vigorous cardiorespiratory fitness training.
- Identify and discuss the effects of exercise training reduction or stoppage on cardiorespiratory endurance.

■ Keywords ■

Caloric expenditure
Cardiorespiratory endurance
Cool-down
Detraining
Duration
Energy expenditure
Fitness-related benefits of activity
Frequency

Health-related benefits of activity
Heart rate reserve
Improvement stage
Initial conditioning stage
Intensity
Maintenance stage
Maximum exercising heart rate
Maximum heart rate

Maximum oxygen uptake
Modality
Progression
Rate of perceived exertion
Rate of progression
Resting heart rate
Reversibility
VO_{2max}
Warm-up

Purpose of the Cardiorespiratory Endurance Exercise Program

The purpose of any Cardiorespiratory (CR) program is to develop the body's ability to deliver oxygen to the working muscles and other tissues. Yet, it is important to remember that when developing the program, the quantity and quality of activity will differ depending on whether the program objectives are fitness-related or health-related. These differences are discussed under separate headers below. In general, unless otherwise delineated, recommendations presented in this text are designed to allow for both health related benefits and improved fitness or increased VO_{2max}.

Health vs. Fitness: Program Considerations

Current knowledge suggests that lower levels of activity may allow for reduced risks of certain degenerative diseases, while allowing for no significant gains in VO_{2max}. For example, reduction in blood pressure, blood lipid profiles, body weight, risk of diabetes and premature mortality have all been linked to moderate levels of activity. It is important to note and restate, *this lowering of disease risk factors can occur without any significant change in an individual's functional capacity.* This means that an individual, by incorporating moderate activity in his/her life, *can lower his/her disease risk without necessarily improving physical fitness.* These types of benefits are referred to as **health-related benefits of activity.**

Fitness-related benefits are achieved at higher levels of activity. Fitness-related benefits are related more to performance levels in sport and higher levels of lifestyle activities. For example, a physically fit individual is more likely able to participate in game activities or take vacations that involve physical activities such as hiking and biking than a person who has only met the lesser health-related fitness standards.

When fitness-related benefits are achieved, health-related benefits are also obtained. But, perhaps surprisingly, significantly greater health benefits are not demonstrated as fitness levels continue to improve. Table 5-1 provides a summary of current recommendations for exercise intensity using a percent of maximum heart rate, heart rate reserve, maximal oxygen uptake, and rate of perceived exertion for health and fitness related benefits.

Table 5-1 ■ Recommended Exercising Intensity for Developing Health-Related and Fitness-Related Benefits

	Recommended Health-Related Benefits	Exercise Intensity Fitness-Related Benefits
% VO_{2max}	40–49 %	40/50–85 %
% Heart Rate Reserve	40–49 %	40/50–85 %
% Maximal Heart Rate	55–64 %	55/65–90 %
Rate of Perceived Exertion (RPE)	11	12–16

Benefits of a Cardiorespiratory Endurance Exercise Program

The Center for Disease Control and Prevention (1997) cites the following benefits of regular physical activity.

- Reduces the risk of dying prematurely
- Reduces the risk of dying from heart disease
- Reduces the risk of developing diabetes
- Reduces the risk of developing high blood pressure
- Helps reduce blood pressure in people who already have high blood pressure

- Reduces the risk of developing colon cancer
- Reduces feelings of depression and anxiety
- Helps control weight
- Helps build and maintain healthy bones, muscles, and joints
- Helps older adults become stronger and better able to move about without falling
- Promotes psychological well-being

Components of a Cardiorespiratory Endurance Exercise Prescription

Modality

The modality or type of exercise is related to change in an individual's VO_{2max}. To increase cardiorespiratory endurance, DeVries (1986) cites the following criteria when selecting activities.

- Involve a large proportion of total muscle mass
- Maximize the use of large muscles
- Minimize the use of small muscles
- Maximize dynamic muscle contraction
- Minimize static muscle contraction
- Be rhythmic, allowing relaxation phases alternating with contraction phases
- Minimize the work of the heart per unit training effect
- Be quantifiable with respect to intensity

Example activities that are consistent with these criteria include, but are not limited to, walking, jogging, stair climbing, and cycling. These activities are readily available and do not require a partner. The exercise intensities are easy to establish and monitor.

Selected game activities (i.e., basketball, soccer) are appropriate if skill levels allow for continuous, intense participation. However, they offer more variability in intensity and heart rate response. Since game activities require others to participate, they may not be readily available on a regular basis. Yet, most individuals find them enjoyable and when available should be considered excellent activities. Because of the variability in heart rate associated with game activities, individuals considered high risk, unstable, or symptomatic should use caution when participating. Some modification of game rules that alters (lowers) the intensity of play may be required for participants presenting lower fitness levels.

There are activities, such as swimming, that are excellent if an individual has the skill to perform the activity. When skills exist, these activities offer benefits similar to walking, jogging or cycling. If, however, proper skill is lacking, it is difficult for an individual to achieve any level of steady state. In this type of situation, inappropriate and unstable heart rates will occur. If this is occurring, this type of activity should be avoided.

One critical criterion must be participant enjoyment. If an activity is not enjoyable, participant attrition will be high. Finally, no activity is substantially better than another. If the exercise session involves similar total energy expenditure, any activity (i.e., walking, swimming, soccer) will produce similar gains in VO_{2max}.

Frequency

The frequency or "How Often" we exercise is related to improvement in cardiorespiratory endurance. The general recommendation is 3 to 5 days per week. Yet, these guidelines are best fitted to normal, healthy individuals. How frequently an individual exercises should be based on his/her current levels of fitness, age, health status, and his/her exercise objectives. Extremely low fit individuals or cardiovascular patients may benefit from several brief daily exercise sessions. As fitness levels improve, more traditional approaches (i.e., 3 to 5 days per week) are warranted. Highly fit individuals may participate in daily activity.

Exercise sessions should be alternated with rest days. "Weekend warriors," or those individuals who employ a Friday, Saturday, Sunday exercise approach, run greater risk of injury and have limited carry over or maintenance of benefits because of the long four day rest period. While this approach allows for an individual to maintain his/her current level of fitness, the additional risk of injury associated would suggest an alternating day approach to be more advisable.

The relationship between level of improvement in cardiorespiratory fitness and frequency of exercise is not linear. Optimal gains are associated with 3 to 5 exercise sessions per week. Exercising less than 2 days per week allows for little positive improvement. Yet, it has been shown that exercising twice a week can maintain levels of fitness if current levels of intensity and duration (total energy expenditure) remain constant. Exercising more than 5 times per week will allow for little additional gains in VO_{2max} and is associated with overtraining and increased rates of musculoskeletal injury.

Finally, it is important to recognize that the above guidelines are recommendations based on improving VO_{2max}. Many individuals choose to exercise as a means of increasing caloric expenditure. These individuals would benefit from more frequent exercise sessions. Precautions should be taken to avoid daily exercise sessions until adequate levels of fitness have been achieved. Pollock and his colleagues (1977) reported the injury rate is three times greater for a 5 day per week approach as compared to a 3 day a week approach. Additionally, when adopting a 5 day a week approach it may be beneficial to lower the intensity of exercise and increase the duration. Table 5-2 provides a summary of recommended exercise frequency based on fitness levels.

Table 5-2 ■ Recommended Exercise Frequency Based on Fitness Level

Fitness Level	Recommended Frequency (days/week)
Low Fitness	3
Average Fitness	3–4
High Fitness	5–7

Intensity

Intensity of exercise or "How Hard" a person exercises is arguably the most important component of a cardiorespiratory exercise prescription and is directly related to the level of improvement in cardiorespiratory improvement. Yet, the level of intensity must be carefully determined and monitored. Intensity has to be hard enough to stimulate physiological adjustments and yet, not be so hard as to potentially induce muscular, skeletal, or articular injury. Less frequently, excessive intensity may induce a negative and potentially a lethal cardiovascular incident.

It is important to note that *intensity is inversely related to duration*. In simple, as the intensity of exercise increases, the more difficult it will be to sustain the activity. The total energy expenditure per exercising session is what is important. Low intensity, high duration activity will allow for similar improvement as compared to high intensity, short duration activity. The biggest difference is, of course, the potential and/or incidence of injury. Low intensity activity has a much lower incidence rate and should be considered as the preferred method of conditioning.

The exact intensities required to be beneficial are specific to the individual. Factors such as fitness level, predisposing injury, will influence exact recommendations. Low functional capacity or low fit individuals may require lower levels of intensity to obtain improvement.

A number of procedures have been suggested as methods of establishing intensity. The methods that are described in this text are:

- Percentage of Maximum Heart Rate
- Percentage of Heart Rate Reserve
- Percentage of Maximum Oxygen Consumption (VO$_{2max}$)
- Rate of Perceived Exertion

These are discussed separately below.

It is important to note that all of these procedures are superior to any method of prescribing intensity of exercise by a predetermined rate and distance (i.e., jogging 5 miles at an 8 minute per mile pace). Any of the suggested methods offer automatic physiological corrections for extraneous variables such as hot, humid environment, the onset of illness, and improvements in cardiorespiratory fitness levels.

For example, on days that are particularly hot and humid, the exercising heart rate when jogging will be reached at a much slower jogging pace than when compared to a cool, dry day. Since the same exercising heart rate is reached even though two different jogging paces are involved, the individual is exercising at the same intensity. In contrast, if this individual were to attempt to jog 5 miles at an 8-minute per mile pace during a hot and humid day, the physiological demand would be much greater and this individual would present a much higher and potentially dangerous heart rate response.

Heart Rate Methods

There are two methods of prescribing intensity of exercise related to the use of heart rates. These include: percentage of maximal heart rate and percentage of heart rate reserve. The use of heart rate methods are quite common and are accepted procedures, provided appropriate heart rate intensities are used for each procedure. It is extremely important to note that these two procedures require the use of different percentages or values to obtain similar levels of work intensity. Table 5-6 provides a comparison of the heart rate intensities for each procedure.

Precaution must be taken to ensure safe use when using heart rate methods. These procedure are safe and reliable when properly implemented. They are not, however, appropriate for all individuals. For example, individuals using certain medications (i.e., beta blockers) will find a drug effect that would reduce resting heart rates and stunt or block elevation in exercising heart rates with increased exertion. In this situation, the use of either heart rate method would be contraindicated. In this example, the altered heart rate response during activity would mean the relationship between heart rate response and intensity of work is lost and the individual would run the risk of exercising at too high of intensity trying to achieve a predetermined exercising heart rate.

While both methods are valid, they differ in how they are computed. The first procedure, percentage of maximum heart rate, uses age only when determining intensity, whereas the second procedure, percentage of heart rate reserve, uses age and resting heart rate when computing intensity. This difference may influence which procedure is more appropriate.

For purposes of illustration, consider the fact that existing fitness levels are reflected in an individual's resting heart rate. Simply stated, individuals presenting higher resting heart rates are less physically fit than those presenting lower resting heart rates. This would mean the percentage of heart rate reserve procedure indirectly factors in an individual's fitness level. In comparison, the procedure for recommending intensity of exercise using a percent of maximal heart rate is computed using only age, and cannot correct for fitness levels.

This difference may be extremely important. Consider the situation of an individual with extremely low functional capacity. In this particular case, you could expect a long-term exercise training effect of a gradual lowering of resting heart rate. This would mean that following a month or two of regular cardiorespiratory endurance training, these individuals would need to recompute their training heart rates to correct for their improved fitness levels. This correction would not be reflected if intensity is only being prescribed by means of a percentage of maximal heart rate.

To numerically illustrate, consider the example of an out of shape, sedentary, 20 year old, college student with an initial resting heart rate of 90 beats per minute. Using the percentage of heart rate reserve procedure, this individual would need to exercise at a sustained heart rate of 136 beats per minute to work at 60% of his/her maximum capacity.

Now consider the situation where this same individual began a program of regular aerobic activity. As a result, his/her resting heart rate is now 70 beats per minute. Again using the percentage of heart rate reserve procedure, this individual would need to exercise at a sustained heart rate of 148 beats per minute to work at 60% of his/her maximum capacity. If this individual failed to recompute his/her training heart rate after his/her fitness levels improved and continued to use the initial heart rate recommendation of 136 beats per minute, he/she would only be working at 50% of his/her maximum capacity, given his/her new and better functional capacity. In essence, he/she would be detraining.

In comparison, if the same situation existed when using the percentage of maximal heart rate procedure, no change in recommended training heart rates would occur as fitness levels improved. This is clearly one of the greatest weaknesses of this procedure and why many fitness professionals prefer the percentage of heart rate reserve procedure. For individuals presenting low functional capacities the percentage of heart rate reserve procedure is the recommended procedure for determining training heart rates.

Maximal Heart Rate

The steps for determining one's exercise intensity using the Maximal Heart Rate method are as follows:

1. Determine Maximum Heart Rate: Maximal heart rate represents the highest achieved heart rate during all out physical exertion. Ideally, maximum heart rate (MHR) would be determined during a medically monitored graded exercise test. This is the safest and most accurate method. Unfortunately, this option is not available for most individuals. Another direct method of measuring maximum heart rate would be to have an individual run a distance of 400 yards as hard as he/she could. When finished, a pulse could be immediately palpated. Because of the potential risks maximal work presents to older, symptomatic populations, this method would only be appropriate for younger, healthy individuals.

    Because of the limitations of direct measurement of maximal heart rate, most individuals use alternative indirect methods for determining MHR. The most common indirect method is to estimate MHR from the equation MHR = 220 – age. For more accurate estimation, a gender specific equation has been developed for females. It is MHR = 226 – age. It is important to recognize that indirect methods only estimate MHR. Reported (ACSM, 1998) potential error using this method is 11 beats per minute. As a result, individuals determining exercising intensities using estimated MHR should be cautioned to watch for abnormal signs and symptoms of fatigue. Symptom limitations may be reached prior to estimated exercising heart rates. In these cases, the determined estimated exercising intensities should be adjusted lower.

2. Determine Appropriate Training Intensity: The American College of Sports Medicine (2000) recommends 55/65% to 90% of maximum heart rate for most individuals. Lower functional capacity individuals or those with symptom limitations will require lower percentages. For example, an extremely sedentary individual, with a limited history of regular physical activity, and limited functional capacity, may respond to exercise intensities of 50% of MHR. Additionally, individuals more interested in using physical activity for health benefits may find lower levels of intensity beneficial. Currently, ACSM (2000) recommendations suggest that 55–64% of MHR are appropriate for establishing health benefits.

3. Determine Recommended Exercising Heart Rates: To determine the recommended exercising heart rate (EHR), multiply the determined training intensity, expressed as a fraction, times the determined MHR.

For example, to determine the recommended exercising heart rate for a 20-year-old individual wanting to exercise at 60% of his/her determined maximum, the following steps would be taken.
- MHR = 220 − 20 or 200 beats per minute.
- EHR = .6 × 200 or 120 beats per minute.

Heart Rate Reserve

The steps for determining exercise intensity using a percentage of heart rate reserve are as follows:

1. Determine Maximum Heart Rate: Determine MHR as described above. The equations are: Male − MHR = 220 − age; Females − MHR = 226 − age.

2. Determine Resting Heart Rate: Resting heart rate (RHR) can be determined by palpating a pulse while at rest. Ideally, RHR should be determined in the morning before a person gets up out of bed and begins his/her day. Yet, reasonably accurate measures can be achieved following 15 to 30 minutes of rest. Procedures for palpating pulse to determine heart rate are discussed below.

3. Determine Heart Rate Reserve: Heart Rate Reserve (HRR) represents the number of beats an individual's heart can increase when changing from a complete resting situation to maximal work. This change is linearly related to the increase in the work of the heart. As we increase in exertion, we will get a corresponding linear increase in heart rate. Heart rate reserve is determined by subtracting RHR from MHR. The equation for determining HRR is HRR = MHR − RHR.

4. Determine the appropriate training intensities: The appropriate training intensity is specific to individual needs. The American College of Sports Medicine (2000) recommends 40/50% to 85% of heart rate reserve. Individuals with symptom limitations or low fitness levels will require a more conservative training intensity. Also, the health benefits of physical activity can be achieved at lower levels of intensity. Current recommendations for establishing health benefits are 40–49% of HRR. Table 5-3 shows recommended exercise percent HRR based on initial fitness levels.

5. Determine the Recommended Exercising Heart Rate (REHR): Use the following equation to determine the recommended exercising heart rate. REHR = [___% (HRR)] + RHR.

Table 5-3 ■ Recommended Exercise Percent HHR Based on Initial Fitness Levels

	Low Fitness	Average Fitness	High Fitness
Minimum HR	40% HRR	60% HRR	70% HRR
Target HR	60% HRR	75% HRR	80% HRR
Do-not-exceed HR	75% HRR	85% HRR	90% HRR

Key: HR = Heart Rate; HRR = Heart Rate Reserve

Adopted from: deVries, H. (1986). *Physiology of Exercise For Physical Education and Athletics*. (4th Ed.). Dubuque, IA: Wm. C. Brown.

Rate of Perceived Exertion

Rate of perceived exertion (RPE) is an alternative method of determining exercise intensity. The procedure is reasonably simple to learn and use. It has virtually no cost associated with it. This procedure is appropriate for most individuals and has rapidly become a standard measure for monitoring and recommending exercise intensity. It is an especially useful procedure for individuals who have difficulty palpating a pulse or who are unable to use standard procedures using heart rates as a measure of monitoring intensity.

Rate of perceived exertion has been shown to be highly related to exercising heart rates, oxygen consumption, blood lactate levels, and other measures of exertion. RPE is based on the perceived effort of an individual during aerobic activity. During activity, individuals monitor or sense their physical effort based on their own physical responses to exercise. Body feedback from muscles, joints, and respiratory patterns are often monitored variables. The common cliché for monitoring is "listening to your body." Verbal expressions related to how hard a person is working are fitted to a numeric scale. Borg's scale (Borg, 1983) shown in Table 5-4, describes various levels of exercise intensity.

Table 5-4 ■ Rate of Perceived Exertion Scale

	Original Scale		Revised Scale
6		0	Nothing at all
7	Very, very light	0.5	Very, very weak
8		1	Very weak
9	Very light	2	Weak
10		3	Moderate
11	Fairly light	4	Somewhat strong
12		5	Strong
13	Somewhat hard	6	
14		7	Very strong
15	Hard	8	
16		9	
17	Very Hard	10	Very, very strong
18		*	Maximal
19	Very, very hard		
20			

From Borg, G. (1982). *Medicine and Science in Sports and Exercise, 22,* 377–387.

To use the RPE scale, individuals are asked to determine or assess how they feel at their current level of activity. Verbal expressions range from no exertion at all to maximal exertion. For example, the verbal expression "somewhat hard" is fitted to the numeric value of 13 on the 6–20 scale and 4 on the 0 to 10 scale.

Initially, RPE should be used in conjunction with some other measure of exercise intensity (i.e., percent of heart rate reserve) to help individuals relate their perceived exertion with actual intensities. Over time, most individuals develop an understanding of how a particular level of exertion feels. Once this level of understanding has been established, the need for frequent heart rate monitoring is diminished. Occasional heart rate monitoring however, is advised.

RPE is not a completely foolproof method and some precautions should be noted. Selected groups of people, particularly the elderly, the young, and the obese may not be able to accurately assess their physical efforts. RPE is also influenced by intensity of activity and from environmental factors. For example, RPE is less reliable when working at lower intensities. Also, RPE values will differ when comparing similar exercising intensities in a laboratory environment and an outside environment. Similarly, reported RPE values in hotter environments tend to be higher than reported values in lower or more moderate climates.

The American College of Sports Medicine (1990) recommends an exercising intensity of 12 to 16 (somewhat hard to hard) on the original scale. Remember, exercise intensities for the less fit are lower. These individuals should initially begin at lower levels (i.e., 11; fairly light) on the scale. Table 5-5 shows the relationship between RPE, VO_{2max}, MHR and HRR based on 20–60 minutes of endurance training.

Table 5-5 ■ Classification of Intensity of Exercise Based on 20–60 Minutes of Endurance Training

Relative Intensity (%)

HR_{max}	VO_{2max} or HRR	RPE	Classification of Intensity
< 35%	< 30%	< 10	Very light
35–59%	30–49%	10–11	Light
60–79%	50–74%	12–13	Moderate
80–89%	75–84%	14–16	Heavy
=> 90%	=> 85%	> 16	Very heavy

Key:
HR_{max} = Maximum Heart Rate; VO_{2max} = Maximum Oxygen Uptake
HRR = Heart Rate Reserve; RPE = Rate of Perceive Exertion

Adopted from Pollock, M. And Wilmore, J. (1990). *Exercise in Health and Disease: Evaluation and Prescription for Prevention and Rehabilitation*, 2nd Ed. Philadelphia, PA: W.B. Saunders.

Percent of VO₂ Maximum

The American College of Sports Medicine (1998) recommends 40/50 to 85% of maximum oxygen uptake. Like heart rate, oxygen uptake is directly related to exercise intensity. The relationship is shown in Table 5-6. As a result of the direct relationship between %HRR and %VO_{2max} exercise recommendations can be made using %HRR when equipment (i.e., treadmill) is not available to control specific levels of oxygen consumption.

Table 5-6 ■ Relationship of Percent of Maximum Heart Rate, Heart Rate Reserve, and Maximal Oxygen Uptake

% VO_{2max}	% HRR	% Max. HR
50	50	65
55	55	68
60	60	72
65	65	76
70	70	79
75	75	83
80	80	87
85	85	91
90	90	94

Key: % VO_{2max} = Percent of Maximal Oxygen Uptake; % HRR = Percent of Heart Rate Reserve; % Max. HR = Percent of Maximal Heart Rate

Adopted from Howley, E. and Franks, B. (1986). *Health/Fitness Instructor's Handbook*. Champaign, Ill. Human Kinetics Press.

Duration

Duration or "How Long" you should exercise in a single exercise session is inversely related to intensity. The American College of Sports Medicine (1998) recommends 20 to 60 minutes of continuous aerobic activity at an appropriate exercise intensity. If intermittent activity is incorporated into the exercise program, a minimum of three 10-minute bouts should be accumulated throughout the day. As is the case with the other components of an exercise prescription (i.e., modality, frequency, intensity, progression), duration is largely based on individual needs. There is really no ideal duration that is appropriate for everyone.

Specific recommendations should be tailored to fitness levels and individual objectives. Beginners will probably be unable to sustain continuous activity even for the minimum recommendation of twenty minutes. In this case, discontinuous activity or multiple activities of short duration (10 minute bouts minimum) may be required. As fitness levels improve, more sustained activity can be expected. Table 5-7 provides a summary of recommended exercise durations based on fitness levels.

Table 5-7 ■ Recommended Exercise Duration Based on Fitness Level

Fitness Level	Recommended Duration (minutes)
Low Fitness	10–20
Average Fitness	20–30
High Fitness	30–60

Recall, the benefits associated with high intensity—short duration activity are similar to those associated with low intensity—long duration activity assuming similar total energy expenditure for each approach. This suggests that a long duration walking program done daily would yield similar cardiorespiratory improvement as compared to an alternating day jogging program, assuming both programs have similar total energy expenditure. ACSM (1990, 1998) recommends an exercise session energy expenditure of approximately 200 kcal for a four day per week program, and 300 kcal for a three day per week program. Therefore, the actual duration of each exercise session would be determined by the intensity of the exercise.

For example, an individual weighing 154 pounds (70kg) with a determined VO_{2max} of 42 ml/kg/min (12 METs) is wanting to exercise on a three day a week program. This individual would need to exercise for 34 minutes at 60% intensity and 25.5 minutes at 80% intensity to expend the recommended 300 kcal. In other words, as the intensity of exercise decreases, more time is needed to expend the same amount of energy.

Progression

The progression or rate at which one advances his/her cardiorespiratory endurance program is specific to the individual. Initial fitness level, age, physical limitations, health status, and individual goals and objectives of the program are only a few of the variables that must be considered. For the non-symptomatic, apparently healthy individual, the ACSM (1998b) recommends a three-stage approach to progression. The three stages include: initial conditioning stage, improvement stage, and maintenance stage. A brief description of each stage follows. Table 5-8 provides an example of a recommended progression of a cardiorespiratory endurance conditioning program for an apparently healthy individual. It is important to recognize that this is only an example. Specific adaptations should be made to fit individual needs, goals, and objectives.

Initial Conditioning Stage

The objective of the initial stage is to introduce the participant to the program. This stage should last approximately one month. Individual differences may shorten or lengthen the period. Low functional capacity participants, or those who have been sedentary for extended periods of time may require six weeks or more to adapt. Older individuals generally require more time to adjust to increased activity. Healthy individuals who have been reasonably active may be introduced to activity and adapt within a few weeks.

Improvement Stage

The purpose of the improvement stage is to progress the participant to a predetermined level of fitness. Since the body has been involved in activity for several weeks (initial stage) it is possible to increase exercise intensities more rapidly. The exact rate of increase will depend on the individual. Again, age, health status, fitness levels, etc., will influence the rate of progress. Typically, the improvement stage should take four to six months. The goal of the stage is to improve the individual's cardiorespiratory fitness levels to a point that he/she may sustain an appropriate exercise intensity for 20 to 30 minutes. Appropriate exercise intensities are between 40/50–85% of VO_{2max} or HRR or 55/65–90% MHR. Individuals with lower functional capacities may start at 40% VO_{2max} or HRR or 50% MHR.

Table 5-8 ■ Example Exercise Progression for an Apparently Healthy 20-Year-Old Student

Name: Joe Example
Age: 20
Body Weight: 154 lbs. (70 kg)
Resting Heart Rate: 70 Beats Per Minute
Estimated MHR: 200 Beats Per Minute
Determined VO_{2max}: 50 ml/kg/min

	Week	Frequency	%VO_{2max} Min.	Target	Max.	Recommended Heart Rates Heart Rate Reserve Min.	Target	Max.	Ex. Time	Sets	Duration
Initial Stage	1	3	40	50	85	122	135	180.5	2	6	12
	2	3	40	50	85	122	135	180.5	2	7	14
	3	3	50	55	85	135	141.5	180.5	2	7	14
	4	3	50	60	85	135	148	180.5	2	8	16
	5	3	50	60	85	135	148	180.5	2	8	16
	6	3–4	50	60	85	135	148	180.5	3	6	18
Improvement Stage	7	3–4	50	60	85	135	148	180.5	3	6	18
	8	3–4	60	65	85	148	154.5	180.5	4	5	20
	9	3–4	60	65	85	148	154.5	180.5	4	5	20
	10	3–4	60	70	85	148	161	180.5	5	4	20
	11	3–4	60	70	85	148	161	180.5	5	4	20
	12	3–4	60	70	85	148	161	180.5	5	5	25
	13	3–4	60	70	85	148	161	180.5	5	5	25
	14	3–4	60	70	85	148	161	180.5	7	4	28
	15	3–4	60	70	85	148	161	180.5	7	4	28
	16	3–4	60	70	85	148	161	180.5	7	4	28
	17	3–4	60	70	85	148	161	180.5	8	4	32
	18	3–4	60	70	85	148	161	180.5	8	4	32
	19	3–4	60	75	85	148	167.5	180.5	8	4	32
	20	4–5	60	75	85	148	167.5	180.5	10	3	30
	21	4–5	60	75	85	148	167.5	180.5	10	3	30
	22	4–5	60	75	85	148	167.5	180.5	10	3	30
	23	4–5	60	75	85	148	167.5	180.5	15	2	30
	24	4–5	60	75	85	148	167.5	180.5	15	2	30
	25	4–5	60	75	85	148	167.5	180.5	15	2	30
	26	4–5	60	75	85	148	167.5	180.5	20/10	2/1	30
	27	4–5	60	75	85	148	167.5	180.5	20/10	2/1	30
Maintenance Stage	28	4–5	60	75	85	148	167.5	180.5	30	1	30

Maintenance Stage

The goal of the maintenance stage is to maintain the previously acquired cardiorespiratory fitness level, not necessarily to improve it. Following reassessment, however, it would be appropriate to establish new goals and objectives.

The maintenance stage begins when an individual can continuously exercise at a predetermined exercising heart rate for 30 minutes or more. Maintenance stage activities can be modified to include a variety of modalities that the participant may enjoy. Group activities are appropriate if participants share similar fitness levels and exercise at similar intensities. This should help in eliminating staleness and boredom. The critical issue is to maintain similar energy costs with whatever exercise modality chosen. This energy cost should be consistent with 30 minutes of continuous activity at the exercising intensity. Any deviation toward a lower level of intensity would allow a detraining effect to occur.

Determination of Heart Rate

Two procedures for determining heart rate are suggested below. Each is safe, valid, and reliable, if proper procedures are followed.

Procedures for Determining Heart Rate Electronically

A number of companies offer reasonably priced heart rate monitors. These devices include a chest monitor and a receiver, usually worn as a watch. When in use, the monitor is worn around the chest over the heart. It has internal electrodes that detect small electrical signals emitted by the heart during contraction and relaxation. The detected signal is then transmitted to the receiver by telemetry. The receiver interprets the signal and provides a continuous display of the existing heart rate.

There are several advantages of electrical monitoring. These include, but are not limited to, accuracy, and continuous display of heart rate. Individuals who have trouble detecting a pulse through palpation or who do not want to stop their activity in order to determine their exercising heart rate, will find electronic monitors especially useful. Depending on the model and the manufacturer, some heart rate monitors allow the user to program minimal and maximal exercising heart rates into the receiver. When in use, the receiver will monitor the heart rate and provide feedback, through an audio sound, to the user when the exercising heart rate drops below or rises above the preprogrammed rates.

Procedures for Palpating Pulse

Resting and exercising heart rates can be monitored by palpating pulse at the carotid artery (see Figure 5.1) or on the radial artery (see Figure 5.2). Initially, it may be difficult to locate the appropriate locations. Upon practice, most develop the skill and can easily incorporate this inexpensive method into their conditioning programs.

Precaution should be taken to only apply light pressure, on one side of the neck, when palpating for pulse. Heavy pressure may occlude blood flow and/or specifically, in the case of the carotid artery, create a vagal effect resulting in a slowed heart rate and decreased blood pressure. This may lead to light-headedness and/or fainting. The exact site of palpation should be one-third of the way between the thyroid cartilage and the angle of the mandible or slightly under the jaw, just to the side of the trachea.

When determining resting heart rate from pulse palpation the following procedural consideration should be followed. As previously mentioned, for the most accurate measurement, resting heart rate should be determined upon wakening. It can, however, be taken with reasonable accuracy after a person has been sitting quietly for 15 to 30 minutes. When determining RHR you should palpate the pulse for 30 seconds and multiply the result by two. Shorter periods of time can be used (i.e., 15 seconds multiplied by 4) but there is greater error in the predicted pulse.

To determine exercising heart rates, the same palpation procedures should be followed as when determining RHR. Most individuals will find they need to slow or stop their activity in order to observe a clock and to feel for a pulse. It is important to recognize that when exercise stops the body will immediately start to recover. It is extremely important to determine the exercising heart rate immediately upon stopping. Any delay is likely to create error. This is especially true for the highly conditioned individual whose heart rate will recover very quickly.

Components of the Daily Cardiorespiratory Exercise Session

The cardiorespiratory exercise session should consist of three distinct components. These include: (1) warm-up, (2) aerobic conditioning, and (3) cool-down. It is important to note, the cardiorespiratory aspect is only part of the total exercise program and should not be thought of as a substitute for flexibility, muscular strength and muscular endurance training.

Warm-Up

The purpose of the warm-up component is to prepare the body for activity. The importance of this component cannot be overstated. Opinions vary as to how to classify warm-up activities. McKardle and colleagues (1991) have suggested the following categories: (1) general warm-up and (2) specific warm-up. Robergs and Roberts (1997) suggest: (1) Active versus passive, (2) general versus specific, and (3) submaximal versus intense. Neither method is uniquely independent of the other. A general understanding of the nature and benefits of warm-up will illustrate this point.

General warm-ups involve light flexibility activity, calisthenics, and low level aerobic activity. These are considered active, non-intensive, non-specific activities. Typically, they are not related to any specific activity, but rather are structured to simply ready the body for elevations in metabolism or increase activity. One of the effects of a proper warm-up is increased muscle temperature. As a result, individuals can use their body temperature as a guide to indicate when they are adequately prepared for activity.

Passive warm-up has been used to increase body or muscle temperature. Passive warm-ups include, but are not limited to, hot showers, whirlpools, and baths. In these cases, the elevations in temperature result from conduction, as opposed to increased metabolism. Passive warming of the body is better when compared to no warm-up but is not as effective as active warm-up (Karlsson, Bonde-Petersen, Henriksson, & Knuttgen, 1975).

Specific warm-ups are focused or related to specific activities. This type of warm-up is associated with activities that rely more on neuromuscular pathways. For example, golf swings and gymnastic maneuvers are high skill activities that require not only general body readiness, but benefit from specific task readiness. In these situations, an individual is readying not only the body, but attempting to prepare psychologically as well.

No matter what type of warm-up is involved, it is important to follow general guidelines. All warm-up activities should allow for gradual physiological changes. Core body temperature, muscle temperatures, heart rate responses and systolic blood pressures should be gradually elevated without creating undue muscle fatigue or exhaustion. Studies indicate this to be particularly true for individuals with compromised coronary blood flow. Gradual warm-ups for these individuals have proven especially beneficial in delaying angina onset or abnormal electrocardiographic changes associated with myocardial ischemia.

Warm-up is highly individualized. For example, a highly trained or conditioned individual may include more activity, at a greater intensity than a low fit individual. In fact, what a conditioned person may consider a proper warm-up could produce fatigue and exhaustion in a low fit individual. In general, the warm-up period should range from 10–15 minutes

Conditioning

The conditioning phase of a daily workout should follow the guidelines for modality, frequency, intensity, duration, and progression described above. The critical issue during the conditioning phase of the daily workout is to sustain the exercising heart rate for 20–60 minutes at the appropriate exercising intensity.

Cool-Down

The purpose of the cool-down is to gradually return the body from an elevated state back to a normal resting state. A cool-down session of 10 to 15 minutes should follow the aerobic conditioning phase of the cardiorespiratory exercise session. Flexibility exercises and slow activity similar to the modality involved in the exercise session (i.e., walking, cycling, or swimming) should be included. For example, for an individual who was jogging, he/she may want to walk during the cool-down. This will help prevent post exertion hypotension, and yet, still allow normal levels of heart rate and blood pressure to return to the body. Precaution should be taken to never abruptly stop the exercise session. This behavior will prevent the needed gradual reduction of body systems back to a normal resting state.

Exercise Prescriptions and Weight Loss

In addition to using exercise as a means of improving health and fitness levels, it is also common for exercise to be used to assist in weight management. It is important to recognize, however, that the levels of activity required to make significant changes in health, fitness levels, and body fatness vary.

The recommendations discussed above represent guidelines, as described by the American College of Sports Medicine, for improving oxygen consumption (VO_{2max}) or cardiorespiratory fitness. Specifically, in terms of caloric expenditure, the guidelines recommend a minimum of 300 kcal per exercise session for a 3 day a week program and 200 kcal per exercise session for a 4-day a week program (ACSM, 1990, 1998b). This represents a total weekly exercise caloric expenditure of 800–900 kcal. While this level of caloric expenditure may be adequate for developing and maintaining cardiorespiratory fitness, it may be too limited for those interested in losing or controlling body fatness. These individuals may need more weekly exercise caloric expenditure to meet individual weight management objectives. This situation presents a number of exercise programming challenges.

How do we tailor the exercise program to address the caloric expenditure needs of an individual? How can the caloric expenditure of an exercise session be determined? More importantly perhaps, how can an exercise program be safely modified to allow for additional caloric expenditure so the objectives of a weight management program can be met without compromising safety and increasing the risk of injury?

The relationships of the components of a fitness program (i.e., frequency, intensity, duration) and energy expenditure can be used to guide the weight management exercise program. Because these variables are related, it is possible to use the weekly exercise caloric expenditure as a guide for helping to establish the frequency, intensity, and duration of an exercise program. Table 5-9 illustrates the relationship of these variables by showing how exercise duration was determined.

The following equations may assist in estimating the energy expenditure of an activity.

- METs × 3.5 × body weight in kg / 200 = kcal/min
- Relative VO_2 (ml/kg/min) × body weight in kg / 200 = kcal/min
- Absolute VO_2 (ml/min) / 200 = kcal/min

Cardiorespiratory Endurance Training Risk

What are the risks of participating in regular and vigorous cardiorespiratory training? How safe or dangerous is exercise? All of us have heard the unfortunate and unexpected traumatic deaths of Jim Fixx, "Pistol Pete" Maravich, and Hank Gathers. What is the relationship between exercise and their deaths? These are fair questions and need to be addressed.

Research indicates that coronary artery disease is the most important factor in contributing to cardiovascular complications that occur during exercise. The risk of exercise is extremely low for younger, apparently healthy, nonsmoking individuals. It is higher for those who possess known coronary risk factors (see Chapter 4). Finally, there is an increased risk of heart attack during or immediately after the actual exercise session. Again, these risks appear to be extremely limited. This risk appears to increase by a factor of 16.9 compared to sedentary periods (Levine, Hanson-Zuckerman, & Cole, 2001). In fact, regular aerobic activity is used as a means of cardiac rehabilitation. To illustrate, Thompson (1982) reported the risk of death is about one in every 7,620 joggers between the ages of 30 and 64 years. ACSM (1998b) estimates an annual risk of death of 1 in 20,000 for healthy men. Nieman (1995) reports that fewer than 10 out of 100,000 men will have a heart attack during exercise. He also cited those individuals who did present incidence: 1) tended to live sedentary lifestyles, 2) had a history of, or were at risk for, heart disease, and 3) participated in extremely intense activity.

Table 5-9 ■ The Relationship of Exercise Frequency, Intensity, Duration and Energy Expenditure

Descriptive Information
Name: Joe Example
VO$_{2max}$: 50 ml/kg/min
Body weight: 70 kg; 154 lbs.
Weekly Exercise Caloric Expenditure: 1000 kcal
Frequency: 3 days per week
Desired Exercise Intensities: 60%; 85%

To determine the energy expenditure (kcal/min) for a given exercise **intensity** use the following:

Formula: Exercise Intensity (expressed as a fraction) × VO$_{2max}$ × Body Weight (kg) /200 = kcal/min

Example:

Exercise Intensity of 60% VO$_{2max}$: .6 × 50 (ml/kg/min.) × 70 (kg) / 200 = 10.5 kcal/min
Exercise Intensity of 85% VO$_{2max}$: .85 × 50 (ml/kg/min) × 70 (kg) / 200 = 14.88 kcal/min

---

To determine daily exercise session caloric expenditure needs based on weekly exercise energy expenditure objectives and **frequency** use the following:

Formula: Daily Exercise Session Caloric Expenditure (kcal) = Weekly Exercise Caloric Expenditure (kcal) / Frequency (days per week)

Example: 1000 kcal / 3 (days per week) = 333.33 kcal/day
1000 kcal / 4 (days per week) = 250 kcal/day

To determine the exercise session **duration** use the following:

Formula: Exercise Session Duration (minutes) = [Weekly Exercise Caloric Expenditure (kcal) / Frequency (days per week)] / Energy expenditure (kcal/min)

Example: 1000 (kcal) /3 (days/wk) / 10.5 (kcal/min) = 31.7 minutes
1000 (kcal)/ 3 (days/wk) / 14.875 (kcal/min) = 22.4 minutes

To determine the **total energy expenditure** (kcal/min) for a given exercise session use the following:

Formula: Exercise Intensity (expressed as a fraction) × VO$_{2max}$ × Body Weight (kg) /200 × Exercise Duration (min) = kcal

Example:

Exercise Intensity of 60% VO$_{2max}$; 60 minutes of activity: .6 × 50 (ml/kg/min) × 70 (kg) / 200 × 30 = 630 kcal
Exercise Intensity of 85% VO$_{2max}$; 30 minutes of activity: .85 × 50 (ml/kg/min) × 70 (kg) / 200 × 30 = 446.25 kcal

---

Risk appears to be correlated with the individual's age and previous health status. For example, incidence of death in younger athletes appears to be linked to congenital cardiovascular defects (Cantu, 1992). In individuals older than 30 years of age, increased risk of death appears to be related to a prior history of coronary heart disease and the intensity of exercise. Extremely intense exercise appears to present significantly higher level of risk for these individuals than lower intensity exercise. This finding is especially true for individuals currently living a sedentary lifestyle (Mittleman, Maclure, Tofler, Sherwood, Goldberg, & Muller, 1993). This finding helps to explain why so many cardiovascular deaths are associated with sedentary individuals suddenly participating in vigorous activity, such as occurs when many of these individuals are forced into shovelling snow. Additionally, it has been shown that occasional participation in vigorous activity presents a 74-fold increase in risk of death.

In summary, it could be argued that there are inherent risks associated with cardiorespiratory endurance training. These risk, however, appear to be extremely limited and should not, for most individuals, serve as a deterrent to regular participation in a cardiovascular endurance training program. The absolute risk of death during vigorous exercise appears to be about 1 death for every 1.51 million episodes of exercise (Levine, Hanson-Zuckerman, & Cole, 2001). When comparing known risks against known health/fitness benefits, the health/fitness benefits of cardiorespiratory endurance training far exceed any associated risk of injury.

Research findings indicate the health risks associated with choosing not to participate in regular cardiorespiratory endurance training, as in the case of living a sedentary lifestyle, are far greater than the risks associated with habitual cardiorespiratory endurance training. It has been reported (Siscovick, et al., 1984) that men who regularly participate in vigorous activity have a 40% risk reduction of sudden cardiac death compared to their sedentary counterparts. The Center for Disease Control reports that sedentary living is as much of a contributor to heart disease in America as hypertension, hypercholesterolemia, and smoking (Powell, Thompson, Caspersen, & Kendrick, 1987). Clearly, the risk of coronary heart disease is reduced from regular participation in activity (Blair, Kampert, Kuhl, et al., 1996).

Detraining: The Effect of Exercise Training Reduction or Stoppage on Cardiorespiratory Endurance

How does aerobic exercise training reduction or stoppage affect cardiorespiratory endurance? The cardiovascular and respiratory systems, like the muscular system, will respond negatively to any form of detraining. This loss in function can be explained by the **principle of reversibility**, which suggest when exercise reduction or cessation occurs, the body will adapt to the new levels of demand. In the case of cardiorespiratory fitness, research suggest that aerobic endurance adaptations are more sensitive to periods of inactivity than muscle tissue (Kraemer, 2000).

Several variables influence the rate and magnitude of loss. One variable appears to be the nature of detraining. Complete exercise cessation appears to have a more traumatic effect than simply exercise reduction. Significant reductions in cardiorespiratory fitness levels can occur after only two weeks of aerobic detraining (Coyle, Martin, Sinacore, Joyner, Hagberg, & Holloszy, 1984). Longer periods of inactivity (several months) will result in losses back to pre-training levels. In cases where individuals have a long-term history of higher levels of aerobic fitness. The loss of fitness appears to be somewhat slower than that which occurs in individuals with short-term histories.

A reduction in training results in less cardiorespiratory fitness loss as compared to complete exercise cessation. It is important to note, however, that the nature of the exercise reduction directly impacts the magnitude of loss (Hickson & Rosenkoetter, 1981; Hickson, Kanakis, Davis, Moore, & Rich, 1982; Hickson, Rosster, Pollock, Galassi, & Rich, 1985). Reduction in exercise intensity will result in more significant losses than the losses associated with reduction in exercise frequency or duration. These findings are important in that they suggest that the occasional missed exercise session or the shortened exercise session will not result in significant cardiorespiratory fitness reduction.

Laboratory Activities

CHAPTER 5

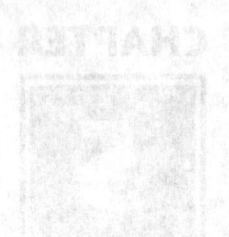

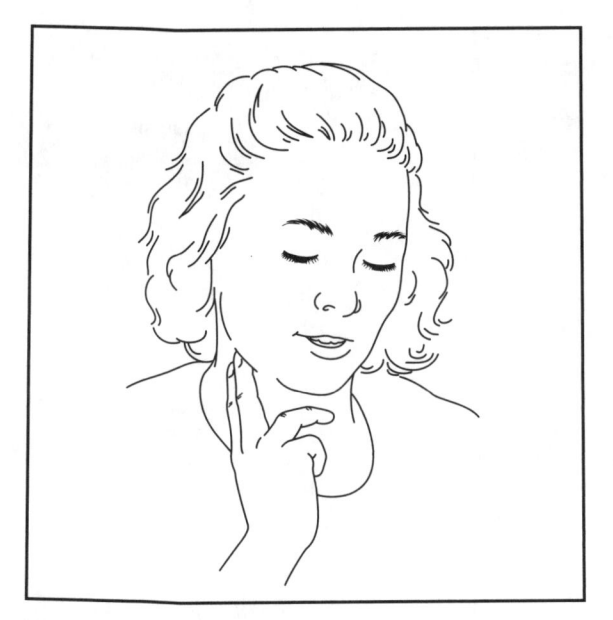

Principles of Cardiorespiratory Endurance ■ 115

Figure 5.1 ■ Pulse Palpation: Carotid

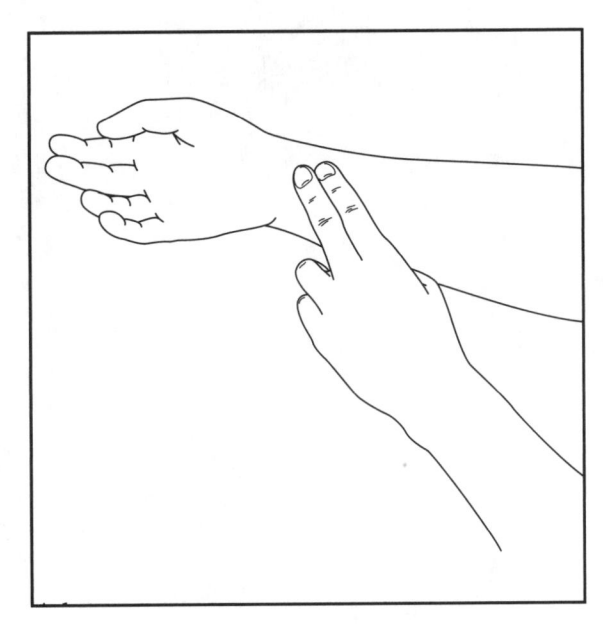

Figure 5.2 ■ Pulse Palpation: Radial

Name: _____ Class Time/Day: _____ Score: _____

LABORATORY 5-B

Cardiorespiratory (VO$_{2Max}$): 1.5-Mile Run Test

- **Purpose:** This test will determine estimated VO$_{2max}$ from a submaximal cardiorespiratory exercise bout (i.e., 1.5-mile jog).

- **Precautions:** Individuals with a history of cardiovascular disease should consult with the class instructor before participating.

- **Equipment:** Stopwatch, heart rate monitor (optional).

- **Procedure:** Each subject should jog exactly one and one-half miles. The pace of the jog should be consistent throughout and should constitute a maximal effort. *Nonmaximal efforts will result in inaccurate estimates*. **Note: This test should be performed by only healthy individuals.**

- **Scoring:** The time at the finish of the 1.5-mile run. Time should be recorded in minutes and seconds. Walk time should be computed according to the following formula: time = minutes + seconds/60. Each subject's body weight should be determined and converted into kilograms (kg). Subject gender is also required. For computational purposes, the following values (0 = female; 1 = male) are used to represent gender. All data should be fitted to the estimation equation provided (ACSM, 2000). Fitness classification based on the estimated oxygen consumption should be determined from Table 5-10 (see Laboratory 5-A).

- **Data/Calculations:**

Name: _____ Date: ___/___/___

Gender: _____ Age: _____ Height: _____ Weight: _____

Age: _____

Gender: _____ (0 = female; 1 = male)

Body Weight (kg): _____ (lbs. × .454)

Run Time: _____ (time = minutes + seconds/60)

Estimated VO$_{2max}$: _____

Fitness Classification: _____

VO$_{2max}$ Percentile Score: _____

Formula: VO$_{2max}$ (ml/kg/min) = [3.5 + (483 / (time in minutes))]

Calculate Estimated VO$_{2max}$: VO$_{2max}$ (ml/kg/min) = [3.5 + (483 / (   ))]

Name: _____ Class Time/Day: _____ Score: _____

LABORATORY 5-C

Three-Mile Walk/Run Test

- **Purpose:** This laboratory is designed to help the student learn the relationship between exercise intensity and exercising heart rate.

- **Precautions:** Individuals with a history of cardiovascular disease should consult with the class instructor before participating.

- **Equipment:** Heart monitor

- **Procedure:**

Step 1: Determine resting heart rate (RHR).

Step 2: Determine estimated maximum heart rate (MHR).

The most common indirect method to determine maximum exercising heart rate is to estimate it. Males can estimate their MHR from the equation MHR = 220 – age. To allow for more accurate estimation, a gender specific equation has been developed for females. It is MHR = 226 – age.

Step 3: Determine heart rate reserve (HRR).

Heart rate reserve is determined by subtracting an individual's RHR from his/her MHR (i.e., MHR – RHR). Heart rate reserve represents the heart's ability to adapt from rest to maximal work.

Step 4: Determine upper and lower exercising heart rates.

Unless otherwise advised by your instructor, use 60% and 85% as lower and upper level exercising intensities, respectively. Use the following formulas: Lower Intensity HR = [.6(HRR)] + RHR and Upper Intensity HR = [.85(HRR)] + RHR.

Step 5: Program the Polar Heart Monitor

To program the Polar Accurex II Heart Monitor press the **SELECT** button until **SET** appears in the lower right hand corner of the clock face. Press the **START*STOP** button on the left side of the watch until **LIM** shows. You are ready to set the upper and lower exercising heart rate limits. The top number represents your upper limit and the bottom number your lower limit. One number on the watch should be flashing. To change the flashing number, press the **SELECT** button to increase the value, or the **SIGNAL** button to decrease the value. When the desired number is flashing, press the **STORE/LAP** button on the bottom of the watch to store the number. Continue to store each digit in the same manner. When all digits are stored and the first number of the upper limit is flashing, press the **START/STOP** button 3 times. You now have the watch set and it is ready to monitor your activity.

119

Step 6: Monitoring the Three-Mile Walk/Jog Exercise Session with the Accurex II

After the polar heart monitor is pre-programmed with an individual's upper and lower exercising heart rate, it is ready to monitor the exercising heart rates. Place the chest strap around the chest at the level of the xiphoid process of the sternum. Position the "electrode" aspect of the strap, directly on the skin, in the center of the chest.

To use the watch to monitor an exercise session, press the **SELECT** button until the word **MEASURE** shows at the lower left corner of the watch face. Press the **START/STOP** button when you want to begin monitoring and the **START/STOP** button when you want to stop the monitoring.

Walk/jog three miles while trying to keep your exercising heart rate within the upper and lower exercising heart rate limits. Adjust your exercising intensity as needed.

■ **Scoring:** The object of this laboratory experience is to teach the relationship of exercise intensity and exercising heart rates. While you are walking or jogging the three miles, you may find that you need to adjust your exercise intensity to keep your heart rate within the predetermined upper and lower limits. If your heart rate is too high, slow your pace. If it falls below the lower exercising heart rate, increase your pace.

At the completion of the walk/jog, record the time, as shown by the heart rate monitor, that your exercising heart rates were above, below, and in the preprogrammed exercising heart rate target zones. Also record the average exercising heart rate as shown on the heart rate monitor.

■ **Data/Calculations:**

Name: Date: /   /

Gender: Age: Height: Weight:

■ **Formulas:**
- Maximum Heart Rate:
    Males: 220 – age = MHR
    Females: 226 – age = MHR
- Heart Rate Reserve:
    MHR – RHR = HRR
- Upper and Lower Exercising Heart Rates:
    .6*(HRR) + RHR = Lower Limit Exercising Heart Rate
    .85*(HRR) + RHR = Upper Limit Exercising Heart Rate

Resting Heart Rate: _____

Maximum Heart Rate: _____

Heart Rate Reserve: _____

Lower Limit Exercising Heart Rate: _____

Upper Limit Exercising Heart Rate: _____

Total run time: _____

Time above target zone: _____

Time within target zone: _____

Time below target zone: _____

Average Heart Rate: _____

6

Principles of Muscular Strength and Endurance

Regular moderate physical activity provides benefits in health and well-being for the vast majority.

U.S. Surgeon General's Report for 2000

■ Chapter Outline ■

Introduction
What Is the Difference between Muscular Strength and Muscular Endurance?
Benefits of Resistive Training
Principle of Overload—Resistive Training
Principle of Specificity of Exercise—Resistive Training
Detraining: The Effects of Resistive Exercise Training Reduction or Stoppage on Skeletal Muscle Tissue
Types of Skeletal Muscular Contraction
    Isometric (Static) Contractions
    Concentric Contractions
    Eccentric Contractions
Skeletal Muscle Actions
Types of Skeletal Muscle Fibers
    Slow Twitch (Type I)
    Fast Twitch (Type IIa and Type IIb)
Factors Effecting Muscular Strength and Endurance Training
    Muscle Size
    Gender
    Age
Muscle Soreness
Basic Techniques of Resistance Training
    Isometric Training

Isotonic (Progressive Resistive Exercise) Training
Isokinetic Training
Principles of Training
    Introduction
        Time Course of Cellular Adaptation and Increased Strength
    Isometric Training Principles
    Isotonic Training Principles
        Training for Muscular Strength
        Training for Muscular Endurance
        Training for Muscular Power
        Training for Hypertrophy
        Inter-Set and Inter-Session Rest Periods
        Practical Guidelines for Isotonic Training
    Isokinetic Training Principles
Additional Resistance Activities
    Circuit Training
    Plyometrics
    Calisthenics
    Body Building
Additional Considerations for Resistive Training Programs

Learning Objectives

The student should be able to:

- Identify the three types of muscle found in the human body.
- Define muscular strength.
- Define muscular endurance.
- Describe the benefits of resistive training.
- Describe the functional characteristics of isometric, isotonic and isokinetic muscle contractions.
- Identify factors that effect muscular strength and endurance.
- Describe the relationship between the principle of overload and the development of muscular strength and endurance.
- Describe the relationship between the principle of specificity and the development of muscular strength and endurance.
- Describe the effects of resistive training reduction or stoppage on skeletal muscle tissue.
- Identify and define the functional characteristics of the three types of muscular contraction.
- Identify and define the metabolic and functional characteristics of Type I and Type II skeletal muscle fibers.
- Describe basic training techniques of isometric, isotonic, and isokinetic resistive training procedures.
- Describe the time course (chronic adaptation) of muscle cell adaptation and increased strength to overload resistive training.
- Describe principles and procedures of isotonic resistive training for muscular strength, endurance, power, and hypertrophy.
- Describe principles and procedures of isometric resistive training for muscular strength and endurance.
- Describe principles and procedures of isokinetic resistive training for muscular strength and endurance.
- Describe the principles and procedures of circuit training.
- Describe the principles and procedures of plyometric training.
- Describe the principles and procedures of calisthenic training.
- Describe the principles and procedures of body building.
- Identify general guidelines and considerations for strength training programs.

Keywords

Atrophy
Body building
Calisthenics
Circuit training
Concentric
Detraining
Dynamic
Eccentric
Extension
Fast-glycolytic
Fast-oxidative-glycolytic
Fast twitch
Flexion
Hypertrophy
Hyperplasia
Isokinetic
Isometric
Isotonic
Load
Muscle endurance
Muscle soreness
Muscle strength
Plyometrics
Principle of overload
Principle of specificity
Progressive resistance exercise (PRE)
Repetitions maximum (RM)
Slow twitch
Static
Tension
Training volume
Type I
Type IIa
Type IIb

Introduction

In the human body there are three types of muscle tissue. These include skeletal muscle, smooth muscle and cardiac muscle. **Skeletal muscle** is the predominant muscle tissue and is found attached to the skeleton of the body. It is under voluntary control. In general, it attaches across the joints of the skeletal system. When skeletal muscle is stimulated, it will contract and generate force. If the force is sufficient, movement at the joint will occur. If the force is insufficient, muscle tension is developed but no movement will occur.

The joints of the body vary in structure and design. As a result, the movement allowed at any particular joint is influenced by its shape. It is this movement that allows our bodies to move. Walking, dancing, and participating in sports are all activities that result from the contraction of skeletal muscle tissue.

Smooth muscle tissue is typically found in hollow organs of the body, such as blood vessels, the stomach and intestines. It is under involuntary control.

Cardiac tissue is found only in the heart. Similar to smooth muscle, it is under involuntary control.

What Is the Difference between Muscular Strength and Muscular Endurance?

Muscular strength is defined as the maximal force that a muscle can generate for a single maximal effort. While a number of procedures exist to measure strength, one of the most practical involves the measurement of dynamic strength using a one-repetition maximum (1-RM) procedure with either free weights or some form of variable resistance weight training machine.

Muscular endurance represents the ability of a muscle to repeatedly generate a submaximal force or to sustain a submaximal force over time. Muscular endurance can be measured with free weights or resistive machines by determining a maximum number of repetitions that can be performed at a submaximal percentage of a person's 1-RM, or absolute strength measurement.

Benefits of Resistive Training

Resistive training has been linked to a number of positive changes in the human body. As a result, the inclusion of some form of resistive training in our daily lives is extremely important. Some of the positive benefits include:

- Increased muscular strength
- Increased muscular endurance
- Increased muscle size (hypertrophy)
- Increased flexibility or range of motion
- Decreased body fat
- Increased lean body mass
- Increased basal metabolism
- Increased performance in daily living activities and potentially sport and game skills
- Maintenance of independent living
- Improved physical appearance
- Assists in the prevention of osteoporosis
- Moderate increases in cardiorespiratory fitness
- Moderate decreases in blood pressure
- Decreased glucose-stimulated plasma insulin concentrations
- Improved blood lipid and lipoprotein profiles

Principle of Overload—Resistive Training

The principle of overload states that a gradual increase in the frequency, duration, or intensity of the activity must occur if any physiological adaptation is going to occur. In the case of resistance training, this principle specifically suggests that for greater gains in muscular strength, endurance, or power to occur, a careful manipulation of these factors must occur.

For example, to improve muscular endurance, an individual may choose to alter his/her resistive training program by including a greater number of repetitions in a set or reducing the recovery time between sets or some combination of both. Someone hoping to increase muscular strength will gradually increase the resistance or load, while restricting the number of repetitions in a set to 10 or lower. In each case, over time, the active muscle tissue will adapt to these program changes and alter its structure and/or function, leading to greater gains in muscular endurance and strength, respectively.

What specific physiological adaptations occur in skeletal muscle tissue as a result of the principle of overload being applied? The initial response is an improvement in neuromuscular function or the body's ability to recruit or stimulate the muscle tissue. This adaptation leads to improved muscular strength and coordination.

The most obvious long-term adaptation is chronic hypertrophy or an increase in muscle fiber diameter (Antonio and Gonyea, 1993). This increase in fiber (muscle cell) size is a direct result of an increase in protein synthesis. The enlargement of the cellular components of a muscle cell, particularly the contractile myofilaments, actin and myosin is a fundamental adaptation to overloading muscle tissue. Cellular hypertrophy has been credited for as much as 95–100% of total muscle organ hypertrophy (Brooks, Fahey, & White, 1996).

There is a high linear relationship between the size of the muscle cell and the force it is capable of producing. Increases in strength ranging from 7 to 45% have been reported resulting from cellular adaptation (Kraemer, 2000). In untrained individuals, strength gains as high as 110% have been reported. These inflated numbers represent both neural and fiber adaptations (Kraemer and Fry, 1995).

Finally, it has also been argued that an increase in the number of fibers or **hyperplasia** occurs as a result of overload. Research findings on this issue remain controversial and inconclusive. It appears that this phenomenon is found to occur more in animals than in the human population (Gonyea, Ericson, & Bonde-Perterson, 1977; Sola, Christensen, & Martin, 1973). It has been reported that hyperplasia may occur in less than 10% of all stimulated *human* skeletal muscle tissue (Ho, Roy, Taylor, Heusner, Van Huss, & Carrow, 1977).

Principle of Specificity of Exercise—Resistive Training

If an individual specifically trains only his/her upper body musculature (chest, back, shoulders, and arms), can he/she expect to gain strength in their legs? If an individual seeks to develop high levels of muscular endurance, should he/she participate in a resistive training program designed to develop anaerobic capacity? If an individual participates in a resistive training program and carefully controls and maintains a slow speed of movement when training, can he/she expect to make significant gains in muscular strength, endurance, and power, that can be later used in both fast and slow speeds of movement?

Can a person who participates in a resistive training program designed to develop muscular endurance expect similar or significant gains in muscular strength? Similarly, can a person who participates in a resistive training program designed to develop muscular strength also expect to make significant gains in muscular endurance?

The answer to these and similar types of questions is no. The human body can only adapt to how it has been trained. Why? The answer is simple and can be explained by the **principle of specificity**.

Recall, the principle of specificity states that systems of the body will physiologically adapt, *specifically to the type and nature of exercise training that are encountered*. Additionally, how the body adapts, and how much it improves, is directly related to how hard, and in what manner, it is trained.

The muscular system, like the other systems of the body responds to the principle of specificity. In other words, how the muscle is trained and conditioned will directly determine exactly how it will adapt. Specific factors such as speed of contraction, the type of muscular contraction, the muscle groups involved and the energy source utilized have been found to directly influence the nature and type of physiological adaptation. From a practical standpoint, this means that programs that do not provide sufficient or appropriate stimulus for adaptation will not be successful in warranting the desired physiological change.

Detraining: The Effects of Resistive Exercise Training Reduction or Stoppage on Skeletal Muscle Tissue

The human body is not like a financial institute or bank. You cannot make a *fitness deposit* and expect the body to store it until you are ready to make a withdrawal. Nor can you expect the body to compound a fitness deposit and increase its value, as would be the case with money and compounding interest.

So, what happens to muscle tissue when resistive training is stopped or is reduced? Obviously, nearly everyone who participates in any form of regular resistive training will, in time, experience some period of reduced training or a period of absolute training cessation. These periods of interruption will vary in length of time and may stem from a number of factors. Common factors interrupting resistive training programs include, but are not limited to, illness, loss of access to equipment as might occur on a family vacation, or simply a desire to "take a break" to restrict resistive training from their lifestyle for a brief period of time.

How the muscular system responds to these periods of detraining has been investigated and can be explained by **principle of reversibility**. The simple answer is that muscle tissue will not retain, for any length of time, any gains in muscular strength or endurance associated with resistive training if training is discontinued or drastically reduced.

The scientific explanation as to why this occurs can be found in looking at the physiological changes that occur as a consequence to detraining. The most obvious change is muscle **atrophy** or muscle size reduction. This loss in size is the result of either reduced cross sectional area of individual muscle cells or a decrease in the number of cells. The latter being more associated with aging. A reduction in muscle size is more common and is usually associated with resistive training cessation, especially during the first few weeks or months following training.

How much actual muscle atrophying occurs as a result of detraining? It has been suggested (Dudley and Ploutz-Snyder, 2001) that the rate of atrophic response to detraining is approximately 1% per week, a level similar to hypertrophic response time. The exact rate of atrophic response, however, is related to the nature and extent of detraining. For example, total bed rest appears to be more damaging than simply the cessation of resistive training while continuing other day-to-day lifestyle activities. In addition to muscular atrophy, other physiological changes to the muscular system that result from detraining include, but are not limited to, neuromuscular impairment and a greater susceptibility to muscle injury and dysfunction.

Types of Skeletal Muscular Contraction

Muscle movement can be categorized into three types of actions (contractions):

- Isometric (Static)
- Concentric
- Eccentric

Isometric (Static) Contractions

Isometric contractions may be defined as contractions that generate muscle tension but involve no appreciable change in the length of the muscle. Subsequently, there is no joint (skeletal) movement. For this reason, isometric contractions are considered static in nature.

Concentric Contractions

Concentric contractions occur when a muscle shortens in length. This is often termed a "positive" contraction. Because joint movement is involved, this contraction is considered a dynamic movement.

Eccentric Contractions

Eccentric contractions are dynamic movements that involve muscle lengthening. They usually occur as muscle tissue is returned from a shortened state to its normal resting length. Eccentric contractions are referred to as negative contractions.

Skeletal Muscle Actions

Skeletal muscle contraction and the resultant movement can be classified broadly as either static or dynamic. In each case, muscle tension is developed. The distinguishing characteristic is the nature of movement.

Static movements occur when *no appreciable change* in muscle tissue length or joint movement occurs. Static contractions can involve either maximal or submaximal muscle tension. In either case, the external load or resistance is greater than the torque generated by the muscle contraction.

Dynamic movements *allow for changes* in muscle tissue length and joint movement. Because muscle tissue can be shortened or lengthened, specific dynamic resistance training procedures have been developed. These basic techniques of resistance training vary depending on the dynamic muscle action and are discussed below. Depending on the particular situation, the tension, or more accurately the torque, generated by the contracting muscle may be greater or less than the external load. In cases where the muscle torque is greater than the external load, muscle length shortens during movement. Conversely, if the external load or resistance is greater than the muscle torque, muscle lengthening occurs during movement.

Types of Skeletal Muscle Fibers

Muscle fibers vary in their structural and functional characteristics. While this may seem scientific in nature, most people have indirectly made this observation without the use of any scientific application. For example, many individuals have observed differences in color of muscle tissue when selecting pieces of chicken. It is not uncommon for someone to prefer light meat, such as that found in the breast of the chicken, while others may choose the dark meat found in the leg and thighs. Obviously, in both selections we are choosing skeletal muscle tissue. The visual difference in color, however, clearly demonstrates some difference in the two muscle tissues exists. This difference stems from the two tissues, functional and structural characteristics.

If we visually compare the breast meat of a duck with the breast meat of a chicken, we find the breast meat of the duck is darker in appearance. The darker color is the same characteristic found in the leg meat of the chicken.

Why do these differences exist? Consider the fact that the chicken is predominantly a weight-bearing animal. While it can fly, it is very inefficient in flight and spends most of its time standing in a weight-bearing situation. As a result, the postural muscles of the chicken's legs are designed to support its body weight for long periods of time without fatiguing.

Now, consider the lifestyle of a duck. The duck is more inclined to fly and is capable of flying for hours without fatigue. During flight, the duck relies heavily on the breast muscles to provide the muscular effort needed to sustain long-term flying. In comparison, the breast tissue of a chicken is not designed for the repeated efforts of wing flapping during long-term flight. As a result, the breast musculature of the chicken fatigues very quickly when flight is attempted.

This simple comparison clearly demonstrates two different functional requirements of the breast musculature. The duck breast musculature is obviously better fitted for a much higher level of muscular endurance than that of the chicken. This difference in functional capacity is visually observed as a difference in the color of the two breast musculatures. This is why the leg musculature of the chicken, which is designed for postural endurance, is visually similar to the darker tissue of the duck breast. In simple, the tissues presenting a dark appearance reflect tissues with greater endurance capacity. Tissues presenting a lighter appearance reflect tissues that are less fatigue resistant.

In humans, these types of differences are also found in skeletal muscle tissue. It is true that in humans, all skeletal muscle fibers share some common characteristics. For example, all skeletal muscle function is under voluntary control or, when observed microscopically, the skeletal muscle fibers will appear striped or striated in appearance. There are, however, differences in the structural and functional characteristics of skeletal muscle fibers.

Skeletal muscle fibers are classified according to these differences. Two major groups or types have been established. These types are based on fiber contractile and metabolic characteristics. The types are commonly referred to as **slow twitch** and **fast twitch** fibers or **Type I** and **Type II**, respectively. Type II fibers (fast twitch) have been further divided into two subdivisions known as **Type IIa** or **fast-oxidative-glycolytic (FOG)** and **Type IIb, fast-glycolytic (FG)**. For reader ease, the different types of tissue have been discussed under the subheaders below.

Wilmore and Costil (1999) indicate that on average, most of the muscles of the body are composed of about 50% slow twitch and 50% fast twitch muscle fibers. The 50% fast twitch fibers are evenly distributed between fast-oxidative-glycolytic and fast-glycolytic fibers.

Individual differences do exist, however, between some of the muscles of the body. For example, a postural muscle, such as the soleus located in the lower leg, will be composed almost entirely of slow twitch fibers. By comparison, the hamstrings and the quadriceps of the upper leg are composed of a mix of fast and slow twitch fibers.

In general, individuals will normally present similar muscle composition in their upper and lower extremities. These structural and functional characteristics appear to be established within the first few years of life and are genetically inherited. All types of skeletal muscle fibers will positively respond and adapt to training and conditioning activities. They do not, however, possess the ability to convert from one Type to another. For example, there is very little evidence that regular participation in an endurance type of an activity, such as long distance running, will allow for muscle fibers to convert from Type II to Type I fibers.

Slow Twitch (Type I)

Slow twitch fibers are also referred to as Type I. Slow twitch fibers possess a high capacity for aerobic energy supply. Metabolically speaking, they are very efficient in producing ATP from the oxidation of carbohydrates and fats. As a result, they possess an especially high level of aerobic endurance and are extremely fatigue resistant. They are limited, however, in their ability to produce anaerobic power. Finally, the speed of contraction of slow twitch fibers is much slower than their fast twitch counterparts.

Type I fibers are particularly adapted for low intensity, long duration (endurance) type activities. For example, activities such as long distance running and cycling rely heavily on slow twitch fibers. Similarly, postural musculature that is extremely fatigue resistant is largely composed of slow twitch muscle fibers.

Fast Twitch (Type IIa and Type IIb)

In comparison to slow twitch fibers, fast twitch fibers possess a higher capacity for rapid force development. McArdle, Katch and Katch (2001) indicated that *fast twitch fibers are capable of shortening and developing tension three to five times faster than slow twitch fibers.* Because they rely almost entirely on anaerobic metabolism for energy, they possess a high level of anaerobic power and have limited aerobic power. Even though they are extremely explosive and powerful, fast twitch fibers fatigue rapidly.

Fast-oxidative-glycolytic (Type IIa) fibers appear to have a greater aerobic capacity than fast-glycolytic (Type IIb). This increase in aerobic potential is still not as high as slow twitch (Type I). Fast-glycolytic (Type IIb) fibers present the highest anaerobic power.

Anaerobic activities rely heavily on both types of fast twitch muscle tissue. Because of the inherent differences in their aerobic and anaerobic potential, specific activities are better fitted to particular fast twitch types. For example, activities that are reasonably short and very high in intensity, such as an 800-meter run, rely heavily on Type IIa fibers. Shorter, extremely intense activities, such as a 50-meter swim or a 100-yard dash, rely on Type IIb fibers.

Factors Affecting Muscular Strength and Endurance Training

Muscle Size

The strength that a skeletal muscle can produce is related to the cross sectional area of that particular muscle. It has been reported that approximately 3 to 8 kg of force per cm^2 of muscle cross section, **regardless of gender** (McKardle, Katch, & Katch, 1991). Simply stated, *the larger the cross sectional area, the stronger the muscle. Strength training does not increase the strength of contraction of the muscle cells, but rather increases in strength result from a proportional increase in the diameter or size of the muscle cell.*

The size of a muscle may be influenced by resistive training and/or disuse. Resistive training increases the size of the muscle by adding contractile proteins, myosin and actin to the myofibrils. Myofibrils are small substructures of a muscle cell. This increase in size is referred to as cellular **hypertrophy.** There is very limited evidence to suggest that increases in muscle size occurs as a result of **hyperplasia**, or the splitting of muscle cells. This finding is particularly true in studies using mammals.

In order to stimulate muscle growth, muscle must be sufficiently overloaded. An increase in demand for muscular force is a prerequisite for muscle cell hypertrophy.

Atrophy, or a decrease in muscle size, occurs when a muscle goes untrained and unused. Clearly, the cliché, *"Use It or Lose It"* is appropriate when summarizing these concepts.

Gender

Women, like men, will experience gains in strength from resistive training. They do not, however, experience as much hypertrophy. This is related to the lower levels of testosterone found in women.

As indicated above, no gender differences exist in strength per squared centimeter of cross sectional area. When comparing men and women, men typically appear stronger. This may be explained by their greater muscle mass. While some differences exist in the ability to recruit muscle fibers, generally speaking, pound for pound, women can produce similar strength.

Age

A loss of skeletal muscle tissue is associated with aging. The greatest losses occur after the age of 50 with an average of a 15% loss occurring in the sixth and seventh decades of life and advancing to as much as a 30% loss every decade thereafter (ACSM, 2001). This loss is highly related to a more sedentary lifestyle and may be preventable and/or reversible. There is overwhelming evidence that resistive training will prevent strength loss and should be a part of an individual's lifestyle throughout his/her life. More specifically, losses appear to be greater in fast twitch fibers than in slow twitch fibers leading to a greater percentage of slow twitch fibers in the elderly.

Age should not be considered a limiting factor in resistive training. In comparison, the muscle tissue of older men or women will respond to resistive training activities similarly to the tissue of younger men and women (Coggan, et. al., 1992).

Muscle Soreness

Muscle soreness can occur late in an exercise session, immediately following exercise, during recovery or several days after exercise. There are several reasons that contribute to this phenomenon and, due to their scientific nature, they are beyond the scope of this manuscript. The most common basic explanation, which makes no attempt to explain tissue damage or repair, would suggest muscle soreness results from structural damage of the muscle tissue or connective tissues associated with the muscle and/or muscle tissue death.

Muscle soreness can be avoided or minimized by taking several precautions during training. Included are:

- Eliminate or minimize eccentric training
- Eliminate or minimize isometric training
- Begin training using low intensities
- Include stretching in warm-up and cool-down activity
- Progress slowly

Surprisingly, one other method shown to help eliminate future muscle soreness is to begin training with a high-intensity, exhaustive session. This approach will result in a great deal of original soreness, but tends to decrease future discomfort (Wilmore & Costill, 1999).

Basic Techniques of Resistance Training

Resistance training techniques include, but are not limited to, isometric, isotonic, and isokinetic procedures. For reader ease, these are described under separate headers.

Isometric Training

With isometric training, the resistive load, or more specifically, resistive torque is greater than the contracting torque of the muscle. An example would include an individual pushing outward on the frame of a door while standing in the doorway. Muscle tension is developed during contraction, but since the doorway doesn't move, there is no appreciable change in active muscle length.

One unique characteristic of isometric training is that it *improves strength only at a given joint angle rather than through a full range of motion.* This is frequently cited as a limitation. There are occasions, however, where improving strength at a single joint angle is desirable. For example, a post-operative or post-injury patient may have a specific joint angle that is associated with muscle weakness. A rehabilitation program that includes isometric training at this particular joint angle may allow for specific strength gains.

Isotonic (Progressive Resistive Exercise) Training

Isotonic or progressive resistive training is dynamic by nature and involves muscle length changes, both shortening and lengthening. In this form of training, the external resistance or weight remains constant. The speed of muscle contraction may vary. For example, consider the movement of the lower arm, at the elbow, during an arm or biceps curl. During flexion, the biceps shortens while contracting concentrically. During extension, the biceps lengthens while contracting eccentrically. During flexion, the torque of the contracting muscle is greater than the torque caused by the resistance load (weight). During extension, the resistive force (weight) exceeds the muscular tension. When an individual works out with free weights or progressive resistance equipment, it could be stated that he/she is involved in isotonic training, the most common and most popular method of strength training.

Isokinetic Training

Similar to isotonic training, isokinetic training requires dynamic muscle contractions. The difference, however, is that the velocity (speed) of the muscular contraction remains constant during contraction, while the resistance (weight) varies. In isotonics, the resistance or external load remains constant and the rate of muscle contraction varies. Isokinetic training requires special equipment that is extremely expensive. While it can be used for muscular strength and endurance development, it is not often found in fitness centers.

The nature of muscle contraction associated with isokinetic training is extremely useful in muscle tissue rehabilitation. As a result, this equipment is more readily found in hospitals and rehabilitation centers.

Principles of Training

Introduction

A review of literature suggests there are numerous beneficial resistive training programs, none of which have been shown to be clearly superior to another. For the purposes of this text and for reader ease, resistive training procedures have been grouped according to type of muscle contraction. Specifics regarding the differing systems or training programs have been avoided.

It is important to recognize, however, that the basic tenets of resistive training that guide all programs are the principles of overload and progressive resistance and the principle of specificity. If these principles are not followed or incorporated into a program, the success of the program will be compromised.

Finally, it is important to understand that it takes the body time to adjust to resistive training. To ensure training benefits, any program should involve a minimum of four to six weeks. A general description of how the body will respond and adapt to a long-term resistive training program follows.

Time Course of Cellular Adaptation and Increased Strength

The time course (chronic adaptation) of muscle cell adaptation to overloading is well established. The rate of adaptation varies and is largely dependent on the individual and his/her previous levels of adaptation. Untrained individuals will present a greater magnitude of adaptation than individuals with a prior history of resistive training.

When beginning a resistive training program, it is common to see rapid, initial gains in strength before cellular adaptations have actually occurred. This phenomenon is especially common in untrained, poorly conditioned individuals. These initial gains in strength, while real, are attributed more to neurological adaptations than to cellular adaptations. As the individual better learns how to recruit muscle fibers for force production, increases in strength are demonstrated. During this period, demonstrated increases in strength are not related to cellular adaptation.

As the training program continues and the muscle tissue is repeatedly overloaded, cellular hypertrophy occurs (see Principle of Overload—Resistive Training and Training for Hypertrophy). Normally, cellular hypertrophy will become noticeable within a couple of months of resistive training (Harris and Dudley, 2000). Gains in strength, at this time, can be attributed to the increase in the size of the muscle fibers and are directly related to the cross-sectional area of the muscle.

In addition to the hypertrophic effect, changes in the muscle fiber type may occur during this time. These changes may include a transition from Type IIb to Type IIa. No transitional change from Type II to Type I has been demonstrated and most likely will never occur. As expected, both Type I and Type II fibers will adapt to resistive training by increasing cross-sectional area.

After a prolonged training, optimal cellular and organ hypertrophy will be achieved. Any additional gains in strength after a maximal hypertrophic response has been reached must be attributed to neural factors.

How strong can an individual get? Initial strength levels largely influence the amount of strength a person can gain. Untrained individuals will demonstrate greater gains in strength as a result of resistive training compared to trained individuals. Typical increases in muscular strength from pretraining values have been reported to be between 7% and 45% (Kraemer, 2000). In some case, the literature will report even higher values have been achieved. These exceptionally high levels of gain may be influenced in part by neural adaptations and may not reflect solely muscular tissue adaptations.

Isometric Training Principles

Isometric muscular strength gains have been reported with a single, maximal voluntary, 1-second isometric contraction or a 6 second contraction at two-thirds maximal effort. Repeating the contraction up to 10 times daily has been shown to allow for greater gains. Because it is difficult for an individual to determine the exact strength of each contraction, maximal contractions are recommended. Holding each contraction for an extended period of time (more than 10 seconds) will not result in increased gains and may result in muscle fatigue and soreness. Also, it is extremely important to practice each isometric contraction at a variety of joint angles. Strength gains have been shown to be angle specific. Isometric strength gains can be maintained with one training session per week.

A couple of precautions should be noted. Extreme elevations in blood pressures occur during the period of isometric muscular contraction. As a result, isometric training should be considered contraindicated for individuals who are hypertensive and/or present other forms of coronary heart disease. Also, to prevent increases in intra-thoracic pressures, individuals should not hold their breath during contraction.

Isotonic Training Principles

Isotonic training consists of dynamic movements against a resistance. Both concentric and eccentric movements should be included in a training program. The most common method of isotonic training incorporates the principle of overload and is known as **progressive resistance training.** This method may include the use of free weights and/or progressive resistive equipment. While variations exist in terms of the recommended number of repetitions, sets, and relative intensity, all progressive resistance training systems stem from the original efforts of Delorme and Watkins (1951). They recommend three sets of ten repetition maximum (10 RM). Ten repetition maximum is defined as the maximum weight that can be successfully lifted 10 times. Intensity of the resistance is varied depending on the set. First set intensity should be at 50% of a 10 RM load. The second set at 75% of 10 RM load, and the third set should be 100% of the weight that can be lifted 10 times.

Muscular strength and muscular endurance training are related. Yet, it must be emphasized that muscle adaptations that occur as a result of training are very specific (i.e., joint angle, rate of contraction). As a result, program variations in the number of sets, repetitions, and load intensity exist. When attempting to obtain optimal strength or endurance, remember the following: (a) develop strength, use heavy weights and limit the number of repetitions, and (b) develop muscular endurance, use lower weights and increase the number of repetitions. No ideal exists.

Since skeletal muscle tissue will respond specifically to how it is trained (see Principle of Specificity—Resistive Training), resistive training programs will vary the load, repetition assignments, and the rest periods in accordance with training program objectives. The appropriate balance between variables is critical in meeting individual training objectives. Specific guidelines for training for strength, endurance, power, and hypertrophy are provided below under separate headers. It should be stressed, however, that any resistive program will result in gains in all three areas, especially in the untrained individual. The guidelines recommended below have been developed to assist the trained individual in meeting specific objectives of improving muscular strength, power, endurance, or organ and cellular hypertrophy. A summary of these guidelines is provided in Table 6-1.

Table 6-1 ■ Recommended Isotonic Training Guidelines Based on Type of Resistive Training

Training Objective	% 1 RM Load	Repetitions	Sets	Inter-set Rest Period
Strength	80–90	3–8	3–6	2–5 minutes
Power	75–95	2–5	2–3	2–5 minutes
Endurance	< 60	> 15	3–5	< 90 seconds
Hypertrophy	50–75	10–20	3–6	< 30 seconds

Training for Muscular Strength

Extremely high resistive loads and a minimal number of repetitions characterize strength training programs. While the perfect training protocol remains controversial, typical programs for muscular strength development prescribe an increase in the resistive load (80–90% of 1RM), use a 3–8 repetitions, and incorporate a minimum of three (3-6) sets. A full recovery period between sets (2–5 minutes) is normally recommended (Stone, O'Bryant, & Garhammer, 1981). Including more than three sets will allow for greater increases in strength, but gains are limited. Additionally, because of the extreme physiological demands placed on the body when training for muscle strength, an increase in sets and, in turn, total training volume, may lead to increased risk of injury.

Training for Muscular Endurance

The relationship between number of repetitions and gains in strength and endurance has been clearly established (Anderson and Kearny, 1982). As the number of repetitions increase, muscular endurance is gained. As a result, resistive training programs designed to improve muscular endurance prescribe a lower resistive load (less than 60% 1-RM) and increased numbers of repetitions (minimum of 15). The specific number of repetitions and resistive load will be inversely related. As lower resistance loads are chosen, greater repetitions should be expected. As a general rule, to determine the appropriate repetitions for any given resistance, repeat the movement to the point of fatigue. Since lower resistive loads are used, total training volume does not become unmanageable and elevated. To prevent full recovery, inter-set rest periods are usually limited to less than 90 seconds. Finally, it should be noted, some gains in muscular endurance are associated with a traditional strength training program (high load, low repetition).

Training for Muscular Power

Training protocols for muscular power and muscular strength are similar, both are characterized by high resistive loads and minimal repetitions. For example, resistive loads used to develop muscular power vary between 75–95% of 1 RM. The main difference between the two is that training for muscular power involves a lower volume (3–5 sets of 2–5 repetitions). This lower volume helps to maximize the quality of exercise. Recall the recommended volume for strength is 3–6 sets of 3–8 repetitions. Because of the intense exercise demand complete inter-set rest periods (2–5 minutes) are warranted.

Training for Hypertrophy

Considerable confusion exists as to how best to develop muscle hypertrophy. In adult mammals, considerable evidence suggests that most (95%–100%) of total muscle hypertrophy can be attributed to cellular hypertrophy (Brooks, Fahey, & White, 1996). Cellular hypertrophy is an increase in the cross sectional area of a muscle cell. This increase in cell size is a direct muscle cell adaptation to progressive resistive training and can be attributed to 1) an increase in protein synthesis, particularly in the contractile proteins actin and myosin, 2) an increase in the number of myofibrils within the muscle cell, and 3) an increase in the size of the myofibrils within the muscle cell. On average, the increase in the diameter of a hypertrophied muscle cell is about 30% (McArdle, Katch, and Katch, 1996). The magnitude of these hypertrophic responses occur over the time course of training and can, in part, be explained by two basic principles; these are: 1) The principle of specificity and 2) The principle of overload.

Programs designed to enhance muscle hypertrophy usually incorporate a lower training intensity (50–75% of 1RM) and a high training volume. High training volume is achieved by incorporating a higher number of repetitions (10–20) and multiple sets (3–6) into the training program. Inter-set rest periods are limited to under 90 seconds to prevent full recovery of the tissue before the next set begins.

High training volume appears to be the critical element of any program attempting to promote or stimulate hypertrophic muscle cell adaptation (McDonagh and Davies, 1984; McArdle, Katch, & Katch, 2001). It is only after long-term adaptation has occurred that muscle fibers will approach genetic limitations. At this point, increased training volume will not result in greater hypertrophic adaptation.

Inter-Set and Inter-Session Rest Periods

Adequate rest and recover, should occur between exercise sets (inter-set), as well as between exercise sessions. There is no specific time established for between set recovering. *Recovery is normally based on the specific training objective.* Several minutes (2–5) of inter-set rest may be necessary during strength and power training. When the objective is muscle hypertrophy, it is common to limit inter-set rest to under 90 seconds. In the case of muscular endurance training, between set recovery time is usually less than 30 seconds.

Between exercise session recovery is influenced by the intensity of the training program and may require an every other day approach (i.e., Monday-Wednesday-Friday). Between exercise session rest days appear critical when attempting to optimize strength improvement (Berger, 1982; Powers and Howley, 1990; Stone and O'Bryant, 1984). Programs involving higher levels of exercise demand will lead to muscle tissue injury if inadequate recovery is allocated between exercise sessions.

Practical Guidelines for Isotonic Training

A number of general or practical guidelines should be followed when developing an isotonic training program. First, it is important to exercise large muscle groups first. Resistive training can be extremely fatiguing to skeletal muscle tissue. If smaller muscle groups are fatigued early in the training session, large muscle group training may be restricted or, if attempted, may lead to injury of the smaller muscles.

Another consideration is to begin the resistive training program slowly using lower weight intensities. Muscle strength gains have been shown with the use of as little as 60% of a 1 RM load. Starting a training program with limited intensity will minimize injury and the risk of muscular soreness.

The principle of specificity of exercise applies to resistive training. Clearly, muscular strength gains closely relate to the nature of the training. Factors such as which muscles are involved, rate of contraction of involved muscles, range of motion, and magnitude of resistance are specifically related to the nature and type of strength gains.

Finally, it is important to recognize that eccentric training is no more effective than concentric training. Many falsely assume they are experiencing a greater training effect because of the larger weights that may be utilized during eccentric movement. For example, a person may have an absolute strength (1 RM) of one hundred pounds for a concentric arm curl. Yet, eccentrically, he/she may be able to "manage," or control the rate of descent, of an eccentric contraction of 120 pounds. As a result of "managing" the greater weight, he/she erroneously assumes a greater training effect. But, in fact, there are no accelerated or increased strength gains occurring during eccentric training than would be accomplished through full range of motion (concentric-eccentric) contractions.

Isokinetic Training Principles

Isokinetic training can only be accomplished using specialized equipment designed to control and maintain a constant predetermined rate of a concentric contraction. In simple, as a muscle generates tension through a full range of motion, the equipment offers an equal and opposite force, thus maintaining a constant speed of contraction. Typically, the rates of contraction will vary between 24 and 180 degrees per second (ACSM, 1993).

The training procedures for isokinetics are similar to those of isotonic training. Three sets of 5 to 10 repetitions are recommended on alternating days. Because of the specific adaptation of muscle to training, speed of contraction should be similar or faster than the activity a person is training for. Bowers and Fox (1988) cite the following when describing the relationship between isokinetics and muscular strength and endurance gains.

- Isokinetic training at slow speeds produces substantial increases in strength only at slow movement speeds.
- Isokinetic training at fast speeds produces increases in strength at all speeds of movement (i.e., rates at and below the training speed).
- Isokinetic training at fast speeds increases muscular endurance at fast speeds more than slow-speed training increases endurance at slow speeds of movement.

Like isotonic training, isokinetic training should occur several days a week, on alternating days.

Additional Resistance Activities

Circuit Training

Circuit training involves the use of a series of weight training exercise stations (12 to 15), combined with additional stations involving aerobic activities and calisthenics. Stations are sequenced to control participant movements. The time spent in physical exertion and the time spent between stations resting are controlled.

Each station is designed to submit the participant to intense work alternated with brief rest periods. By way of illustration, a participant may work for one minute on the leg press (at sub-maximal resistance), then quickly proceed to 30 to 40 seconds of jogging in place (or perhaps doing leg lifts) before proceeding to the next weight station.

Depending on the circuit's size, participants typically will rotate through an entire circuit several times. Some aerobic endurance may be developed (approximately 8%) as well as, strength and endurance. The limiting factor for increases in aerobic performance appears to be the amount of recovery between stations. Recovery time should be limited to a maximum of 30 seconds if any aerobic fitness gains are desired. More traditional aerobic fitness programs may be required for individuals seeking to significantly increase cardiorespiratory fitness.

Plyometrics

Plyometric training involves depth jumping, bounds, and hops. It is often used in athletics, especially in drills involving jumping on and off a series of boxes. The underlying theory is to rapidly lengthen or stretch a muscle (eccentric contraction) followed by an immediate subsequent concentric contraction. The magnitude of the muscle lengthening is not the critical component, but rather the rate at which the muscle is lengthened. Rapid muscle lengthening induces muscle proprioceptive (muscle spindle) activity causing a violent, forceful concentric contraction. This is referred to as the stretch/shortening cycle.

Plyometrics are used to develop muscle power or explosive forceful contractions. Plyometric activities, inherently traumatic by nature, require a significant strength base before being included into a fitness program. Because plyometric activities rely heavily on the elastic and stretching properties of muscle tissue, they carry an increased risk of injury. These activities are recommended for only the highly fit individual. Plyometrics should be considered contraindicated for individuals presenting low levels of fitness, particularly in muscular strength, over-weight individuals, and persons with a known history of joint pain.

Calisthenics

Calisthenics are activities that require body movements and rely on the weight of the body and its extremities as resistance. Leg lifts, crunches, and pushups are all examples. These are excellent beginning fitness program activities, warm-up and cool-down activities, and supplemental activities to muscular strength and endurance training.

Body Building

Body building is a sport in which the participants attempt to change the morphology (form and structure) of their bodies. Similar to an artist working with clay to form and shape his/her creations, the body builder is attempting to shape and form his/her body by controlling specific muscle development. Any activity that is included in the workout is designed to develop body mass, definition, and symmetry or balance. While muscle strength and endurance gains may accompany training, this is not necessarily the objective. Likewise, specific skill acquisition is not considered an objective.

Generally, body builders follow resistive training programs that incorporate a very high training volume. The training intensity is usually low and varies between 50–75% 1RM. High training volume is achieved by incorporating high repetitions (10–20) and multiple sets (3–6) into the training program. Inter-set rest periods are usually limited to less than 90 seconds. The limited recovery period prevents complete recovery of the tissue before the next set begins. Finally, most body builders incorporate multiple exercises per muscle group designed to vary the training angle to allow for maximal muscle fiber stimulation and adaptation

This high training volume appears to be the critical factor when attempting to stimulate hypertrophic muscle cell adaptation (McDonagh and Davies, 1984; McArdle, Katch, & Katch, 2001). Optimal muscle organ and cellular growth appears to be associated with higher training volume. It is only after long-term adaptation has occurred that a muscle fiber will approach its genetic hypertrophic limitation and high training volume will no longer result in greater hypertrophic adaptation.

Additional Considerations for Resistive Training Programs

A number of universal considerations or guidelines should be followed in any resistive training program. These considerations apply to any type of resistive training program. They are appropriate for the highly trained, as well as the untrained or poorly conditioned. For reader ease, they are itemized below.

- Always warm up and cool down.
- Begin with exercises for the lower body.
- Exhale on exertion.

- Strengthen your weak side.
- Work arms and legs independently.
- Use proper lifting techniques or form to reduce injury.
- Always protect the lower back (no hyperextension).
- Isolate activities by muscle group.
- Work larger muscle groups first.
- Work through a full range of motion.
- Periodically reassess needs.

Laboratory Activities

CHAPTER 6

Name: _____ Class Time/Day: _____ Score: _____

LABORATORY 6-A

Muscular Endurance: One-Minute Bent Knee Sit-Up Test

- **Purpose:** This test measures abdominal muscular strength and endurance.

- **Precautions:** Individuals with lower fitness levels may experience limited post-test muscle soreness. Individuals should warmup properly before participating.

- **Equipment:** Mat and stopwatch.

- **Procedure:** Each subject should be allowed to warm-up and become familiar with the sit-up procedure. The subject is placed on his/her back with hands interlocked over the chest touching the shoulders. The legs should be bent at the knees so that their heels are 12–8 inches from the buttocks. An assistant should hold the ankles to keep the feet firmly on the ground and to provide support (see Figure 6.1). Within a one-minute period, the subject performs as many correct sit-ups as possible. A correct sit-up is performed when a subject sits up and touches his/her elbows to his/her knees while keeping the buttocks on the mat and the hands/arms in contact with his/her chest and shoulders. To complete the sit-up, the subject must return to the mat and make full contact with the back and shoulders. The subject should not hold his/her breath during this test, but should breathe freely with each repetition.

- **Scoring:** The number of correctly executed sit-ups performed in one minute is counted as the score. Determine normative rating by using Table 6-2.

- **Data/Calculations:**

Name: _____   Date: ___/___/___

Gender: _____ Age: _____ Height: _____ Weight: _____

Total number of sit-ups completed in one minute's time: _____

Fitness Rating: _____

Table 6-2 ■ Normative Values by Age and Gender for 1-Minute Sit-Up Muscular Strength and Endurance Test

Rating	20–29	30–39	40–49	50–59	60+
Men					
Excellent	> 47	> 39	> 34	> 29	> 24
Good	43–47	35–39	30–34	25–29	20–24
Average	37–42	29–34	24–29	19–24	14–19
Fair	33–36	25–28	20–23	15–18	10–13
Poor	< 33	< 25	< 20	< 15	< 10
Women					
Excellent	>43	>35	>30	>25	>20
Good	39–43	31–35	26–30	21–25	16–20
Average	33–38	25–30	19–25	15–20	10–15
Fair	29–32	21–24	16–18	11–14	6–9
Poor	< 29	< 21	< 16	< 11	< 6

Source: Pollock, M., Wilmore, J., and Fox, S. 1978. *Health and Fitness through Physical Activity.* New York: John Wiley & Sons.

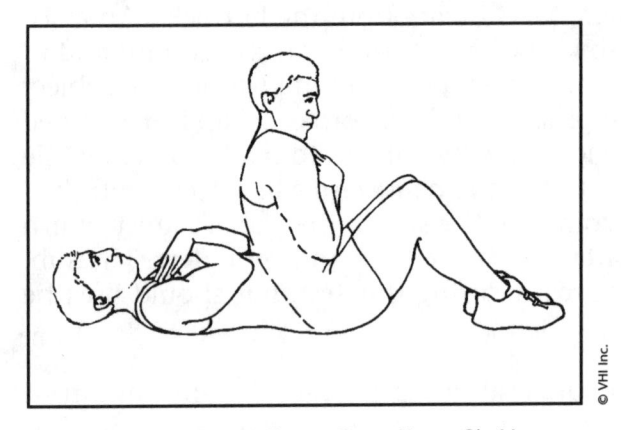

Figure 6.1 ■ One-Minute Bent Knee Sit-Up

Name: _____ Class Time/Day: _____ Score: _____

LABORATORY 6-B

Muscular Strength: Upper Leg Press

- **Purpose:** This test measures one repetition maximum (1 RM) absolute leg strength.

- **Precautions:** Individuals with lower fitness levels may experience limited post-test muscle soreness. Hypertensive individuals should consult with the class instructor before participating. Individuals should warmup properly before participating.

- **Equipment:** Isotonic resistive training equipment.

- **Procedure:** Each subject should be allowed to properly warmup and become familiar with the leg press equipment and procedure. Position yourself by sitting down on the seat provided and place your feet, perpendicular on the footpad, directly in front of the hips (see Figure 6.2). Adjust the seat to the appropriate position. The distance between the footpad and the seat is critical. Never assume a position that bends the knees greater than 90 degrees. Lightly grasp the handgrips to stabilize the body during the leg press. The action of the concentric phase of the leg press is to press or push the footpad forward until the legs are fully extended. Do not lock the knees out at extension. During the eccentric phase, slowly return the legs and footpad to their original position. In leg pressing, the subject has a series of trials to determine the greatest weight that can be lifted just once for that particular movement. The test starts with a low weight that can be easily and safely lifted. Weight is added gradually until the lift cannot be performed correctly. The subject should breathe freely with each lift and be discouraged from holding his/her breath. The maximal weight that a subject can lift for a single repetition represents the subject's 1 RM score.

- **Scoring:** After the 1RM score is obtained for the leg press test, the 1RM weight in pounds is divided by the subject's body weight in pounds. Determine normative ratings by using Table 6-3.

- **Data/Calculations:**

Name: _____   Date: / /

Gender: _____   Age: _____   Height: _____   Weight: _____

Maximum Single Repetition Leg Press Score (lbs.): _____

Fitness Classification: _____

Leg Press Percentile Score: _____

Calculate leg press weight ratio by dividing maximum leg press (lbs.) by body weight (lbs.).

Leg Press Weight Ratio = _____ (Maximum Weight in pounds) / _____ (Body Weight in pounds)

Table 6-3 ■ Normative Values by Age and Gender for 1 RM Absolute Upper Leg Strength Normalized by Body Weight

Classification	Percentile	20–29	30–39	40–49	50–59	60+
			Age			
			Men			
Excellent	90	2.27	2.07	1.92	1.80	1.73
	80	2.13	1.93	1.82	1.71	1.62
Above Average	70	2.05	1.85	1.74	1.64	1.56
	60	1.97	1.77	1.68	1.58	1.49
Average	50	1.91	1.71	1.62	1.52	1.43
	40	1.83	1.65	1.57	1.46	1.38
Below Average	30	1.74	1.59	1.51	1.39	1.30
	20	1.63	1.52	1.44	1.32	1.25
Poor	10	1.51	1.43	1.35	1.22	1.16
			Women			
Excellent	90	1.82	1.61	1.48	1.37	1.32
	80	1.68	1.47	1.37	1.25	1.18
Above Average	70	1.58	1.39	1.29	1.17	1.13
	60	1.50	1.33	1.23	1.10	1.04
Average	50	1.44	1.27	1.18	1.05	.99
	40	1.37	1.21	1.13	.99	.93
Below Average	30	1.27	1.15	1.08	.95	.88
	20	1.22	1.09	1.02	.88	.85
Poor	10	1.14	1.00	.94	.78	.72

From: *ACSM's Guidelines For Exercise Testing and Prescription*, 6th Edition. 2000. Philadelphia: Lippincott, Williams, & Wilkins.

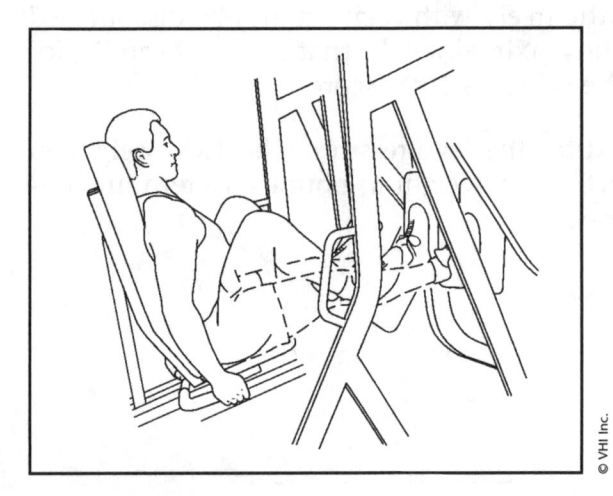

Figure 6.2 ■ Leg Press

Name: _____ Class Time/Day: _____ Score: _____

LABORATORY 6-C

Muscular Strength: Bench Press

- **Purpose:** This test measures one repetition maximum (1 RM) absolute upper body strength.

- **Precautions:** Individuals with lower fitness levels may experience limited muscle soreness. Hypertensive individuals should consult with the class instructor before participating. Individuals should warmup properly before participating.

- **Equipment:** Isotonic resistive training machines.

- **Procedure:** Each subject should be allowed to properly warmup and become familiar with the bench press equipment and lifting procedure. The subject should breathe freely with each lift and be discouraged from holding his/her breath. The lifting procedure calls for the subject to lie on the bench, facing up. The head, back, and hips should be in contact with the bench. He/she should grasp the bar with the hands approximately shoulder width apart. The weight should be pushed upward, while the subject exhales, until the arms are fully extended at the elbow. Full extension of the elbows must be achieved to constitute a correct lift (see Figure 6.3). The subject is allowed multiple trials to establish the greatest weight that he/she can lift. The maximal weight a subject can lift for a single repetition represents the subject's 1 RM score.

- **Scoring:** The subject's bench press weight ratio score is determined by dividing the subject's 1 RM score (weight in pounds) by the subject's body weight in pounds. Determine the normative ratings by using Table 6-4.

- **Data/Calculations:**

Calculate leg press weight ratio by dividing maximum leg press (lbs.) by body weight (lbs.).

Bench Press Weight Ratio = _____ (Maximum Weight in pounds) /
                          _____ (Body Weight in pounds)

Name: Date: / /

Gender: Age: Height: Weight:

Maximum Single Repetition Bench Press: _____

Fitness Classification: _____

Bench Press Percentile Score: _____

Table 6-4 ■ Normative Values by Age and Gender for 1 RM Absolute Bench Press Strength Normalized by Body Weight

Classification	Percentile	20–29	30–39	40–49	50–59	60+
			Men			
Excellent	90	1.48	1.24	1.10	.97	.89
	80	1.32	1.12	1.00	.90	.82
Above Average	70	1.22	1.04	.93	.84	.77
	60	1.14	.98	.88	.79	.72
Average	50	1.06	.93	.84	.75	.68
	40	.99	.88	.80	.71	.66
Below Average	30	.93	.83	.76	.68	.63
	20	.88	.78	.72	.63	.57
Poor	10	.80	.71	.65	.57	.53
			Women			
Excellent	90	.90	.76	.71	.61	.64
	80	.80	.70	.62	.55	.54
Above Average	70	.74	.63	.57	.52	.51
	60	.70	.60	.54	.48	.47
Average	50	.65	.57	.52	.46	.45
	40	.59	.53	.50	.44	.43
Below Average	30	.56	.51	.47	.42	.40
	20	.51	.47	.43	.39	.38
Poor	10	.48	.42	.38	.37	.33

From: *ACSM's Guidelines For Exercise Testing and Prescription,* 6th Edition. 2000. Philadelphia: Lippincott, Williams, & Wilkins.

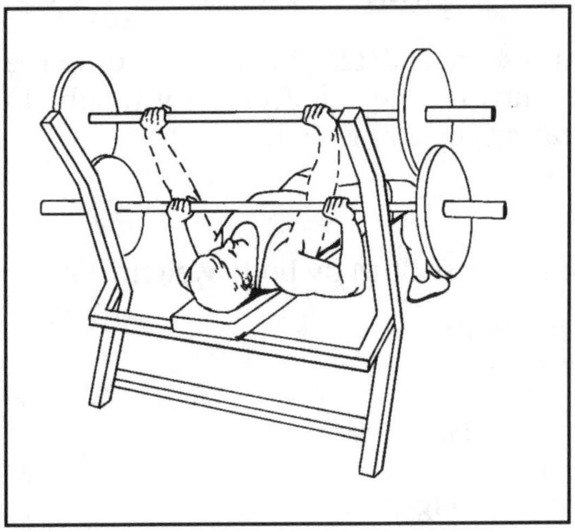

Figure 6.3 ■ Bench Press

7

Resistive Training Activities

People do not lack strength; they lack will.
Victor Hugo

By too much sitting still the body becomes unhealthy, and soon the mind.
Henry Wadsworth Longfellow

■ Chapter Outline ■

General Considerations When Performing Resistance Training Exercises
    Breath Control (Breathing) during Resistive Training
        Valsava Maneuver
    Weight Belts
    Knee Wraps
    Hand Grips and Placement
    Body Positioning
    Spotting

Machines vs. Free Weights
    Advantages/Disadvantages of Variable Resistance Machines
    Advantages/Disadvantages of Free Weights
Progressive, Variable, and Cable Resistance Machine Exercises
Free Weight Barbell Exercises
Free Weight Dumbbell Exercises
Resistance Training Without Free Weights or Resistance Machines

■ Learning Objectives ■

The student should be able to:

- Describe proper breathing procedures and techniques used during resistance training.
- Define and discuss the physiological implications of valsava maneuver.
- Discuss the advantages and disadvantages of weight belts.
- Identify and discuss the advantages and disadvantages of knee wraps.
- Identify and describe proper hand grips and hand placements used in resistance training with either free weights or resistive training machines.
- Identify and describe proper body positions used in resistance training with either free weights or resistive training.
- Define and describe the roles of a spotter when resistive training with free weights.
- Identify and discuss the advantages of variable or progressive resistance machines.
- Identify and discuss the biomechanical difference between variable and progressive resistance machines.

- Identify and discuss the advantages and disadvantages of free weights.
- Identify and discuss proper lifting techniques for common resistance training procedures, by selected body regions or segments, using progressive, variable, or cable machines.
- Identify and discuss proper lifting techniques for common resistance training procedures, by selected body regions or segments, using barbells.
- Identify and discuss proper lifting techniques for common resistance training procedures, by selected body regions or segments, using dumb bells.
- Identify and discuss proper training procedures and mechanics for common resistance training activities that do not require the use of free weights or resistance machines.

■ Keywords ■

Body position	Progressive resistance machines	Supinated grip
Breath control	Pronated grip	Valsava maneuver
Hand grip	Spotter	Variable resistance machines
Knee wraps	Spotting	Weight belt
Neutral grip		

General Considerations When Performing Resistance Training Exercises

When participating in any resistive training activity several factors should be considered. These variables are common whether participating in free weight activities or machine activities. For reader ease, subheaders have been used. They include:

- Breath Control (Breathing) During Resistive Training
- Weight Belts
- Knee Wraps
- Hand Grips and Placement
- Body Position
- Spotting

Breath Control (Breathing) during Resistive Training

Controlled breathing patterns are critical to safe, resistive training. Unfortunately, it is common for participants to hold their breath, particularly during strenuous lifting. This type of breathing pattern or behavior results in a phenomenon known as **Valsava maneuver.** Valsalva maneuver is discussed under a separate header below.

When lifting free weights, the recommended breathing procedure is to **exhale during the strenuous positions** and to **inhale during less strenuous positions.** Normally, this equates to exhaling during the concentric or shortening phase, and inhaling during the eccentric or muscle-lengthening phase.

For example, during an arm curl, the participant should exhale as the arm is flexed, especially as the arm moves through the 90 degree position, and inhale as the arm is returned from the flexed position to its original position. During a bench press, the most strenuous phase is lifting the weight off the chest. As a result, the participant should exhale as the arms extend and inhale as the weight is returned to the chest.

When working with variable resistance machines, the participant will notice a more constant load through the range of motion. This helps to eliminate the specific positions where greater or less tension is experienced. This should not indicate the lack of need to control breathing. The recommended procedure is to exhale during the concentric phases and to inhale during the eccentric movements.

Valsava Maneuver

By description, **valsava maneuver** is *forced expired air against a closed glottis.* The glottis is a flap of tissue that covers or protects the air passageway (trachea) to the lungs by covering the trachea during swallowing. During resistive training, it has been observed that if the glottis remains closed, it blocks or obstructs air escaping from the lungs. This results in a variety of physiological responses. The most prominent response is an increase in intrathoracic pressure that affects venous flow and cardiac output. The severity of impairment is related to the length and intensity of the valsava maneuver. The more strenuous the activity and the more severe the physical straining associated with the lift and breath holding, the more pronounced or severe the physiological response.

The most pronounced physiological response is a significant reduction of blood flow returning to the heart (venous return) from the body. This reduction in venous return leads to a substantial decrease in cardiac output. This decrease occurs mostly during the most strenuous aspects of the lift and may result in light-headedness or black out. When the physical strain of the lift is removed, blood flow is no longer restricted and rapidly returns to the heart, leading to a large after-load being placed on the heart. The dramatic rise in returned blood causes an increase in myocardial contractility or strength of contraction of the heart and higher blood pressures.

Valsava maneuver may be used advantageously by highly trained lifters. When properly utilized, breathe holding during the strenuous part of the lift will help to maintain proper alignment in the vertebral column and provide additional support to the vertebral discs. This is especially beneficial and helps reduce the risk of injury to the lower back during maximal or near maximal lifts.

This procedure, however, is associated with increased thoracic pressure, resulting in diminished venous return or blood flow back to the heart. As previously mentioned, this will lead to an increased **risk of blackout, disorientation, or dizziness** for the lifter. As a result, the use of the valsava maneuver is **not recommended** for most individuals. For those attempting to incorporate the valsava maneuver into their lift, precaution should be taken to restrict all breath holding to under 2 seconds.

Weight Belts

Weightlifting belts are used by many individuals to increase intraabdominal pressure. This helps to protect the lower back region and improve lifting safety. Precaution must be taken, however, *not to rely completely on the weight belt during training*. This practice will contribute to weakened abdominal musculature and may lead to injury. This is especially true for individuals attempting lifts without the use of weightlifting belts who are accustomed to lifting with the use of a belt. These individuals would be advised to lift submaximally, without the belt, until he/she has properly conditioned the back and abdominal musculature.

Additionally, if the weight belt is used, it should only be used on lifts that place unusually high levels of stress on the lower back, such as maximal or near maximal dead lifts. Activities such as lat pulls that do not present high levels of stress on the lower back should be performed without the use of the belt.

It should be stressed that proper training and conditioning of the abdominal and back musculature will allow for musculature development. Properly trained and conditioned back and abdominal musculatures are capable of generating enough intraabdominal pressure to protect and support the vertebral column, particularly in the lower back region during lifting. For these individuals, the use of weightlifting belts is not required. Should weightlifting belts be indicated, however, the following guidelines should be followed (Baechle & Earle, 2000):

- Use of the weightlifting belt should be restricted to activities or exercises that directly involve the lower back region.
- Use of the weightlifting belt should be restricted to near maximal and maximal lifts only.
- Train and condition the deep abdominal musculature to assist in generating needed intraabdominal pressure.

Knee Wraps

Many individuals, particularly power lifters, use knee wraps to protect the knees. However, *there is, no evidence available that suggests wrapping the knee prevents knee injury.* In fact, knee wraps may actually increase the risk of, or actually cause, knee injury (Harman, 2000). Given these findings, **the use of knee wraps is contraindicated and should be avoided.**

Hand Grips and Placement

The nature of how to grasp a barbell, dumbbell, or the handgrip of a variable resistance weight machine is critical to proper lifting procedure and technique. While differences exist between the grips, all are used universally with the differing pieces of resistive training equipment. For purposes of this text, the following grips, as described by Earle and Baechle (2000), will be considered when describing specific resistive training activities:

- **Pronated Grip:** The pronated grip may also be referred to as an overhand grip. In the pronated grip, the hand is positioned so the palms are facing down.

- **Supinated Grip:** The supinated grip may also be referred to as an underhand grip. In the supinated grip, the hand is positioned so the palms are facing upward.
- **Neutral Grip:** In the neutral grip, the hands are positioned half way between a pronated and supinated position or perpendicular to the ground. The hand position would resemble the position of the hand during a traditional handshake.

Hand placement is normally controlled by the nature or specific design of the handgrips provided on most variable resistance weight machines. In the case of a barbell however, hand placement or grip width may be varied. Grip widths can range from a narrow to a wide grip. The most common grip or hand placement requires the hands to be placed approximately shoulder width apart. The critical consideration in all grips is to have the weight of the bar balanced and evenly distributed on each hand. Unless otherwise indicated, all resistive training activities using a barbell presented in this text will require the more traditional shoulder width handgrip arrangement.

Body Positioning

Body position before and during a resistive training activity is critical to the safety of the participant. Proper body position helps to ensure proper lifting techniques. In the case of weight machines, adjustable components such as seat backs, seat heights, and roller pads will need to be positioned or fitted specifically to the participant. *Appropriate equipment fitting ensures that the active body segments are in line with the axis of rotation of the machine.* Additionally, proper body positioning ensures proper body alignment promoting maximal stability and support throughout a full range of motion when lifting. There are three frequently used body positions when lifting with either a bench or a variable resistance machine. These include:

- **Supine Position:** Normally, the supine position requires participants to lie face up on a bench with their head, back, shoulders, and hips resting on the bench. Both feet are placed flat on the floor.
- **Prone Position:** The prone position requires participants to lie face down on a bench with their head, back, shoulders, and hips resting on the bench. Normally, the legs are fully extended and the feet may be hooked on a roller pad.
- **Seated Position:** The seated or sitting position requires participants to sit upright on a seat or bench. When seat backs are provided as part of the seat, the head, back, and hips should be in contact with, and be supported by, the seat back. Both feet are placed flat on the floor.

Variations in these positions are possible and may be required depending on the specific nature of the resistive training activity. The critical consideration when varying any of the described positions is to provide adequate support for the head, shoulders, back, hips, and feet.

Many free weight activities and cable system activities require the participant to assume a **standing position**. Normally, when standing, both feet should be flat on the floor. Body weight should be evenly distributed between the feet. The participant's center of gravity should lie between the balls of the feet and the heels, with his/her weight and center of gravity shifted slightly forward toward the balls of the feet. To provide an adequate base of support, the feet should be positioned about shoulder width apart.

Spotting

By definition, a spotter is a resistive training partner who assists in the execution of a weight training activity. Therefore, spotting may be defined as any process or action taken by a spotter to assist a lifter when resistive training. The specific roles of the spotter are several-fold. For brevity, these may be summarized as follows:

- Protect the lifter from injury.
- Assist the lifter in forced (spotter-assisted) repetitions.

- Assist the lifter when participating in negative training lifting procedures.
- Provide motivation.

The number of spotters and the specific spotting technique required vary according to the type and nature of the resistive training activity. For example, overhead activities require different spotting techniques than those required for over-the-face activities. Activities that involve larger loads require a greater number of spotters than lighter load activities.

Finally, the role of the spotters will change slightly when assisting with variable resistance equipment. Typically, the role of protecting the lifter from being pinned by a bar is eliminated. Normally, the design of the equipment will protect the lifter should an untoward event such as a muscle tear, muscle spasm, or muscle cramp occur. Additionally, in resistive training activities where multiple spotters are required the need to have spotters of similar strength is not required.

Machines vs. Free Weights

Opinions vary between individuals as to the value of progressive resistance machines and free weights. *It is the position of this author that both types of resistive training equipment are warranted and should be included in any resistive training program.* Each type of equipment offers unique and positive features that allow for the development of muscular strength and endurance. Fleck and Kraemer (1987) demonstrated that similar gains in muscular strength can occur using either type of equipment for resistive training.

It should also be noted that differences exist in the types and features of progressive resistance machines. Some pieces are designed using only round pulleys or bars with fixed lengths. A single, round pulley, or a fixed bar length, can only change the direction or line of pull of the resistive force. They cannot change the magnitude of the resistive load. As a result, this type of equipment is not designed to correct for differences in muscular tension or torques that result from the body's joint and lever arrangements. These pieces of equipment act only as isotonic, constant resistant machines.

In contrast, variable resistance machines incorporate the use of specifically designed cams that serve to change the line of pull or direction of the resistive force, as well as its magnitude. The change in load is designed to match the body's ability to produce force at any given joint.

For reader ease, the advantages and disadvantages of variable resistance machines and free weights are discussed under separate headers below. With the exception of the ability to alter the magnitude of the resistive load, pulley and fixed bar machines offer the same advantages and disadvantages as variable resistance machines. As a result, no additional discussion on the advantages and disadvantages of single pulley or fixed bar length machines will be offered.

Advantages/Disadvantages of Variable Resistance Machines

Variable resistance machines are specifically designed resistance training equipment that, like free weights, rely on gravity for resistance. Specific advantages and disadvantages are discussed below and are itemized in Table 7-1.

Variable resistance machines are designed to correct for the differences in muscular tension or torques that result from the body's joint and lever arrangements as a body segment moves through a range of motion. This is accomplished by incorporating a cam-shaped pulley arrangement into the equipment. This arrangement allows the resistance offered by the machine to vary and match the changes in muscle torque relative to specific joint angles. In positions where greater levels of muscle torque can be generated by the lifter, greater resistance is offered. Similarly, when joint angles change leverage and allow for lower levels of muscle torque to be generated, the machine offers lower resistance.

The ability of the machine to vary resistance allows the lifter to experience a relatively **constant load, throughout the entire range of motion,** on the muscles involved in the lift.

The lifter experiences little or no sensation of weak or strong positions. Because of this arrangement, variable resistance training is extremely efficient.

Selecting a resistance is a simple matter of moving a pin in a stack of weights. It requires no effort and a limited amount of time. Like free weights, variable resistance machines offer positive and negative resistance throughout a full range of motion.

Variable resistance machines offer safe, convenient exercises. They provide a controlled range of motion and require no spotters. The elimination of the risk of being pinned by a weight helps many individuals to feel more comfortable and secure when using machines. The controlled movements of the machines help to eliminate users from needing to develop or learn specific lifting techniques.

Variable resistance machines isolate muscle groups well and as a result, allow for very specific muscular development. In many cases, specific machines have been developed to create resistive movement patterns that are difficult to mimic with free weights. For example, most manufacturers offer hip flexor, hip abductor, and hip adductor machines. To offer resistance to these movements with free weights is extremely difficult.

The major disadvantages of variable resistance machines are cost and space. Because of the large numbers of machines required for a full body workout, a large floor space will be required. By comparison, variable resistance machines are far more expensive than free weights.

Table 7-1 ■ Advantages and Disadvantages of Variable Resistance Weight Machines

Advantages
- Provide positive and negative resistance
- Rapid (saves time), effortless change of resistance
- Controlled range of motion
- Safe, convenient, no spotters required
- Variable resistance (The cam shaped oval used on many machines allows for a relatively constant load throughout the range of motion.)
- More efficient (constant resistance through a full range of motion)
- Easy to use (require no specific lifting techniques)
- Large number of machines are available for a wide variety of movements
- Isolate muscle groups well

Disadvantages
- Expensive
- Require a large amount of space

Advantages/Disadvantages of Free Weights

Barbells and dumbbells are the most common free weights. The advantages and disadvantages of free weights are discussed below and summarized in Table 7-2. Barbells require both hands to manipulate and allow for simultaneous limb movements. Dumbbells are designed for one-handed usage and allow for single limb movements. Between the two, a large number of variations of lifting activities or exercises are possible.

Free weights are relatively inexpensive compared to variable resistance machines and require minimal space. They offer both positive and negative resistance and can be used by most everyone to successfully develop muscular strength and muscular endurance.

Barbells and dumbbells are considered fixed resistance equipment. It is important to recognize, however, that as a result of the lever system of the human body, they do not offer a constant resistance throughout a range of motion. There will be points in the range of motion where the load offers greater or less resistive torque than at other points. Similarly, there will be points, or selected limb positions, in any range of motion that favor the muscle contraction and allow for greater muscular torque than other points. As a result, as a barbell or dumbbell is moved through a range of motion, there will be times where the weight feels lighter than at other times. Conversely, most individuals will also experience a "sticking point" in the range of motion where the resistance seems greatest.

By way of example, consider an individual attempting to flex the lower arm at the elbow during a simple arm curl. The period of greatest resistance, or the "sticking point," is when the lower arm is at a 90-degree angle with the upper arm. The bench press represents another example. Even though the barbell weight is fixed and remains constant throughout the range of motion during the bench press, the lifter will sense it is more difficult to lift the weight when it is closer to the chest as compared to positions where the arms are more fully extended.

Because of the free, uncontrolled range of motion provided during lifting, spotters may be required. Spotters help to reduce the risks of falling weights or injury to the lifter when the lifter is unable to successfully manage the load. The uncontrolled range of motion allows for a more whole-body approach. Where variable resistance machines isolate muscle groups, the use of free weight encourages multiple muscle groups to work together.

Selecting the resistance on barbells does require manipulation of the weight plates on barbells. The process is time-consuming and does require physical effort. Typically, dumbbells come in a variety of fixed weights so in most cases weight adjustment is limited. Selecting the appropriate resistive load simply requires selecting the appropriate dumbbell.

Table 7-2 ■ Advantages and Disadvantages of Free Weights

Advantages
- Barbells and dumbbells are the most common free weights and are readily available
- Inexpensive
- Allow for a free range of motion
- Versatile
- Provide positive and negative resistance
- Require a number of muscle groups to work together when lifting
- Allow for sport specific exercises that mimic particular sport movements

Disadvantages
- Risk of injury from falling weights or being pinned by a weight
- May require spotters
- Require time and effort to adjust resistance
- Fixed resistance (Offers maximal resistance only at a joint specific angle. At any other point in the range of motion, the resistance may be submaximal.)

Progressive, Variable, and Cable Resistance Machine Exercises

There are many appropriate progressive, variable, and cable resistance machine training activities that could be recommended. If properly incorporated into a regular muscular strength and endurance training program each would allow for positive gains in both muscular strength and muscular endurance. To illustrate and describe such a large number of procedures is beyond the scope of this manuscript. As a result, a sampling of the more common procedures have been provided. For reader ease, procedures have been grouped by body segment.

Chest

Bench Press

Action

The action of the machine bench press is similar to all machine bench press variations. When performing a bench press, the subject should position him or herself in a supine position on a flat bench. The sacrum, head, and shoulders should all touch the bench. The subject's feet should be placed flat on the floor or on the foot platform if provided. The knees should be bent at approximately 90-degree angles. If a foot platform is used, the subject may find slightly more knee bend and slight hip flexion will occur. Set the machine to the appropriate resistance. In the initial position, grasp the handgrips using a pronated grip. The bar height should be adjusted so the hands are slightly higher than the chest. During the upward or concentric phase, the bar is pressed upward and the arms are fully extended. Do not lock the elbows during arm extension. The arms should be externally rotated so that the elbows are positioned or pointed outward. During the downward or eccentric phase, the handgrips are lowered toward the chest while keeping the wrists extended and directly above the elbow. During the action of the arms, precaution should be taken to keep the back flat on the bench. Arching of the back should be avoided. Proper breath control is strongly recommended. Inhale during the eccentric phase of the lift and exhale during the concentric phase. The action of the bench press using a progressive resistance bench press machine is shown in Figure 7.1.

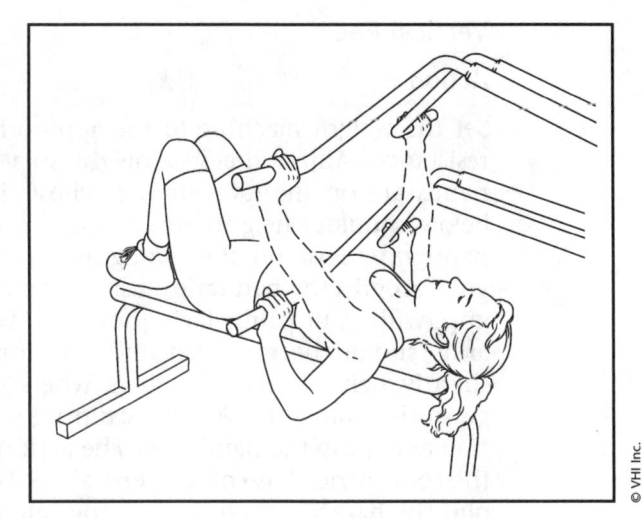

Figure 7.1 ■ Machine - Bench Press

Major Muscles Conditioned

Pectoralis Major, Deltoid (anterior), Triceps

Vertical Chest Press

Action

Set the weight machine to the appropriate resistance. Adjust the seat position so your hands are on the level of your chest (just below shoulder height) when seated and grasping the handgrips. Assume a sitting position. The action of the concentric phase of the vertical chest press is to lightly grasp the handgrips, using a pronated handgrip and push the bar forward and away from your chest until your arms are extended in front of you. Do not lock out the elbows during arm extension. It should also be noted that some variable resistance machines provide handgrips that allow for a neutral grip. During the eccentric phase, slowly return the arms to their original position. Proper breath control is strongly recommended. Inhale during the eccentric phase of the lift and exhale during the concentric phase. The action of the vertical chest press using a progressive resistance vertical chest press machine is shown in Figure 7.2.

Major Muscles Conditioned

Pectoralis Major, Deltoid (anterior), Triceps

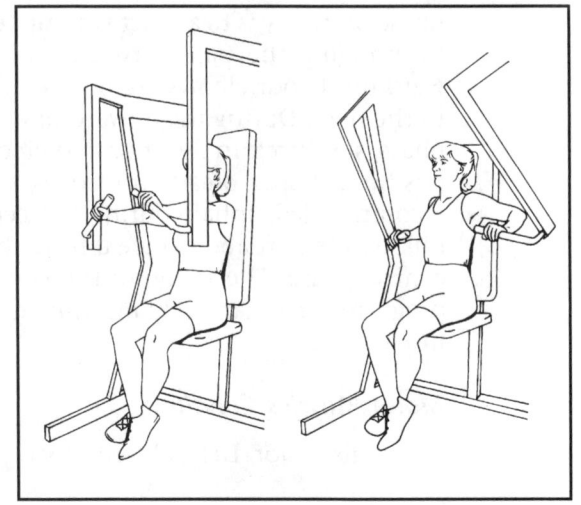

Figure 7.2 ■ Machine - Vertical Chest Press

Vertical Pec

Action

Set the weight machine to the appropriate resistance. Adjust the seat height so your hands are on the level of your chest (just below shoulder height) when grasping the handgrips. Position the handgrips so that you can grip the handgrips, using a neutral grip, with your palms facing forward. Your arms should be extended and positioned slightly behind your shoulders when you grasp the handgrips. Assume a sitting position and grasp the handgrips. The action of the concentric phase of the vertical pec is to pull the hands forward toward the midline of your body (transverse adduction) until the hands almost touch in front of the chest. During the eccentric phase, slowly return the arms to their original position. Proper breath control is strongly recommended. Inhale during the eccentric phase of the lift and exhale during the concentric phase. The action of the vertical pec exercise using a progressive resistance vertical pec machine is shown in Figure 7.3.

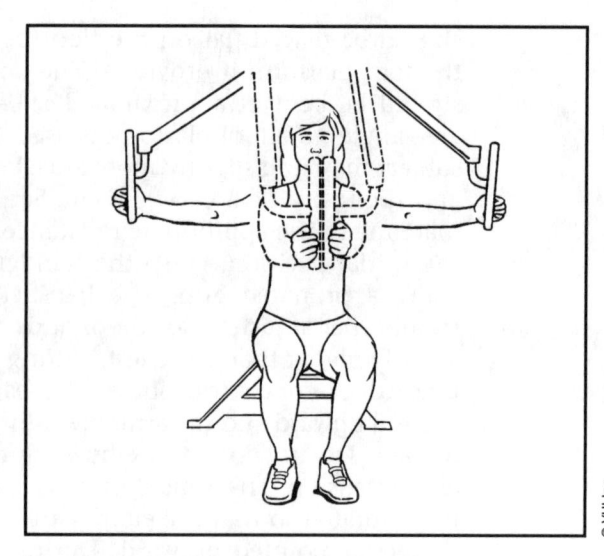

Figure 7.3 ■ Machine - Vertical Pec

Major Muscles Conditioned

Pectoralis Major, Deltoid (anterior)

Fly

Action

Set the weight machine to the appropriate resistance. Adjust the seat position so your shoulders are in line with the roller pads. In the initial position, assume a sitting position and reach your arms over the top of the roller pads. Your upper arm should be resting on the top of the pad with the pad positioned at the bend in your elbow. The elbows should be bent to approximately 90-degrees. The concentric phase of the Fly is to adduct your upper arms by bringing the pads forward and downward until your elbows are pointed directly to the floor. During the upward or eccentric phase, slowly return the arms to their original position. Proper breath control is strongly recommended. Inhale during the eccentric phase of the lift and exhale during the concentric phase. The action of the Fly using a progressive resistance Fly machine is shown in Figure 7.4.

Major Muscles Conditioned

Pectoralis Major, Deltoid (anterior)

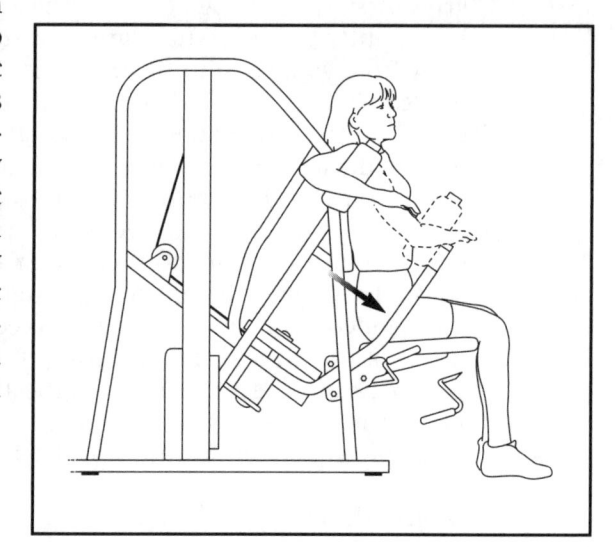

Figure 7.4 ■ Machine - Fly

Assisted Dips

Action

Assisted dip machines have been developed to allow individuals to control the magnitude of resistance when participating in dipping activities. Unlike most resistance training equipment, however, the greater the load selected, the less muscular effort required by the participant. To perform an assisted dip, begin by selecting the appropriate resistance. Then, adjust the handgrips so they are approximately shoulder width apart. Initially, you should grasp each handgrip with a neutral grip. While keeping your arms fully extended, step off the platform onto the machine's knee bar. Allow your body weight to push the foot bar downward until your legs are fully extended at the hip. The eccentric phase is the first action. To perform the eccentric phase, lower your body by flexing the lower arms at the elbows and abducting the upper arms at the shoulders. The body should be lowered until the upper chest is even with the bars. During the concentric phase, return the body to its original position by pressing downward on the bars and extending the arms. Continue to kneel on the knee bar and allow the selected resistance to assist in lifting your body upward. Once the activity has been completed, precaution should be taken to step off the foot bar only when the weight plates are resting on the weight stack. Proper breath control is strongly recommended. Inhale during the eccentric phase of the lift and exhale during the concentric phase. The action of the assisted dip is shown in Figure 7.5.

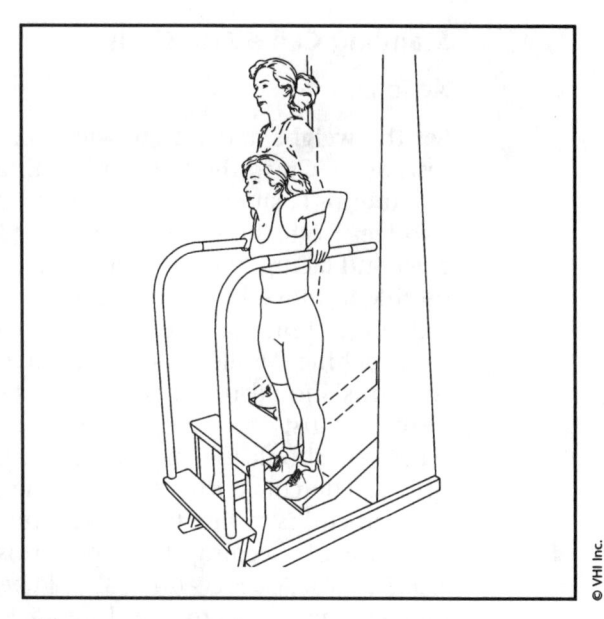

Figure 7.5 ■ Machine - Assisted Dips

Major Muscles Conditioned

Pectoralis Major, Pectoralis Minor, Triceps, Deltoid (anterior), Latissimus Dorsi, Teres Major

Upper Arms – Anterior

Seated Arm Curls

Action

Set the weight machine to the appropriate resistance. Adjust the seat back and seat height so the triceps are parallel with the restraint pads when the arms are resting on the restraint pads. Grasp the handgrips with a supinated grip (palms facing upward). The elbows should be in line with the axis of rotation of the machine when sitting down. The concentric phase of the arm curl is to flex the lower arm at the elbow. Precaution should be taken to move through a full range of motion. During the downward or eccentric phase, slowly return the lower arms to their original position. Proper breath control is strongly recommended. Inhale during the eccentric phase of the lift and exhale during the concentric phase. The action of the seated arm curl is shown in Figure 7.6.

Major Muscles Conditioned

Biceps Brachii, Brachialis, Brachioradialis

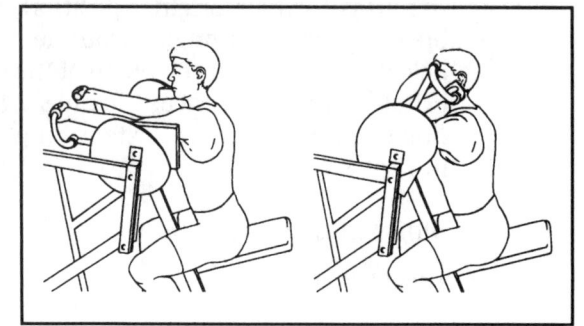

Figure 7.6 ■ Machine - Seated Arm Curls

Standing Cable Arm Curls

Action

Set the weight machine to the appropriate resistance. Grasp the hand bar with a supinated grip. Position yourself approximately two feet from the machine when standing erect and facing the equipment. You should be able to move your lower arms through a full range of motion without interference of the machine. While holding the hand bar, the arms should be externally rotated and rested against the sides of the trunk. The hand bar should be in contact with your thighs. The concentric phase of the standing arm curl is to flex the lower arms at the elbows while keeping the upper arms fixed against the sides. Precaution should be taken to keep the body erect and avoid leaning backward, particularly when the lower arms are moving through the 90-degree angle. During the downward or eccentric phase, extend the lower arms at the elbows back to their original position. Proper breath control is strongly recommended. Inhale during the eccentric phase of the lift and exhale during the concentric phase. The action of the standing cable arm curl is shown in Figure 7.7.

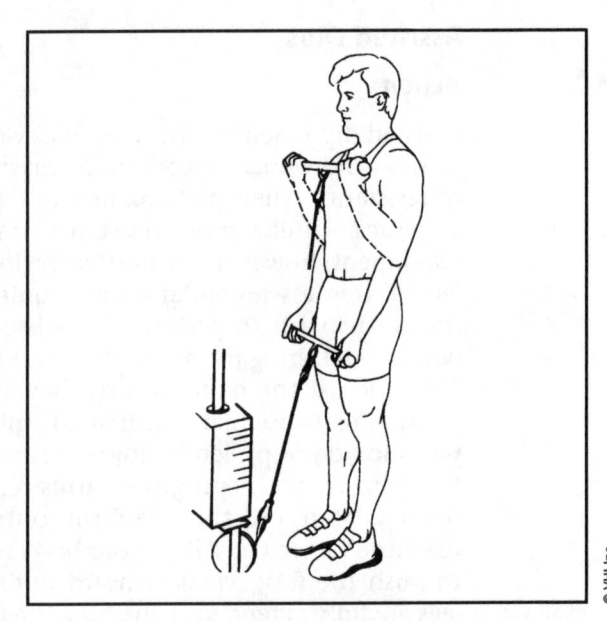

Figure 7.7 ■ Machine - Standing Cable Arm Curls

Major Muscles Conditioned

Biceps Brachii, Brachialis, Brachioradialis

Upper Arms – Posterior

Seated Triceps Extension

Action

Set the weight machine to the appropriate resistance. Adjust the seat back and seat height so the triceps are parallel with the restraint pads when the arms are resting on the restraint pads. Grasp the handgrips using a neutral grip (palms facing inward). The elbows should be in line with the axis of rotation of the machine when sitting down. The concentric phase of the triceps extension is to extend the lower arm at the elbow. During the upward or eccentric phase, slowly return the arms to their original position. Proper breath control is strongly recommended. Inhale during the eccentric phase of the lift and exhale during the concentric phase. The action of the seated triceps extension is shown in Figure 7.8.

Major Muscles Conditioned

Triceps Brachii

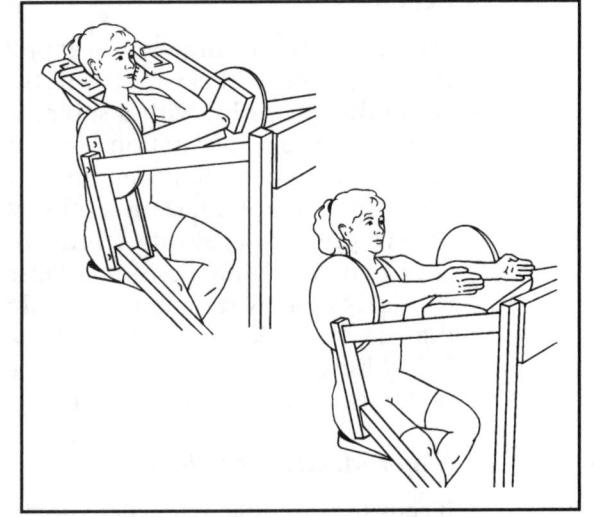

Figure 7.8 ■ Machine - Seated Triceps Extension

Standing Triceps Extension

Action

Set the weight machine to the appropriate resistance. Grasp the hand bar with a pronated grip. The hands should be approximately shoulder width apart. Position yourself approximately two feet from the machine when standing erect and facing the equipment. You should be able to move your lower arms through a full range of motion without interference of the machine. While holding the hand bar, the arms should be flexed a minimum of 90 degrees. The concentric phase of the standing triceps extension is to fully extend the lower arms at the elbows while keeping the upper arms fixed against the sides. Precaution should be taken to keep the body erect and avoid leaning forward. During the upward or eccentric phase, flex the lower arms, at the elbows, back to their original position. Proper breath control is strongly recommended. Inhale during the eccentric phase of the lift and exhale during the concentric phase. The action of the standing triceps extension is shown in Figure 7.9.

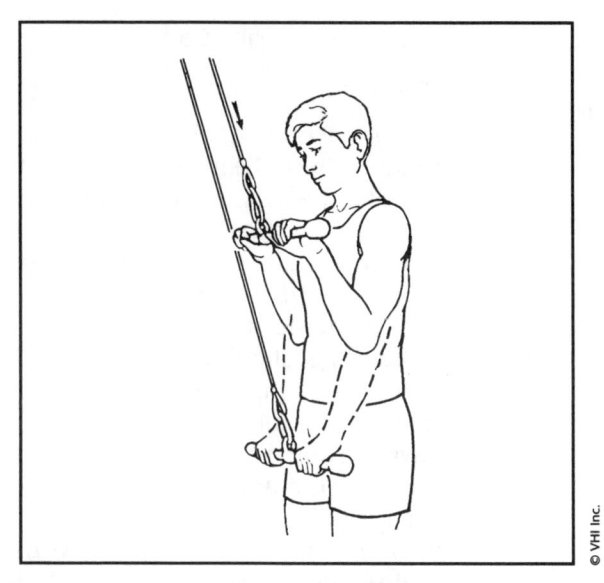

Figure 7.9 ■ Machine - Standing Triceps Extension

Note: Some standing triceps extension machines provide a pad to rest the hips and back. When using this type of equipment, assume a standing position, facing away from the equipment, with the back and hips leaning back while being supported by the back pad. The hips should be slightly flexed, so the feet are positioned slightly in front of the body with the legs fully extended.

Major Muscles Conditioned

Triceps Brachii

Shoulders

Overhead Press

Action

Set the weight machine to the appropriate resistance. Adjust the seat position so your shoulders are even with the hand bars. Assume a sitting position. Lightly grasp the handgrips using a pronated grip (palms facing out). The concentric phase of the overhead press is to push upward to a point that the arms are fully extended. Do not lock the elbows out during extension. It should also

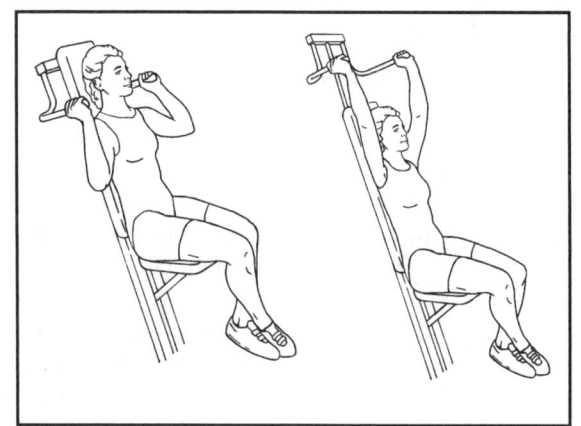

Figure 7.10 ■ Machine - Overhead Press

be noted that some variable resistance equipment provide handgrips that allow for a neutral grip. During the overhead press, precaution should be taken to keep the back straight, with the head, shoulders, and hips in contact with the seatback (if provided). During the downward or eccentric phase, slowly return the arms to their original position. Proper breath control is strongly recommended. Inhale during the eccentric phase of the lift and exhale during the concentric phase. The action of the overhead press using a progressive resistance machine is shown in Figure 7.10.

Major Muscles Conditioned

Deltoid (anterior, medial), Triceps Brachii, Trapezius (upper)

Standing Upright Cable Row

Action

Set the machine to the to the appropriate resistance. Grasp the handgrip with a pronated grip. Hand placement or grip width should be inside the shoulders. Assume a standing position and allow the handgrip to rest comfortably on the thigh. In order to provide a more stable stance, position the feet slightly outside the shoulders and turn the toes slightly out. During the concentric or upward phase, pull or lift the handgrip directly upward against the abdomen and chest toward the chin until the handgrip is approximately on the level with the clavicles. During the lifting motion, keep the elbows high. Precaution should be taken to keep the back straight and the head up during the lifting motion. During the downward or eccentric phase, extend the elbows and adduct the upper arms toward the side lowering the barbell back to its original position. Proper breath control is strongly recommended. Inhale during the eccentric phase of the lift and exhale during the concentric phase. The action of the standing upright cable row is shown in Figure 7.11.

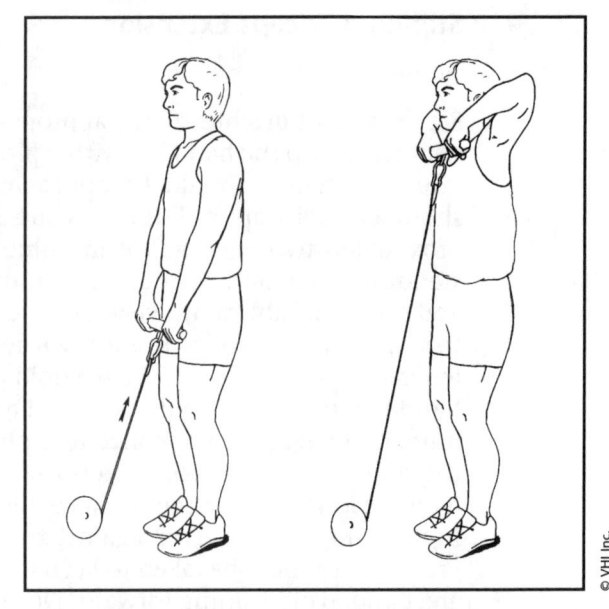

Figure 7.11 ■ Machine - Standng Upright Cable Row

Major Muscles Conditioned

Deltoid (anterior, medial, posterior), Trapezius (upper)

Seated Lateral Raise (Abduction)

Action

Set the weight machine to the appropriate resistance. Adjust the seat position so your shoulders are in line with the axis of motion of the machine when you are seated. Assume a sitting position and place your arms inside the pads. Lightly grasp the handgrips. The concentric phase of the seated lateral raise is to lift the pads just above the horizontal by abducting your upper arms at the shoulders. During the downward or eccentric phase, slowly return the arms to their original position. Proper breath control is strongly recommended. Inhale during the eccentric phase of the lift and exhale during the concentric phase. The action of the seated lateral raise is shown in Figure 7.12.

Major Muscles Conditioned

Deltoid (middle), Trapezius (upper)

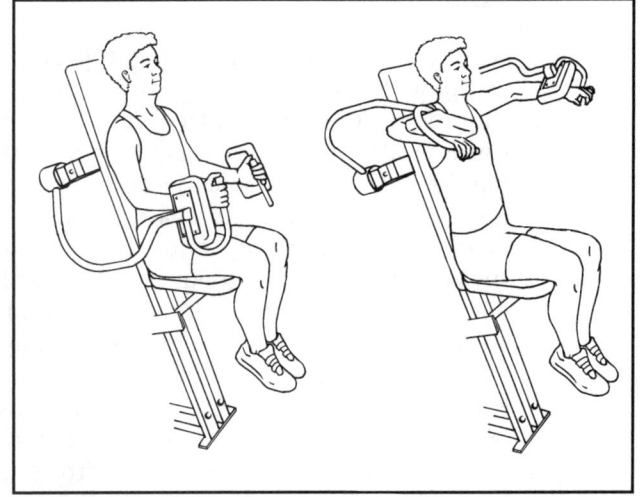

Figure 7.12 ■ Machine - Seated Lateral Raise (Abduction)

Seated Posterior Deltoid

Action

Set the weight machine to the appropriate resistance. Adjust the seat height so your hands are on the level of your chest (just below shoulder height) when grasping the handgrips. Position the handgrips so you can grip the handgrips with your palms facing inward. Your arms will be extended and positioned directly in front of your shoulders when you grasp the handgrips. The action of the concentric phase of the seated posterior deltoid is to pull the hands backward away from the midline of your body (transverse abduction) until the hands are extended behind your shoulders. During the eccentric phase, slowly return the arms to their original position. Proper breath control is strongly recommended. Inhale during the eccentric phase of the lift and exhale during the concentric phase. The action of the seated posterior deltoid is shown in Figure 7.13.

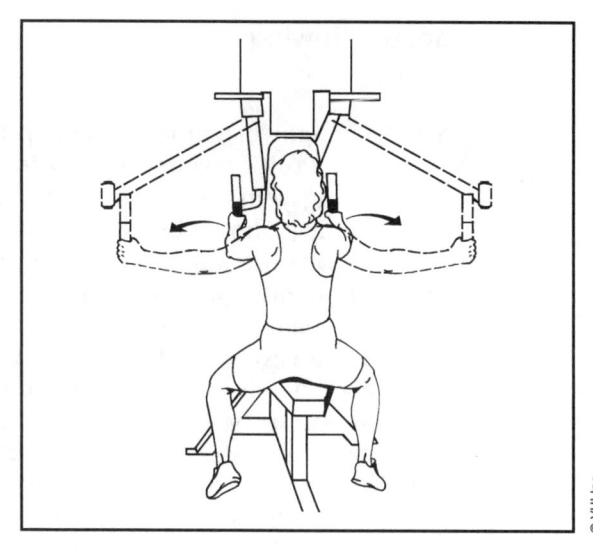

Figure 7.13 ■ Machine - Seated Posterior Deltoid

Major Muscles Conditioned

Deltoid (posterior), Trapezius (upper, middle)

Upper Back

Lat Pull Down

Action

Set the machine to the appropriate resistance. Adjust the seat height to allow for full extension of the arms. Adjust the seat roller pads so they comfortably rest on the tops of the thighs and knees. The roller pads should secure the hips and body to the seat during movement. Grasp either the handgrips or the outer aspect of the bar (if provided), with a pronated grip (palms facing away). When using a bar, hand placement should position the hands approximately shoulder width apart. The concentric phase of the lat pull down is to pull the handgrips or bar down toward the chest with moderate backward lean. During the upward or eccentric phase, slowly return the arms to their original position. Do not lock the elbows out on full extension. Proper breath control is strongly recommended. Inhale during the eccentric phase of the lift and exhale during the concentric phase. The action of the lat pull down is shown in Figure 7.14.

Major Muscles Conditioned

Latissimus Dorsi, Teres Major, Trapezius (middle, upper), Rhomboids, Deltoid (posterior), Biceps, Triceps, Pectoralis Major, Pectoralis Minor

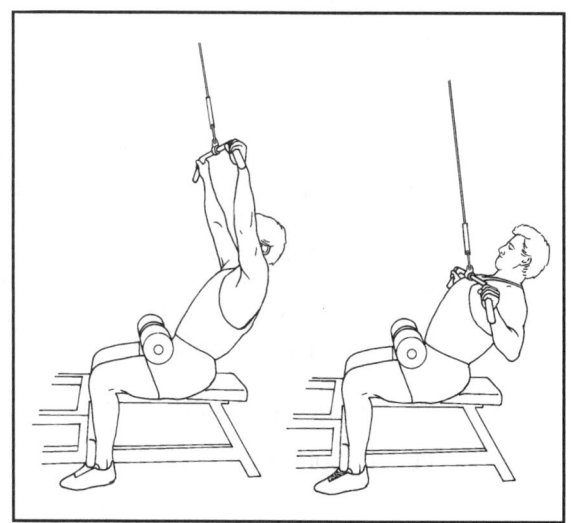

Figure 7.14 ■ Machine - Lat Pull Down

Seated Rowing

Action

Set the weight machine to the appropriate resistance. Position yourself by sitting down and placing your feet parallel on the footpad. Your legs should be fully extended. Do not lock out the knees. Lean forward and grasp the handgrips using a pronated grip, with the palms facing inward. You may bend the knees during this action. Holding the bar or handgrips, sit either upright or with a moderate backward lean keeping your arms extended. Straighten your legs back out if you bent the knee when grasping the handgrips. The action during the concentric phase of the seated row is to pull the handgrips to the chest. Variations allow the elbows to be positioned either upright or kept down by the sides. Precaution should be taken to limit the movement occurring at the hips. During the eccentric phase, slowly return the arms to their original position. Do not return the weight back to the stack by leaning forward until the full set of repetitions is completed. To return the weights to the stack, you should slowly lean forward at the hips while bending the knees. Proper breath control is strongly recommended. Inhale during the eccentric phase of the lift and exhale during the concentric phase. The action of seated rowing is shown in Figure 7.15.

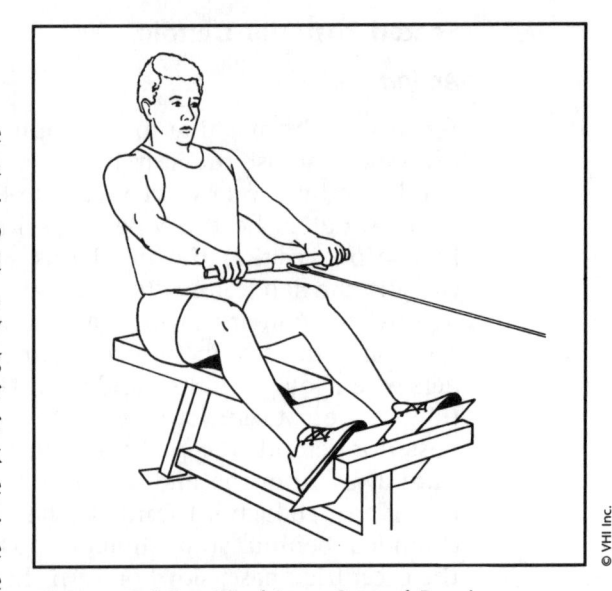

Figure 7.15 ■ Machine - Seated Rowing

Note: Some seated rowing equipment provides a chest pad to support the upper body. When using this type of equipment, position the seat height and chest pad so the arms are parallel and fully extended when grasping the handgrips. The upper body should be upright when resting on the chest pad.

Major Muscles Conditioned

Latissimus Dorsi, Trapezius (middle), Teres Major, Rhomboids, Biceps, Deltoids (rear)

Lower Back

Back Extension

Action

Set the weight machine to the appropriate resistance. Set the seat height so the navel is in line with the axis of rotation of the machine. Set the footrest so that it positions the knees higher than the hips. Position yourself by leaning forward and sitting on the seat. The back and shoulders should be in contact with the back pad of the machine. Place your feet parallel on the footpad. Lightly grip the handgrips to stabilize the body during muscular contraction. The action during the concentric phase of the back extension is to push backward as if sitting upright by contracting the musculature of the lower back. During the eccentric phase, slowly return to the original position by leaning forward. The action of the back extension is shown in Figure 7.16.

Major Muscles Conditioned

Erector Spinae

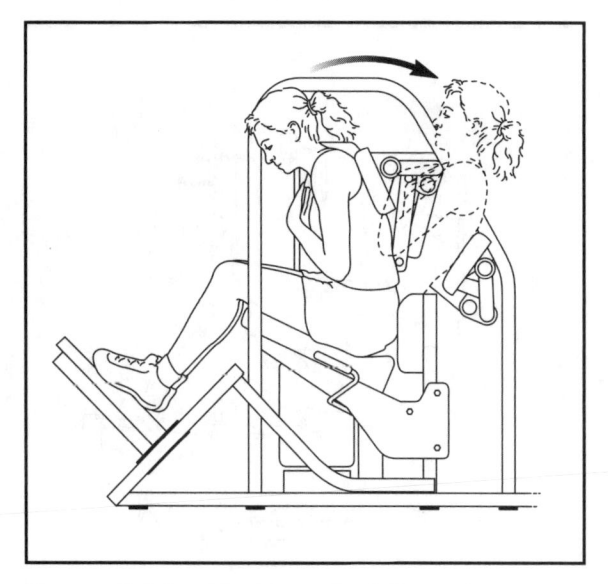

Figure 7.16 ■ Machine - Back Extension

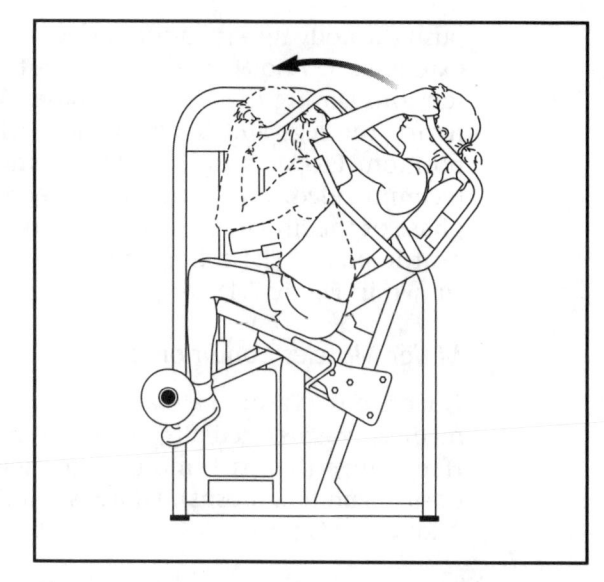

Figure 7.17 ■ Machine - Abdominals

Abdominals

Abdominal Machine

Action

Set the weight machine to the appropriate resistance. Adjust the seat height so the subject's navel is in line with the axis of rotation of the machine. Raise the arms so the elbows and posterior upper arm (triceps) rest on the machine's arm rests. Hook your feet behind the leg restraint so the roller pad of the leg restraint is positioned where it rests on the shin and tops of your feet. The action during the concentric phase is to contract the abdominals, lowering your chest toward your knees. Precaution should be taken to keep your hips and back in contact with the seat and seat back during the concentric phase. Your head should be kept upright. Do not tuck the chin toward the chest. During the upward or eccentric phase, slowly return the upper body to its original position. Proper breath control is strongly recommended. Inhale during the eccentric phase of the lift and exhale during the concentric phase. The action of the abdominal machine is shown in Figure 7.17.

Major Muscles Conditioned

Rectus Abdominis, External Abdominal Oblique, Internal Abdominal Oblique

Gluteal

Hip Sled

Action

There are several variations of hip sled weight machines available. The primary difference between equipment is the moving segment. In some sleds the resistance moves while the body remains stationary, while in others the body moves. The action discussed below assumes the footpad remains fixed and the body moves. Set the weight machine to the appropriate resistance. Position yourself by sitting down on the chair provided and place your feet, perpendicular on the footpad, directly in front of the hips. Adjust the seat to the appropriate position. The distance between the footpad and the seat is critical. Never assume a position that bends the knees greater than 90 degrees. Lightly grasp the handgrips to stabilize the body during the leg press. The action of the concentric phase of the leg press is to press or push the body upward until the legs are fully extended. Do not lock the knees out at extension. During the eccentric phase, slowly return the legs and body to their original position. Proper breath control is strongly recommended. Inhale during the eccentric phase of the lift and exhale during the concentric phase. The action of the hip sled is shown in Figure 7.18.

Major Muscles Conditioned

Quadriceps (Vastus Lateralis, Vastus Intermedius, Vastus Medialis, Rectus Femoris), Hamstrings (Biceps Femoris, Semimembranosus, Semitendinosus), Gluteus Maximus, Adductor Magnus

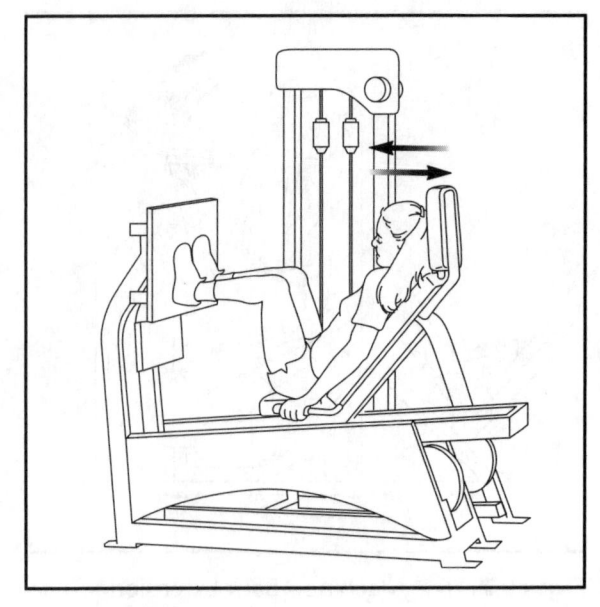

Figure 7.18 ■ Machine - Hip Sled

Leg Abduction

Action

Set the weight machine to the appropriate resistance. Position yourself by sitting upright with the outside of your knees and thighs on the inside of the leg pads. Adjust the pads so the legs are fully adducted (knees together), in a transverse plane, in front of you. Lightly grasp the handgrips to stabilize the body during muscle contraction. The action during the concentric phase of the leg abductor is to abduct the legs outward using a slow, controlled movement through a full range of motion. Precaution should be taken to to keep the back in contact with the seat back during muscle contraction. During the eccentric phase, slowly return the legs by adducting the upper legs to their original position. Proper breath control is strongly recommended. Inhale during the eccentric phase of the lift and exhale during the concentric phase. The action of the leg abduction machine is shown in Figure 7.19.

Major Muscles Conditioned

Gluteus Medius, Gluteus Minimums, Tensor Fasciae Latae

Seated Leg Press

Action

Set the weight machine to the appropriate resistance. Position yourself by sitting down

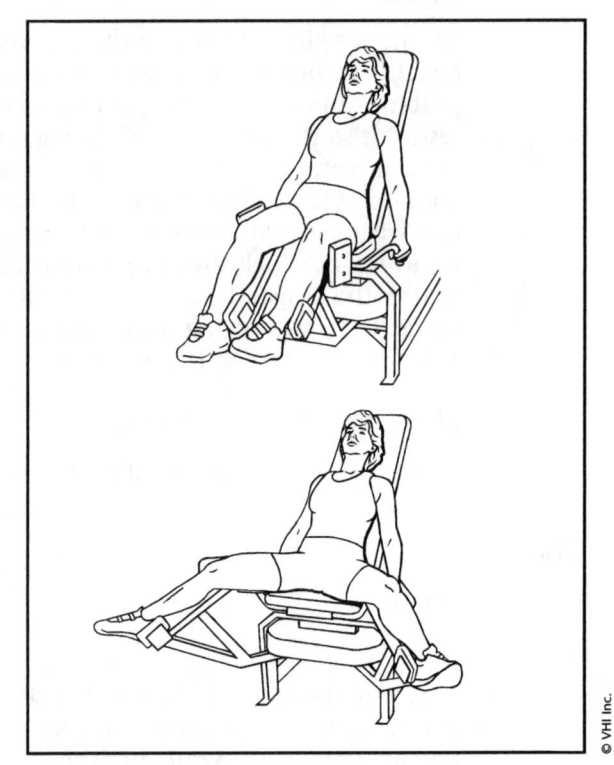

Figure 7.19 ■ Machine - Leg Abduction

on the chair provided and place your feet, perpendicular on the footpad, directly in front of the hips. Adjust the seat to the appropriate position. The distance between the footpad and the seat is critical. Never assume a position that bends the knees greater than 90 degrees. Lightly grasp the handgrips to stabilize the body during the leg press. The action of the concentric phase of the leg press is to press or push the footpad forward until the legs are fully extended. Do not lock the knees out at extension. During the eccentric phase, slowly return the legs and footpad to their original position. Proper breath control is strongly recommended. Inhale during the eccentric phase of the lift and exhale during the concentric phase. The action of the seated leg press is shown in Figure 7.20.

Major Muscles Conditioned

Quadriceps (Vastus Lateralis, Vastus Intermedius, Vastus Medialis, Rectus Femoris), Hamstrings (Biceps Femoris, Semimembranosus, Semitendinosus), Gluteus Maximus, Adductor Magnus

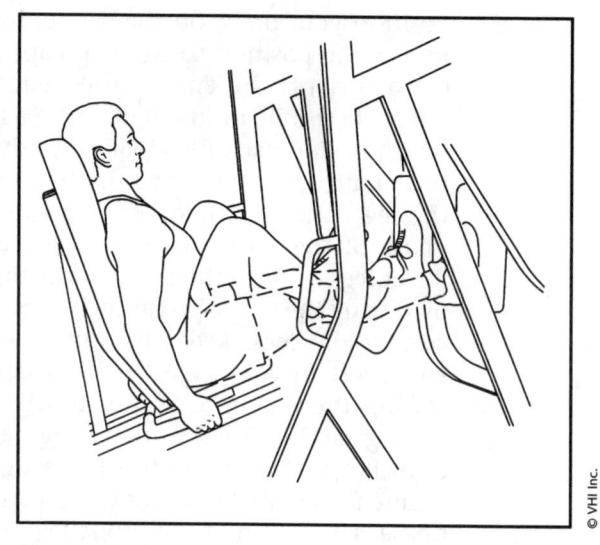

Figure 7.20 ■ Machine - Seated Leg Press

Upper Legs – Anterior

Seated Leg Extension

Action

Set the weight machine to the appropriate resistance. Adjust the lower leg roller pad so it rests on the anterior aspect of the lower legs (shins) just above the feet. The top of the feet should be in contact with the bottom of the roller pad. Adjust the seat back so the knees are in line with the axis of motion of the machine when the hips are in contact with the seat back. Lightly grasp the handgrips to stabilize the body during leg extension. The action of the concentric phase of the seated leg extension is to extend the lower legs at the knees lifting the roller pad. When extending the legs, keep the hips, stomach, and chest in contact with the bench pad. During the eccentric phase, slowly return the legs and footpad to their original position. Proper breath control is strongly recommended. Inhale during the eccentric phase of the lift and exhale during the concentric phase. The action of the seated leg extension is shown in Figure 7.21.

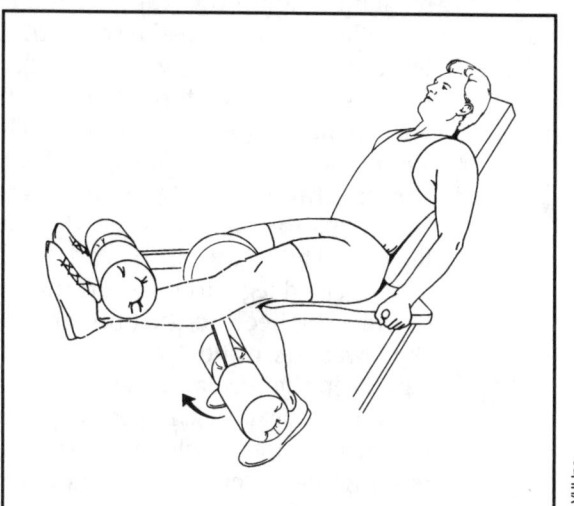

Figure 7.21 ■ Machine - Seated Leg Extension

Muscles Conditioned

Quadriceps (Vastus Lateralis, Vastus Intermedius, Vastus Medialis, Rectus Femoris)

Upper Legs – Posterior

Prone Leg Curl

Action

Set the weight machine to the appropriate resistance. Adjust the lower leg roller pad so the pad rests on the Achilles tendons of each leg while laying in a prone position on the bench.

Position your body, on the bench, by lying in a prone position so the kneecaps are located just off the end of the bench. The knees should be in line with the axis of rotation of the machine. Finally, lightly grasp the handgrips to stabilize the body during the leg curl. The action of the concentric phase of the prone leg curl is to curl the lower legs or draw the heels to the buttocks by flexing the lower legs at the knees. When curling the legs, keep the hips, stomach, and chest in contact with the bench pad. During the eccentric phase, slowly return the legs and footpad to their original position. Proper breath control is strongly recommended. Inhale during the eccentric phase of the lift and exhale during the concentric phase. The action of the prone leg curl is shown in Figure 7.22.

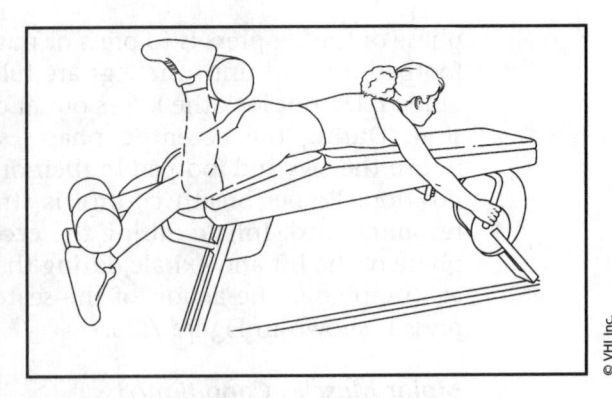

Figure 7.22 ■ Machine - Prone Leg Curl

Major Muscles Conditioned

Hamstrings (Semimembranosus, Semitendinosus, Biceps Femoris)

Seated Leg Curl

Action

Set the weight machine to the appropriate resistance. Adjust the seat back and the lower leg roller pad so the pad rests on the Achilles tendons of each leg with the legs almost fully extended. The top roller pad should be located just below the kneecap. The knees should be in line with the axis of rotation of the machine. Finally, lightly grasp the handgrips to stabilize the body during the leg curl. The action of the concentric phase of the seated leg curl is to curl the lower legs or draw the heels to the buttocks by flexing the lower legs at the knees. When curling the legs, keep the hips and back in contact with the seat and seat back, respectively. During the eccentric phase, slowly return the legs by extending the lower legs at the knees to their original position. Proper breath control is strongly recommended. Inhale during the eccentric phase of the lift and exhale during the concentric phase. The action of the seated leg curl is shown in Figure 7.23.

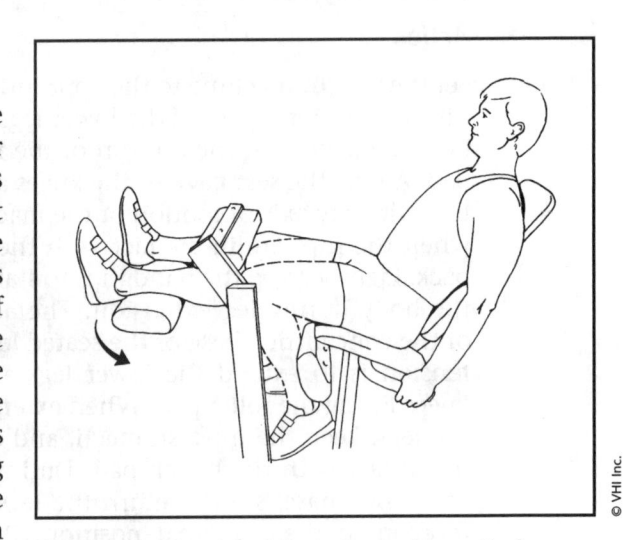

Figure 7.23 ■ Machine - Seated Leg Curl

Major Muscles Conditioned

Hamstrings (Semimembranosus, Semitendinosus, Biceps Femoris)

Upper Legs – Medial

Leg Adduction

Action

Set the weight machine to the appropriate resistance. Position yourself by sitting upright with the inside of the knees and thighs on the outside of the leg pads. Adjust the leg pads so the legs are fully abducted, in a transverse plane, out to the side. Lightly grasp the handgrips to stabilize the body during muscle contraction. The action during the concentric phase is to adduct the legs forward by drawing the knees together, using a slow controlled movement. Precaution should be taken to sit erect and to keep the back in contact with the seatback during muscle contraction. During the eccentric phase, slowly return the legs by abducting the upper legs to their original position. Proper breath control is strongly recommended. Inhale during the eccentric phase of the lift and exhale during the concentric phase. The action of the leg adduction in shown is Figure 7.24.

Major Muscles Conditioned

Adductor Magnus, Adductor Longus, Adductor Brevis

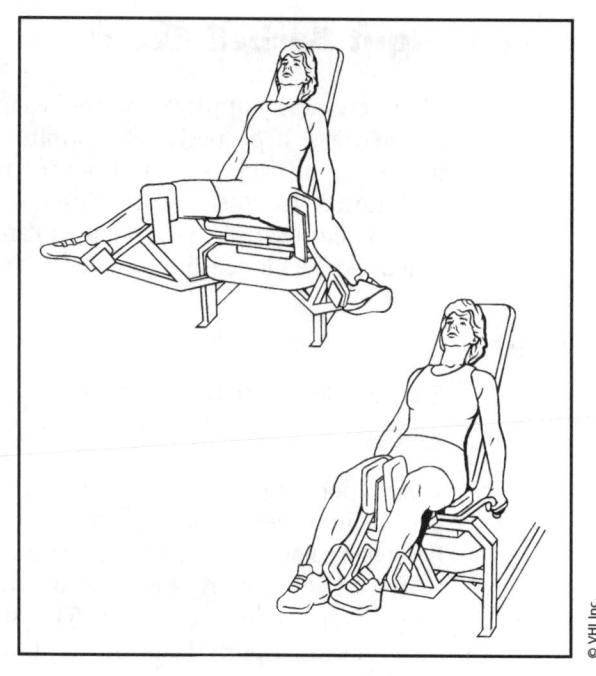

Figure 7.24 ■ Machine - Leg Adduction

Lower Legs – Posterior

Foot Plantar Flexion

Action

To exercise the posterior lower legs, you may elect to use the Leg Press weight machine or a Seated Calf machine. When using a leg press machine, set the weight machine to the appropriate resistance. Position yourself by sitting down and placing your feet perpendicular on the foot pad directly in front of the hips. The distance between the footpad and the seat is critical. Never assume a position that bends the knees greater than 90 degrees. Lightly grasp the handgrips to stabilize the body during the leg press. Press the footpad forward until the legs are fully extended. Do not lock the knees out at extension. When using a seated calf machine, position yourself by sitting down with you back and hips fully supported by the seat back. Adjust the seat so the legs are extended. Do not lock the legs out. Position your feet on the foot platform so the heels are resting on the bottom lip of the platform. To exercise the posterior lower leg, the action of the concentric phase is to press or push the footpad forward by plantar flexing (pointing the toes) the foot. During the eccentric phase, slowly return the feet to a dorsi flexed position. Proper breath control is strongly recommended. Inhale during the eccentric phase of the lift and exhale during the concentric phase. The action of foot plantar flexion using a seated calf machine is shown in Figure 7.25.

Major Muscles Conditioned

Gastrocnemius, Soleus

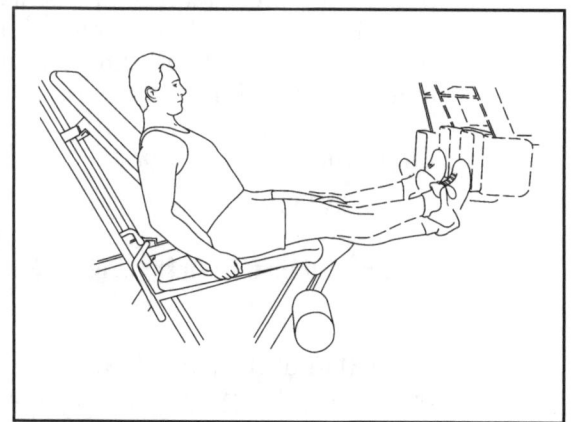

Figure 7.25 ■ Machine - Foot Plantar Flexion

Free Weight Barbell Exercises

There are many appropriate free weight barbell resistive training activities that could be recommended. If properly incorporated into a regular muscular strength and endurance training program each would allow for positive gains in both muscular strength and muscular endurance. To illustrate and describe such a large number of procedures is beyond the scope of this manuscript. As a result, examples of the more common procedures have been provided. For reader ease, procedures have been grouped by body segment.

Chest

Barbell Bench (Chest) Press

Action

When performing a barbell bench (chest) press, the subject should position himself or herself in a supine position on the inclined bench. The sacrum, head, and shoulders should all touch the bench. The subject's feet should be placed flat on the floor with the knees bent at approximately 90-degree angles. In the initial position, the barbell is grasped with a pronated grip, slightly outside the shoulders. The arms are raised and fully extended. The upper arms should be internally rotated so the elbows are positioned or pointed outward. During the downward or eccentric phase, the barbell is lowered toward the chest while keeping the wrists extended and directly above the elbow. The barbell should be lowered until the upper arms are parallel with the floor. The lower arms should continue to extend upward forming a 90-degree angle at the elbows. During the upward or concentric phase, the barbell is pressed back upward to its original position. Do not externally rotate your upper arm at the shoulder during extension or when the arm is fully extended. During the action of the arms, precaution should be taken to keep the back flat on the bench. Arching the back should be avoided. Proper breath control is strongly recommended. Inhale during the eccentric phase of the lift and exhale during the concentric phase. The action of the barbell bench (chest) press is shown in Figure 7.26.

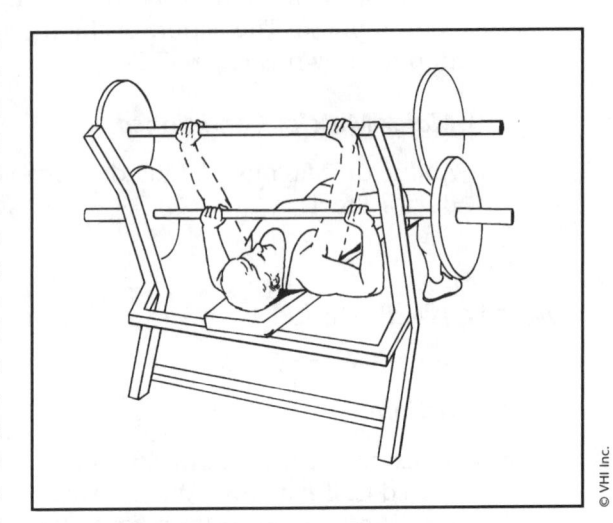

Figure 7.26 ■ Free Weight Barbell - Barbell Bench (Chest) Press

Major Muscles Conditioned

Pectoralis Major, Triceps

Barbell Incline Bench (Chest) Press

Action

The action of the barbell incline bench (chest) press is similar to the barbell bench or chest press. The primary difference is that the bench used is elevated as opposed to a standard flat bench. This change in bench position allows for a different line of action or muscular pull during movement. *In comparison, a bench press on a flat bench emphases the lower and mid-chest, whereas a bench press on an incline bench emphases the upper chest and shoulders.* When performing a barbell incline bench press, the subject should position himself or herself in a supine position on the inclined bench. The sacrum, head, and shoulders should all touch the bench. The subject's feet should be placed flat on the floor or the bench footpad with the knees bent at approximately 90-degree angles. In the initial position, the barbell is grasped with the hands facing outward, slightly outside the shoulders. The arms are raised and fully extended. The upper arms should be internally rotated so the elbows are positioned or pointed outward. During the downward or eccentric phase, the barbell is lowered toward the chests while keeping the wrists extended and directly above the elbow. The barbell should be lowered until the upper arms are parallel with the floor. The lower arms should continue to extend upward forming a 90-degree angle at the elbows. During the upward or concentric phase, the barbell is pressed back upward to its original position. Do not internally rotate your upper arm at the shoulder during the lift or when the arm is fully extended. During the action of the arms, precaution should be taken to keep the back flat on the bench. Arching of the back should be avoided. Proper breath control is strongly recommended. Inhale during the eccentric phase of the lift and exhale during the concentric phase. The action of the barbell incline bench (chest) press is shown in Figure 7.27.

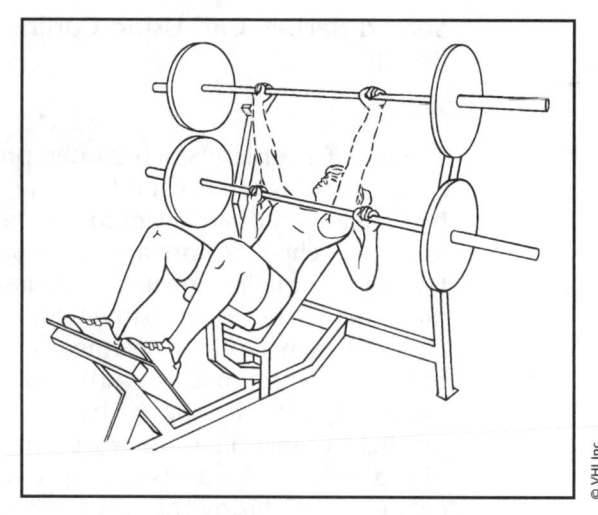

Figure 7.27 ■ Free Weight Barbell - Barbell Incline Bench (Chest) Press

Major Muscles Conditioned

Pectoralis Major, Triceps

Upper Arms – Anterior

Standing Barbell Curl

Action

The standing barbell curl can be performed with a flat bar or a "curling bar." A curling bar is a specifically shaped bar that allows for slight pronation at the wrist. This particular position helps to isolate specific musculature used during the curl and to reduce stress on the wrists. To perform the standing barbell curl, prepare the selected barbell to the appropriate resistance. Grasp the barbell with a closed, supinated grip. While holding the barbell, the arms should be fully extended. The barbell should be resting comfortably on the thigh. The concentric phase of the standing barbell curl is to flex the lower arms at the elbows while keeping the upper arms fixed against the sides. Precaution should be taken to keep the body erect and avoid leaning backward, particularly when the lower arms are moving through the 90-degree angle. During the downward or eccentric phase, extend the lower arms at the elbows back to their original position. Proper breath control is strongly recommended. Inhale during the eccentric phase of the lift and exhale during the concentric phase. The action of the standing barbell curl is shown in Figure 7.28.

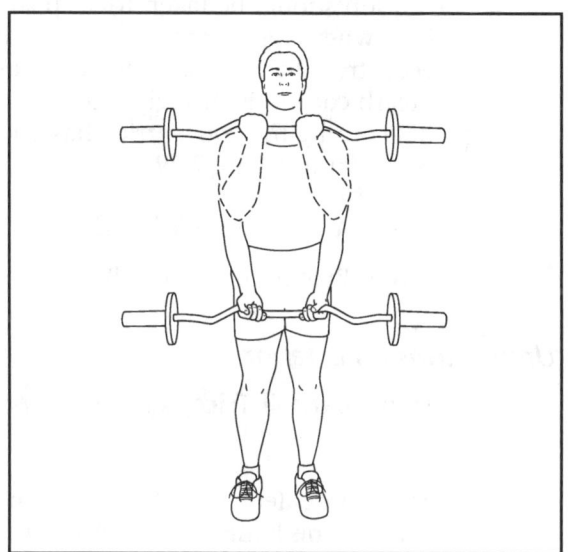

Figure 7.28 ■ Free Weight Barbell - Standing Barbell Curl

Major Muscles Conditioned

Biceps Brachii, Brachialis, Brachioradialis

Seated Barbell Curl Using Curling Bench

Action

The use of a curling bench is often preferred because of the stability it offers. The curling bench allows the participant to rest the upper arms and chest against a padded support, thereby eliminating any upper arm and body movement. The seated barbell curl using a curling bench can be performed with a flat bar or a "curling bar." A curling or angled bar is a specifically shaped bar that allows for slight pronation at the wrist. This particular position helps to isolate specific musculature used during the curl and to reduce stress on the wrist. To perform the seated barbell curl using a curling bench, prepare the barbell to the appropriate resistance. Adjust the support pad height so the arms can extend comfortably over the top of the support with the chest resting against the pad.

Figure 7.29 ■ Free Weight Barbell - Seated Barbell Curl Using Curling Bench

A spotter may be used to hand the barbell to the seated participant. Grasp the barbell with a closed, supinated grip. While holding the barbell, lean forward and rest the chest on the support pad, fully extending the arms over the top of the bench support. The upper arm (triceps) should be resting on the pad. The concentric phase of the seated barbell curl is to flex the lower arms at the elbows while keeping the upper arms fixed against the support pad. Precaution should be taken to keep the upper body still and fixed against the support, particularly when the lower arms are moving through the 90-degree angle. During the downward or eccentric phase, extend the lower arms at the elbows back to their original position. Proper breath control is strongly recommended. Inhale during the eccentric phase of the lift and exhale during the concentric phase. The action of the seated barbell curl using a curling bench is shown in Figure 7.29.

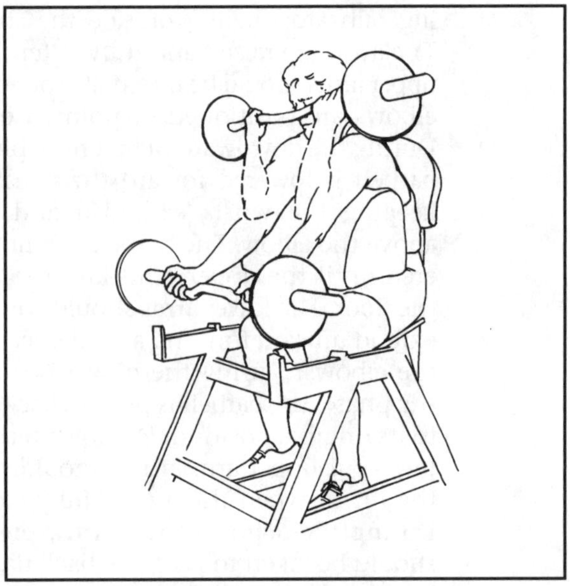

Major Muscles Conditioned

Biceps Brachii, Brachialis, Brachioradialis

Upper Arms – Posterior

Lying Barbell Triceps Extension

Action

To ensure safety, as well as assist in positioning the barbell, a spotter is required to properly execute the lying barbell triceps extension. To perform the lying barbell triceps extension, prepare the barbell to the appropriate resistance. To prevent unnecessary stress at the wrist, the use of an angled bar may be warranted. Assume a supine position on a flat bench with the head, shoulders, back, and hips resting on the bench. The feet should be placed flat on the floor with the knees bent at approximately 90-degree angles. Grasp the bar directly over the chest with a narrow, pronated grip. The arms should be fully extended. A spotter may assist in positioning the bar. The eccentric phase is the first action. To perform the eccentric phase, flex the arms at the elbows and lower the bar toward the face. The elbows should remain elevated above the chest, perpendicular to the floor, and be pointed toward the feet. Precaution should be taken to prevent the elbows from turning out to the sides. During the concentric phase, the bar is returned to its original position. Proper breath control is strongly recommended. Inhale during the eccentric phase of the lift and exhale during the concentric phase. The action of the lying barbell triceps extension is shown in Figure 7.30.

Major Muscles Conditioned

Triceps Brachii

Sitting Triceps Extension

Action

The sitting triceps extension is also referred to as a French press. To ensure safety, as well as assist in positioning the barbell, a spotter is required to properly execute the sitting triceps extension. To perform the sitting triceps extension, select a barbell of appropriate resistance and assume a sitting position, on a flat bench, with both feet flat on the floor. Grasp the end of the barbell, directly behind the head. The arms should be flexed at the elbow while keeping the upper arms extended overhead, directly over the shoulders. The concentric phase is the first action. During the concentric phase, lift the barbell overhead by extending the lower arms at the elbows. Precaution should be taken to keep the upper arms stable. Additionally, care should be taken to keep the upper body erect and avoid leaning backward particularly when lowering the arms. To perform the eccentric phase, slowly lower the barbell back to its original position by flexing the elbows until the hands are directly behind the head. Proper breath control is strongly recommended. Inhale during the eccentric phase of the lift and exhale during the concentric phase. The action of the sitting triceps extension is shown in Figure 7.31.

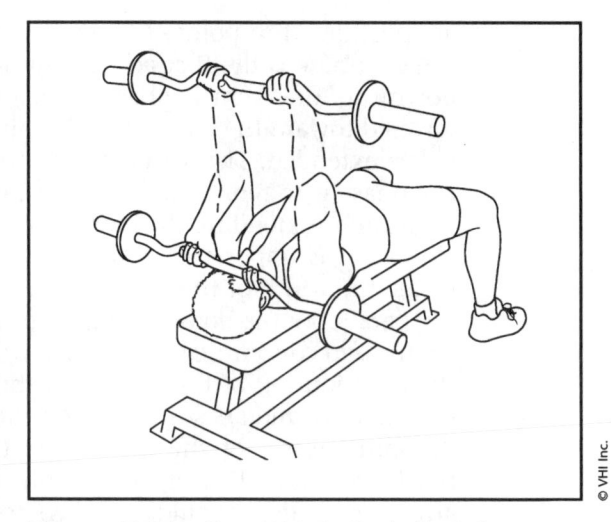

Figure 7.30 ■ Free Weight Barbell - Lying Barbell Triceps Extension

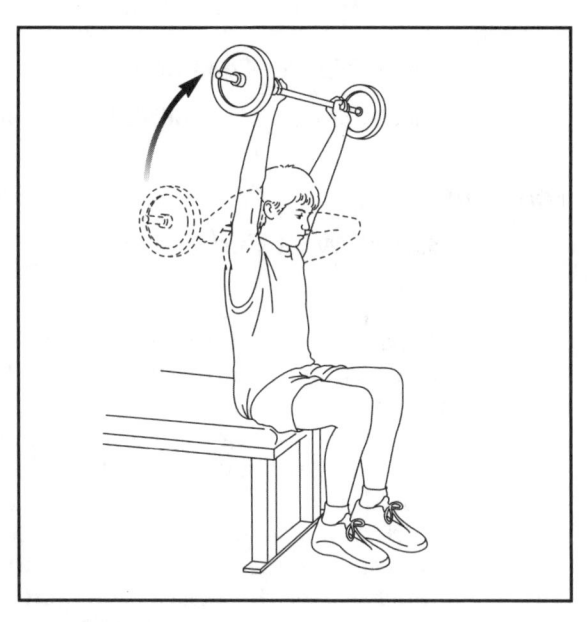

Figure 7.31 ■ Free Weight Barbell - Sitting Triceps Extension

Major Muscles Conditioned

Triceps Brachii

Lying Closed Grip Bench Press

Action

The lying closed grip bench press is performed similar to a bench press. As a result, the muscles of the chest and shoulder are also conditioned. Because of the extremely narrowed grip, however, the lying closed grip bench press offers excellent conditioning to the triceps brachii musculature. Typically, an angled bar is the preferred bar when performing the lying closed grip bench press. This is because its shape helps to reduce stress on the wrist during movement. To perform the lying closed grip bench press, prepare a barbell to the appropriate resistance. Assume a supine position on a flat bench. The head, shoulders, back and hips should be in contact with the bench. The feet should be placed flat on the floor with the knees bent at approximately 90-degree angles. In the initial position, the barbell is grasped with a narrow, pronated grip. The distance between the hands should be no greater than a few inches. The arms are raised and fully extend. The upper arms should be internally rotated so the elbows are positioned or pointed outward. The eccentric phase is the first action. During the downward or eccentric phase, the barbell is lowered toward the chest while keeping the wrists extended. The action of the concentric phase is to return the bar to its original position by extending the lower arms at the elbows. It is important to keep the elbows inside the width of the shoulders and moving parallel to the body during both the eccentric and concentric phases. This will limit the contribution of the chest and shoulder musculature and assist in focusing the conditioning aspect of the lift on the triceps brachii muscles. During the action of the arms, precaution should be taken to keep the back flat on the bench. Arching the back should be avoided. Proper breath control is strongly recommended. Inhale during the eccentric phase of the lift and exhale during the concentric phase. The action of the lying closed grip bench press is shown in Figure 7.32.

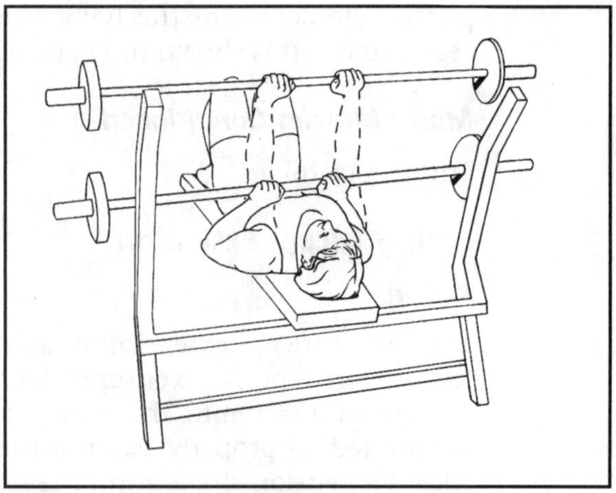

Figure 7.32 ■ Free Weight Barbell - Lying Closed Grip Bench Press

Major Muscles Conditioned

Triceps Brachii, Pectoralis Major, Deltoid (anterior)

Forearms

Barbell Wrist Curl

Action

Prepare the barbell to the appropriate resistance. Assume a sitting position on the end of a flat bench. Position the feet and legs directly in front of the hips. Grasp the barbell, with a supinated grip. Hand placement should be approximately shoulder width apart. While holding the barbell, lean forward and rest the forearms and elbows on the upper legs so the wrists are hyperextended just beyond the knees. Open the supinated grip slightly so the fingers hold the barbell. The concentric phase of the barbell wrist curl is to lift the barbell by flexing the fingers and the wrist. Precaution should be taken to keep the forearms and elbows in contact with the thigh when curling the barbell. During the downward or eccentric phase, extend the wrist so the barbell returns to its original position. Proper breath control is strongly recommended. Inhale during the eccentric phase of the lift and exhale during the concentric phase. The action of the barbell wrist curl is shown in Figure 7.33.

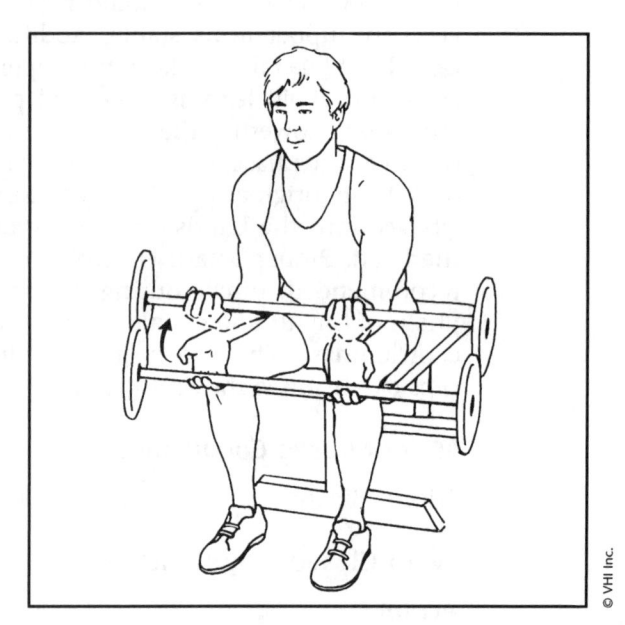

Figure 7.33 ■ Free Weight Barbell - Barbell Wrist Curl

Major Muscles Conditioned

Flexor Carpi Radialis, Flexor Carpi Ulnaris

Barbell Wrist Extensions

Action

Prepare the barbell to the appropriate resistance. Assume a sitting position on the end of a flat bench. Position the feet and legs directly in front of the hips. Grasp the barbell, with a pronated grip. Hand placement should be approximately shoulder width apart. While holding the barbell, lean forward and rest the forearms and elbows, on the upper legs, so the wrists are flexed just beyond the knees. The concentric phase of the barbell wrist extension is to lift the barbell by extending the wrist. Precaution should be taken to keep the forearms and elbows in contact with the thigh when extending the wrist. During the downward or eccentric phase, flex the wrist so the barbell returns to its original position. Proper breath control is strongly recommended. Inhale during the eccentric phase of the lift and exhale during the concentric phase. The action of the barbell wrist extension is shown in Figure 7.34.

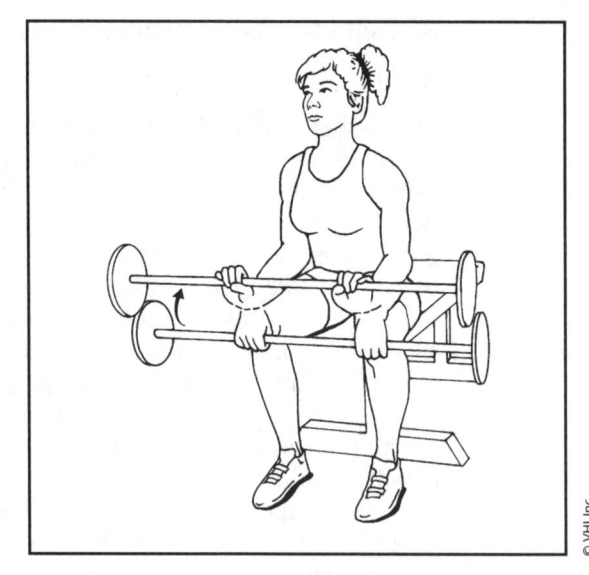

Figure 7.34 ■ Free Weight Barbell - Barbell Wrist Extension

Major Muscles Conditioned

Extensor Carpi Radialis, Extensor Carpi Ulnaris

Shoulders

Overhead Barbell Press

Action

The overhead barbell press requires the use of a vertical shoulder press bench. Additionally, a spotter may be required to assist in moving the barbell off the bench supports. Prepare the barbell to the appropriate resistance. Assume a sitting position on the vertical shoulder press bench. Precaution should be taken to keep the back, shoulders, head, and hips in contact with the seat back. Lightly grasp the barbell using a pronated grip. Handgrip width should be slightly larger than shoulder width. Unrack the barbell and position the barbell directly overhead with the arms fully extended. Do not lock the elbows out during extension. The wrists should be fixed and extended above the elbows. The first action of the overhead barbell press is the eccentric phase. The downward or eccentric phase requires the elbows to be flexed, lowering the barbell toward the chest. Stop the downward movement when the barbell is even with the clavicles. During the upward or concentric phase, return the barbell directly overhead by pressing the barbell upward to a point where the arms are fully extended. Again, do not lock the elbows out during extension. During both the concentric and eccentric phases, the head and neck will have to be tilted slightly backward, in order to allow the barbell to pass in front of the face. Proper breath control is strongly recommended. Inhale during the eccentric phase of the lift and exhale during the concentric phase. The action of the overhead barbell press is shown in Figure 7.35.

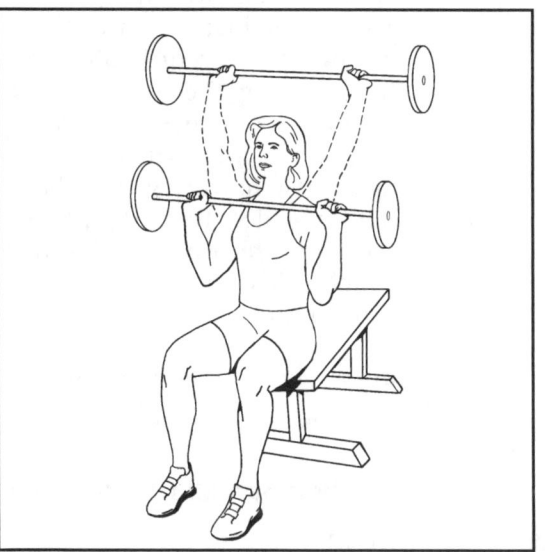

Figure 7.35 ■ Free Weight Barbell - Overhead Barbell Press

Major Muscles Conditioned

Deltoid (anterior, medial)

Barbell Inclined Overhead Press

Action

The barbell inclined overhead press is similar to the overhead barbell press. The primary difference is that the use of the inclined bench allows for different musculature to be emphasized during lifting activity. *The higher the incline, the more emphasis placed on the shoulder musculature. Lower inclines place greater emphasis on chest musculature.* To perform the barbell inclined overhead press, prepare the barbell to the appropriate resistance. Assume a sitting position on an inclined bench. The bench should be set at a high incline. Precaution should be taken to keep the back, shoulders, head, and hips in contact with the seat back. Grasp the barbell using a pronated grip. Handgrip width should be slightly larger than shoulder width. Unrack the barbell and position the barbell directly overhead with the arms fully extended. Do not lock the elbows out when assuming this position. The wrists should be fixed and extended above the elbows. The first action of the barbell inclined overhead press is the eccentric phase. The downward or eccentric phase requires the elbows to be flexed, lowering the barbell toward the chest. Stop the downward movement when the barbell is even with the clavicles. During the upward or concentric phase, return the barbell directly overhead by pressing the barbell upward to a point where the arms are fully extended. Again, do not lock the elbows out during extension. During both the concentric and eccentric phases, the head and neck will have to be extended, tilted slightly backward, in order to allow the barbell to pass in front of the face. Proper breath control is strongly recommended. Inhale during the eccentric phase of the lift and exhale during the concentric phase. The action of the barbell inclined overhead press is shown in Figure 7.36.

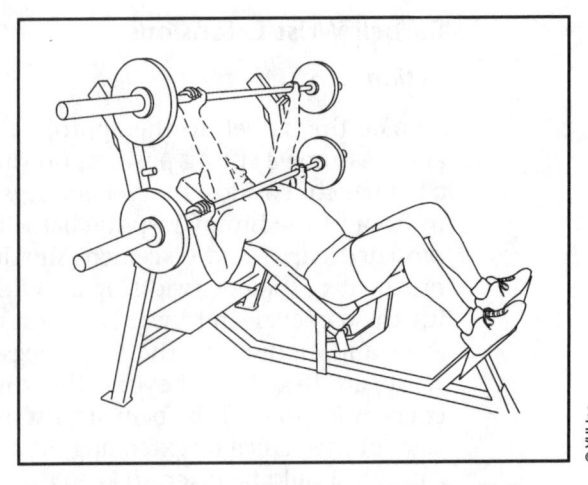

Figure 7.36 ■ Free Weight Barbell - Barbell Inclined Overhead Press

Major Muscles Conditioned

Pectoralis Major, Deltoid (anterior), Triceps

Standing Barbell Upright Row

Action

Prepare the barbell to the appropriate resistance. Grasp the barbell with a pronated grip. Hand placement or grip width should be inside the shoulders. Assume a standing position and allow the barbell to rest comfortably on the thigh. In order to provide a more stable stance, position the feet slightly outside the shoulders and turn the toes slightly out. During the concentric or upward phase, pull or lift the barbell directly upward against the abdomen and chest toward the chin until the barbell is approximately on the level with the clavicles. During the lifting motion, keep the elbows high. Precaution should be taken to keep the back straight and the head up during the lifting motion. During the downward or eccentric phase, extend the elbows and adduct the upper arms toward the side, lowering the barbell back to its original position. Proper breath control is strongly recommended. Inhale during the eccentric phase of the lift and exhale during the concentric phase. The action of the standing barbell upright row is shown in Figure 7.37.

Major Muscles Conditioned

Deltoids (anterior, middle, Posterior), Trapezius (upper)

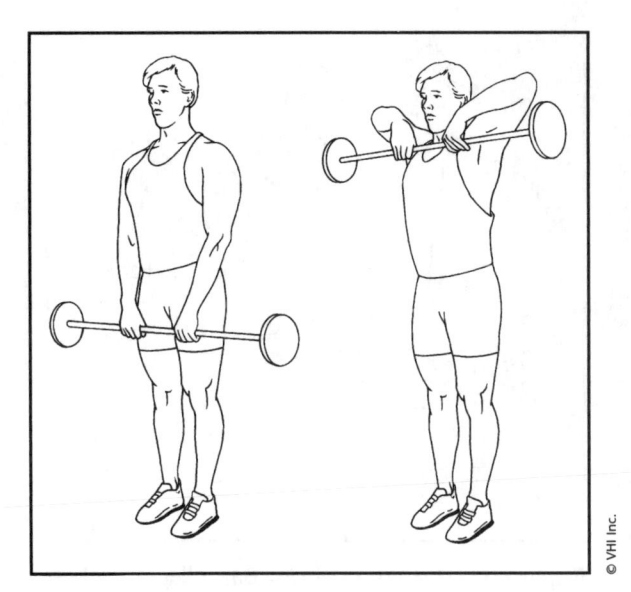

Figure 7.37 ■ Free Weight Barbell - Standing Barbell Upright Row

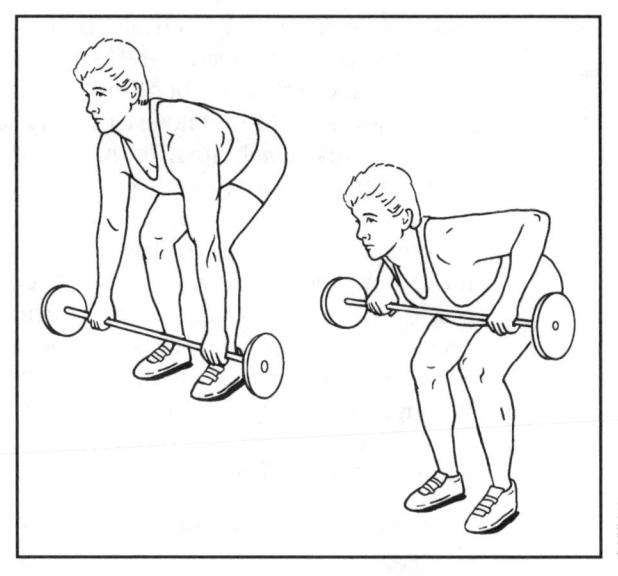

Figure 7.38 ■ Free Weight Barbell - Barbell Bent Over Row

Upper Back

Barbell Bent Over Row

Action

Prepare the barbell to the appropriate resistance. Assume a standing position so the bar is almost touching the anterior aspect (chins) of the lower leg. The feet should be placed approximately shoulder width apart with the toes turned slightly outward. Squat down keeping the hips slightly lower than the shoulders and grasp the bar with a wide, pronated grip. Grip width should be outside the shoulders. Precaution should be taken to keep the back flat and the head up with the eyes focused ahead. Do not tuck the head and look downward. Keeping the back flat, lift the bar slightly off the floor by slightly extending the hips and knees. Do not stand erect. The arms should remain extended and hang straight down. The concentric phase of the barbell bent over row is to pull the barbell up toward the lower chest and upper abdominal area of the trunk. Keep the elbows high during this movement. The back should continue to remain flat with little or no movement occurring outside of the area of the shoulder and shoulder girdle. During the downward or eccentric phase, slowly extend the arms, at the elbows, and allow the shoulders to flex until the arms are fully extended below the shoulders. Proper breath control is strongly recommended. Inhale during the eccentric phase of the lift and exhale during the concentric phase. The action of the barbell bent over row is shown in Figure 7.38.

Major Muscles Conditioned

Latissimus Dorsi, Teres Major, Trapezius (middle), Rhomboids

Barbell Pull-Over

Action

To perform the barbell pull-over, prepare a barbell to the appropriate resistance. Assume a supine position on a flat bench with the head, shoulders, back, and hips resting on the bench. The feet should be placed flat on the floor with the knees bent to approximately 90-degree angles. Grasp the barbell with a pronated grip with the hands approximately shoulder width apart. In the original position the barbell is rested on the chest. The first action of the barbell pull-over is the eccentric phase. During the eccentric phase, lift the bar off the chest and move it over the face. When the arms are extended over the head, carefully lower the bar toward the floor by bending the elbows. Precaution should be taken to slowly lower the bar. This will help in controlling how far the musculature is stretched. During the concentric phase, the barbell is pulled back up and over the face until it is returned to its original position. Proper breath control is strongly recommended. Inhale during the eccentric phase of the lift and exhale during the concentric phase. The action of the barbell pull-over is shown in Figure 7.39.

Major Muscles Conditioned

Latissimus Dorsi, Deltoid (posterior), Triceps

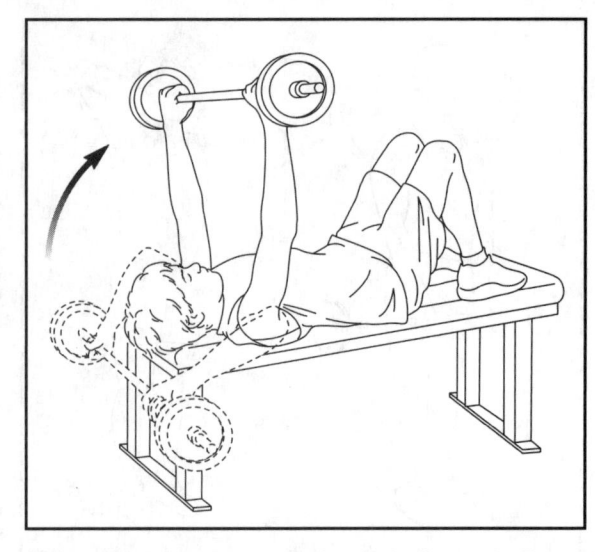

Figure 7.39 ■ Free Weight Barbell - Barbell Pull-Over

Lower Legs – Posterior

Standing Barbell Heel Raise

Action

To perform the standing barbell heel raise, prepare a barbell with the appropriate resistance and place it approximately shoulder height on a rack. Step under the bar and grasp it with a pronated grip. Grip width should be outside of the shoulders. Facing away from the bar, position yourself so the bar rests across the shoulders, neck, and upper back (posterior deltoids and trapezius) musculature. Assuming a standing position, place the toes and balls of the foot on an elevated platform or board. Platform height should not exceed more than a couple of inches. The heels of the foot should rest comfortably on the ground when the toes are elevated. Unrack the bar by lifting up and allow it to rest on the shoulders, back, and neck musculature. Use the hands to stabilize the bar. The concentric phase of the standing barbell heel raise is the first action. During the concentric phase, plantar flex the toes and lift the heels off the ground. To complete the eccentric phase, return the heels back to the ground. Proper breath control is strongly recommended. Inhale during the eccentric phase of the lift and exhale during the concentric phase. The action of the standing barbell heel raise is shown in Figure 7.40.

Major Muscles Conditioned

Soleus, Gastrocnemius

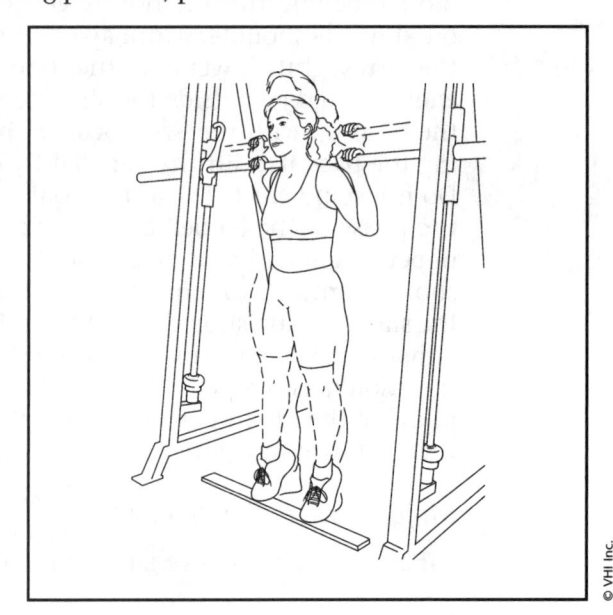

Figure 7.40 ■ Free Weight Barbell - Standing Barbell Heel Raise

Free Weight Dumbbell Exercises

There are many appropriate free weight dumbbell resistive training activities that could be recommended. If properly incorporated into a regular muscular strength and endurance training program, each would allow for positive gains in both muscular strength and muscular endurance. To illustrate and describe such a large number of procedures is beyond the scope of this manuscript. As a result, examples of the more common procedures have been provided. For reader ease, procedures have been grouped by body segment.

Chest

Dumbbell Fly

Action

Dumbbell fly, dumbbell bench or chest press, and dumbbell chest adduction are terms used to describe the same lift. The action for this activity is described under dumbbell bench (chest) press. The action of the dumbbell fly is shown in Figure 7.41.

Major Muscles Conditioned

Pectoralis Major, Triceps

Dumbbell Chest Adduction

Action

Dumbbell fly, dumbbell bench or chest press, and dumbbell chest adduction are terms used to describe the same lift. The action for this activity is described under dumbbell bench (chest) press. The action of the dumbbell chest adduction is shown in Figure 7.41.

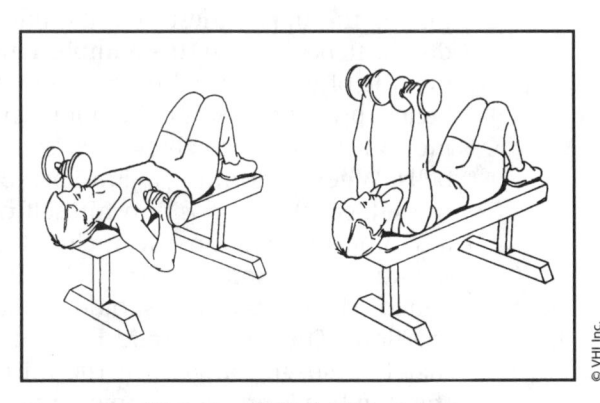

Figure 7.41 ■ Free Weight Dumbbell - Dumbbell Fly, Chest Adduction, Bench (Chest) Press

Major Muscles Conditioned

Pectoralis Major, Triceps

Dumbbell Bench (Chest) Press

Action

The action of the dumbbell bench (chest) press is similar to all bench press variations. The dumbbell bench press, however, is often a preferred activity when compared to a barbell bench press, because of the additional range of motion that can be achieved when using dumbbells. When performing a dumbbell bench press, the subject should position himself or herself in a supine position on a standard bench. The sacrum, head, and shoulders should touch the bench. The subject's feet should be placed flat on the floor. The knees should be bent at approximately 90-degree angles. In the initial position, the dumbbells are raised upward with the arms fully extended. Do not lock the elbows out during extension. The arms should be externally rotated so the elbows are positioned or pointed outward. During the downward or eccentric phase, the dumbbells are lowered toward the chest while keeping the wrists extended and directly above the elbows. The dumbbells should be lowered until the upper arms are at least parallel with the floor. The lower arms should continue to extend upward forming a 90-degree angle at the elbows. During the upward phase or concentric phase, the dumbbells are pressed back upward to their original position. Do not externally rotate your upper arm at the shoulder during the lift or when the arm is fully extended. During the action of the arms, precaution should be taken to keep the back flat on the bench. Arching of the back should be avoided. Proper breath control is strongly recommended. Inhale during the eccentric phase of the lift and exhale during the concentric phase. The action of the dumbbell bench (chest) press is shown in Figure 7.41.

Major Muscles Conditioned

Pectoralis Major, Triceps

Dumbbell Incline Bench (Chest) Press

Action

The action of the dumbbell incline bench press is similar to the dumbbell bench press. The primary difference is that the bench used is elevated as opposed to a standard flat bench. This change in bench position allows for a different line of action or muscular pull during movement. In comparison, a dumbbell bench press on a flat bench emphases the lower and mid-chest, whereas a dumbbell bench press on an incline bench emphases the upper chest and shoulders. Like the dumbbell bench press, the dumbbell incline bench press is often preferred over an inclined barbell bench press because of the additional range of motion that can be achieved when using dumbbells. When performing a dumbbell bench press, the subject should position himself or herself in a supine position on the inclined bench. The sacrum, head, and shoulders should touch the bench. The subject's feet should be placed flat on the floor. The knees should be bent at approximately 90-degree angles. In the initial position, the dumbbells are raised upward with the arms fully extended. Do not lock the elbows out during extension. The arms should be externally rotated so the elbows are positioned or pointed outward. During the downward or eccentric phase, the dumbbells are lowered toward the chests while keeping the wrists extended and directly above the elbow. The dumbbells should be lowered until the upper arms are at least parallel with the floor. The lower arms should continue to extend upward forming a 90-degree angle at the elbows. During the upward or concentric phase, the dumbbells are pressed back upward to their original position. Do not externally rotate your upper arm at the shoulder during the lift or when the arm is fully extended. During the action of the arms, precaution should be taken to keep the back flat on the bench. Arching of the back should be avoided. Proper breath control is strongly recommended. Inhale during the eccentric phase of the lift and exhale during the concentric phase. The action of the dumbbell incline bench (chest) press is shown in Figure 7.42.

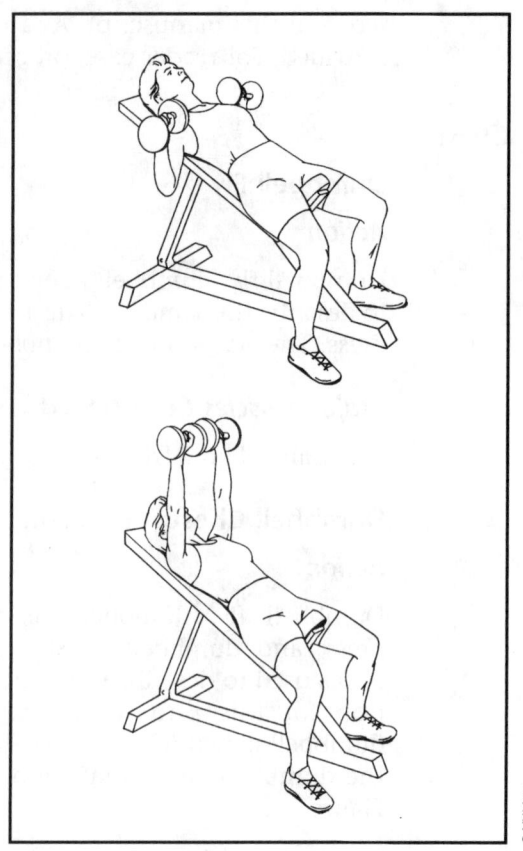

Figure 7.42 ■ Free Weight Dumbbell - Dumbbell Incline Bench (Chest) Press

Major Muscles Conditioned

Pectoralis Major, Triceps

Upper Arms – Anterior

Standing Dumbbell Curl

Action

Because dumbbells offer greater range of motion, they are often preferred when compared to the standing barbell curl. The greater range of motion is particularly helpful in reducing stress that occurs at the wrist when using a flat bar. Select the dumbbells of the appropriate resistance. Grasp and position each dumbbell with a closed, supinated grip. While holding the dumbbells, the fully extended arms should be externally rotated and rested against the sides of the trunk. The dumbbells should be resting comfortably in contact with the thighs. The concentric phase of the standing dumbbell curl is to flex the lower arms at the elbows while keeping the upper arms fixed against the sides. Precaution should be taken to keep the body erect and avoid leaning backward, particularly when the lower arms are moving through the 90-degree angle. During the downward or eccentric phase, extend the lower arms at the elbows back to their original position. It should be noted that alternating arm movements is a viable option. When working arms individually, it is important to maintain an erect posture and keep the active arm fixed at the side during movement. Proper breath control is strongly recommended. Inhale during the eccentric phase of the lift and exhale during the concentric phase. The action of the standing dumbbell curl is shown in Figure 7.43.

Major Muscles Conditioned

Biceps Brachii, Brachialis, Brachioradialis

Figure 7.43 ■ Free Weight Dumbbell - Standing Dumbbell Curl

Standing Hammer Curl

Action

Select the dumbbells of the appropriate resistance. Grasp each dumbbell with a closed grip. While holding the dumbbells, the arms should be fully extended. The lower arms should be pronated so the hands are positioned in a neutral grip position or with the palms of the hands facing inward toward the thighs. The dumbbells should rest comfortably in contact with the thighs. The concentric phase of the standing hammer curl is to flex the lower arms at the elbows while keeping the upper arms fixed against the sides. Precaution should be taken to keep the body erect and avoid leaning backward, particularly when the lower arms are moving through the 90-degree angle. During the downward or eccentric phase, extend the lower arms at the elbows back to their original position. It should be noted that alternating arm movements is a viable option. When working arms individually, it is important to maintain an erect posture and keep the active arm fixed at the side during movement. Proper breath control is strongly recommended. Inhale during the eccentric phase of the lift and exhale during the concentric phase. The action of the standing hammer curl is shown in Figure 7.44.

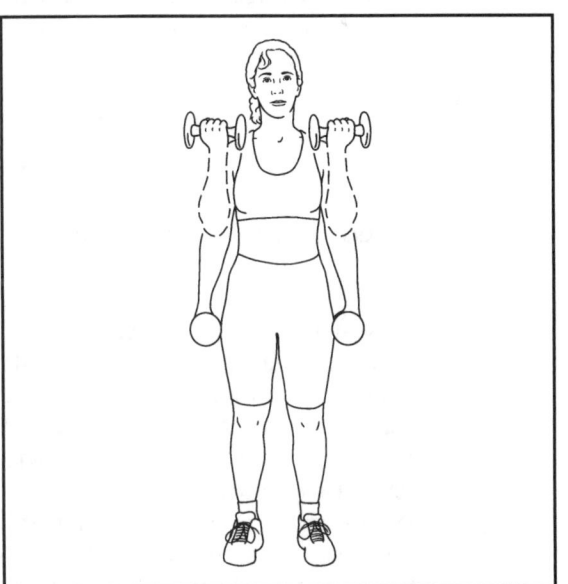

Figure 7.44 ■ Free Weight Dumbbell - Standing Hammer Curl

Major Muscles Conditioned

Biceps Brachii, Brachialis, Brachioradialis

Seated Dumbbell Curl

Action

The seated dumbbell curl is often preferred over standing curls using either the barbell or dumbbells. This is because sitting on a bench helps to eliminate the tendency to lean backward; a behavior that frequently occurs with standing activities. Additionally, because dumbbells offer greater range of motion, they are often preferred over barbell activities. In curling activities, the greater range of motion is particularly helpful in reducing stress occurring at the wrist, associated with curling a flat bar. To perform the seated dumbbell curl, select the dumbbells of the appropriate resistance. Grasp and position each dumbbell with a closed, supinated grip. While holding the dumbbells, the fully extended arms should be externally rotated and hanging straight down off the sides of the bench. The concentric phase of the seated dumbbell curl is to flex the lower arms at the elbows while keeping the upper arms fixed against the sides. Precaution should be taken to keep the upper body erect and avoid leaning backward, particularly when the lower arms are moving through the 90-degree angle. During the downward or eccentric phase, extend the lower arms at the elbows back to their original position. It should be noted that alternating arm movements is a viable option. When working arms individually, it is important to maintain an erect posture and keep the active arm fixed at the side during movement. Proper breath control is strongly recommended. Inhale during the eccentric phase of the lift and exhale during the concentric phase. The action of the seated dumbbell curl is shown in Figure 7.45.

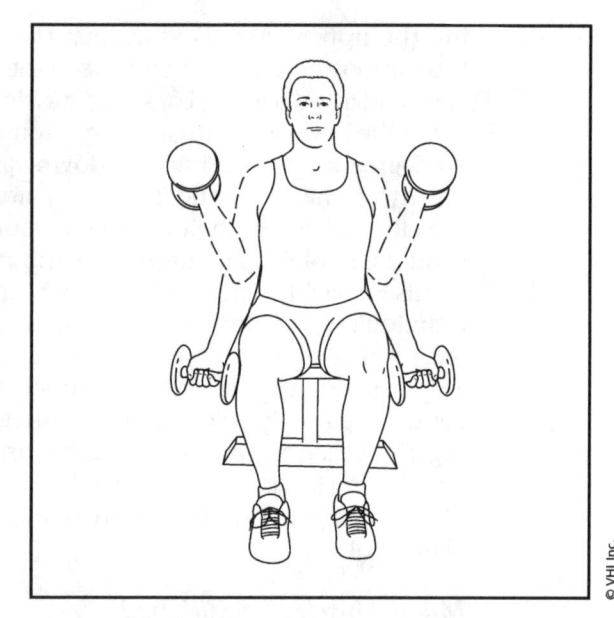

Figure 7.45 ■ Free Weight Dumbbell - Seated Dumbbell Curl

Major Muscles Conditioned

Biceps Brachii, Brachialis, Brachioradialis

Seated Thigh Dumbbell Curl

Action

The seated thigh dumbbell curl is similar to the seated dumbbell curl in that it is often preferred over standing curls using either the barbell or dumbbells. This is because sitting on a bench helps to eliminate the tendency to lean back. Additionally, because dumbbells offer greater range of motion, they are often preferred over barbell activities. In curling activities, the greater range of motion is particularly helpful in reducing stress occurring at the wrist, associated with curling a flat bar. The action of the seated thigh dumbbell curl is similar to the seated dumbbell curl other than it utilizes the inside of the thigh to stabilize the upper arm. This position offers almost as much control as found when using a curling bench. Because of this unique position, only one arm can be active. To perform the seated dumbbell curl, select the dumbbell of the appropriate resistance. Grasp and position the dumbbell with a closed, supinated grip. While holding the dumbbell, the fully extended arm should be externally rotated and hanging straight down between your legs. Lean forward so the posterior aspect of the upper arm is resting against the inside of the thigh. The concentric phase of the seated dumbbell curl is to flex the lower arms at the elbows while keeping the upper arm fixed against the inside of the leg. Precaution should be taken to keep the body still during the lifting movement, particularly when the lower arm is moving through the 90-degree angle. During the downward or eccentric phase, extend the lower arm at the elbow back to its original position. Proper breath control is strongly recommended. Inhale during the eccentric phase of the lift and exhale during the concentric phase. The action of the seated thigh dumbbell curl is shown in Figure 7.46.

Major Muscles Conditioned

Biceps Brachii, Brachialis, Brachioradialis

Seated Dumbbell Curl Using Curling Bench

Action

The use of a curling bench is often preferred because of the stability it offers. The curling bench allows the participant to rest the upper arms and chest against a padded support thereby eliminating any upper arm and body movement. Like all the seated curling activities, the seated dumbbell curl using a curling bench is often preferred over standing curls using either the barbell or dumbbells. Additionally, because dumbbells offer greater range of motion, they are often preferred over barbell activities. In curling activities, the greater range of motion is particularly helpful in reducing stress occurring at the wrist, associated with curling a flat bar. To perform the seated dumbbell curl using a curling bench, select the dumbbells of the appropriate resistance. Adjust the support pad height so the arms can extend comfortably over the top of the support with the chest resting against the pad. Grasp and position each dumbbell with a closed, supinated grip. While holding the dumbbells, lean forward and rest the chest on the support pad, fully extending the arms over the top of the bench support. The concentric phase of the seated dumbbell curl is to flex the lower arms at the elbows while keeping the upper arms fixed against the support pad. Precaution should be taken to keep the upper body still and fixed against the support, particularly when the lower arms are moving through the 90-degree angle. During the downward or eccentric phase, extend the lower arms at the elbows back to their original position. It should be noted that alternating arm movements is a viable option. When working arms individually, it is important to maintain correct posture and minimize any movement other than that occurring in the active arm. Proper breath control is strongly recommended. Inhale during the eccentric phase of the lift and exhale during the concentric phase. The action of the seated dumbbell curl using a curling bench is shown in Figure 7.47.

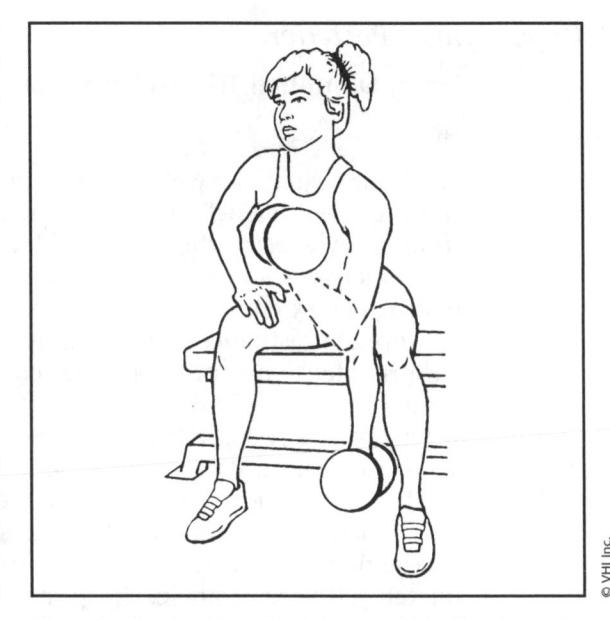

Figure 7.46 ■ Free Weight Dumbbell - Seated Thigh Dumbbell Curl

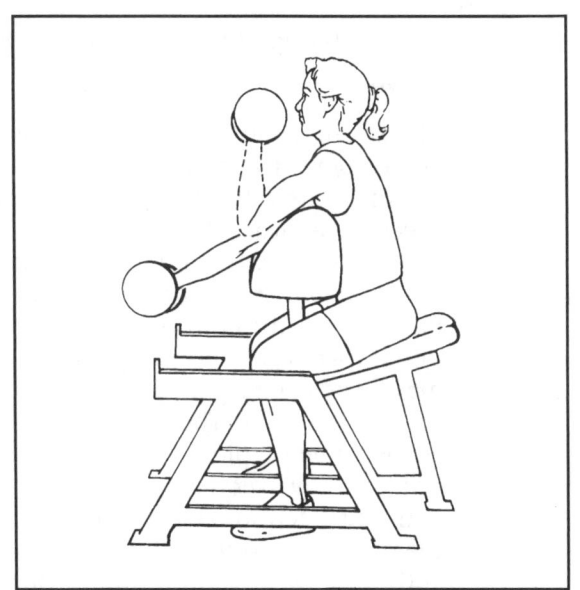

Figure 7.47 ■ Free Weight Dumbbell - Seated Dumbbell Curl Using Curling Bench

Major Muscles Conditioned

Biceps Brachii, Brachialis, Brachioradialis

Upper Arms – Posterior

Lying Dumbbell Triceps Extension

Action

To ensure safety, as well as assist in positioning the dumbbell, a spotter is required to properly execute the lying dumbbell triceps extension. To perform the lying dumbbell triceps extension, select a dumbbell of appropriate resistance. The lying dumbbell triceps extension is often a preferred activity over the lying barbell triceps extension when only a straight bar is available. Assume a supine position on a flat bench with the head, shoulders, back, and hips resting on the bench. The feet should be placed flat on the floor with the knees bent to approximately a 90-degree angle. Grasp the end of the dumbbell, directly over the chest. The

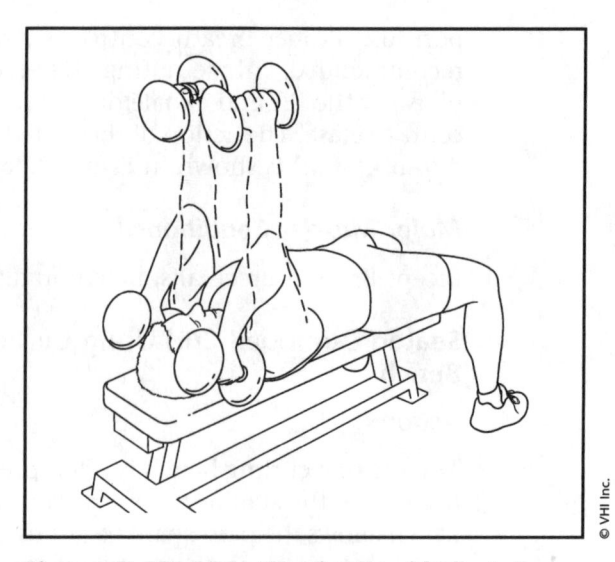

Figure 7.48 ■ Free Weight Dumbbell - Lying Dumbbell Triceps Extension

arms should be fully extended. A spotter may assist in positioning the dumbbell. The eccentric phase is the first action. To perform the eccentric phase, flex the arms at the elbows and lower the dumbbell toward the face. Because the dumbbell is held on end, the length of the dumbbell will require the dumbbell to be lowered to the side of the face. The elbows should remain elevated above the chest, perpendicular to the floor, and be pointed toward the feet. Precaution should be taken to prevent the elbows from turning out to the sides. During the concentric phase, the dumbbell is returned to its original position. Proper breath control is strongly recommended. Inhale during the eccentric phase of the lift and exhale during the concentric phase. The action of the lying dumbbell triceps extension is shown in 7.48.

Major Muscles Conditioned

Triceps Brachii

Sitting Triceps Extension

Action

The sitting triceps extension is also referred to as a French press. To ensure safety, as well as assist in positioning the dumbbell, a spotter is required to properly execute the sitting triceps extension. To perform the sitting triceps extension, select a dumbbell of appropriate resistance and assume a sitting position, on a flat bench, with both feet flat on the floor. In situations where lower back support is warranted a chair may be used. Grasp the end of the dumbbell, directly behind the head. The arms should be flexed at the elbow while keeping the upper arms extended overhead, directly over the shoulders. The concentric phase is the first action. During the concentric phase, lift the dumbbell overhead by extending the lower arms at the elbows. Precaution should be taken to keep the upper arms stable. Additionally, care should be taken

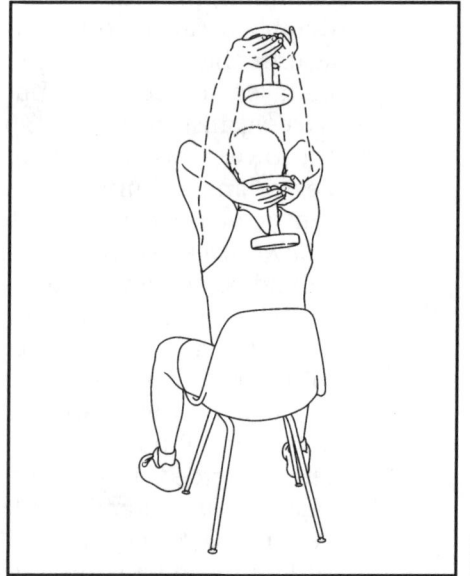

Figure 7.49 ■ Free Weight Dumbbell - Sitting Triceps Extension

to keep the upper body erect and avoid leaning backward particularly when lowering the arms. To perform the eccentric phase, slowly lower the barbell back to its original position by flexing the elbows until the hands are directly behind the head. Proper breath control is strongly recommended. Inhale during the eccentric phase of the lift and exhale during the concentric phase. The action of the sitting triceps extension is shown in Figure 7.49.

Major Muscles Conditioned

Triceps Brachii

Forearms

Dumbbell Wrist Curl

Action

Select the dumbbells of appropriate resistance. Assume a sitting position on the end of a flat bench. Position the feet and legs directly in front of the hips. Grasp the dumbbells, with a supinated grip. While holding the dumbbells, lean forward and rest the forearms and elbows on the upper legs so the wrists are hyperextended just beyond the knees. Open the supinated grip slightly so fingers hold each dumbbell. The concentric phase of the dumbbell wrist curl is to lift the dumbbell by flexing the fingers and the wrist. Precaution should be taken to keep the forearms and elbows in contact with the thigh when curling the dumbbells. During the downward or eccentric phase, extend the wrist so the dumbbells return to their original position. Proper breath control is strongly recommended. Inhale during the eccentric phase of the lift and exhale during the concentric phase. The action of the dumbbell wrist curl is shown in Figure 7.50.

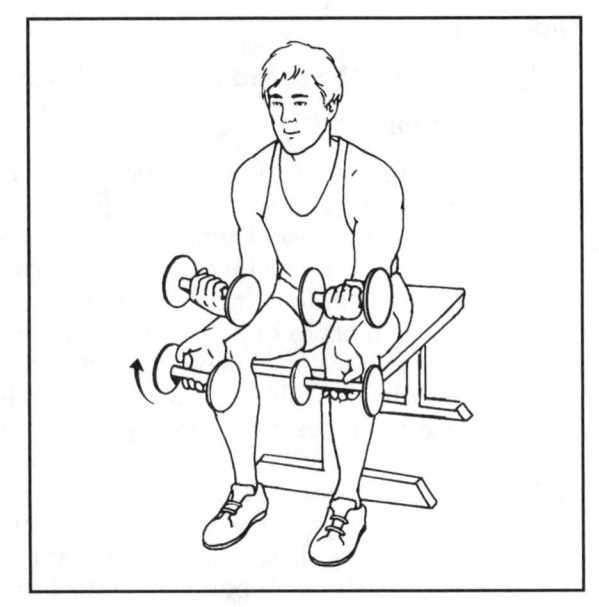

Figure 7.50 ■ Free Weight Dumbbell - Dumbbell Wrist Curl

Major Muscles Conditioned

Flexor Carpi Radialis, Flexor Carpi Ulnaris

Dumbbell Wrist Extensions

Action

Select the dumbbells of appropriate resistance. Assume a sitting position on the end of a flat bench. Position the feet and legs directly in front of the hips. Grasp the dumbbells, with a pronated grip. While holding the dumbbells, lean forward and rest the forearms and elbows on the upper legs so the wrists are flexed just beyond the knees. The concentric phase of the dumbbell wrist extension is to lift the dumbbells by extending the wrists. Precaution should be taken to keep the forearms and elbows in contact with the thigh when extending the wrists. During the downward or eccentric phase, flex the wrists so the dumbbells return to their original position. Proper breath control is strongly recommended. Inhale during the eccentric phase of the lift and exhale during the concentric phase. The action of the dumbbell wrist extension is shown in Figure 7.51.

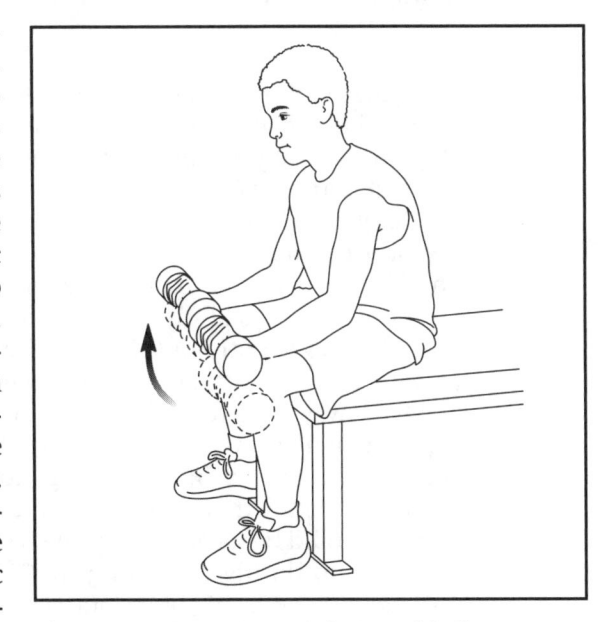

Figure 7.51 ■ Free Weight Dumbbell - Dumbbell Wrist Extension

Major Muscles Conditioned

Extensor Carpi Radialis, Extensor Carpi Ulnaris

Shoulders

Seated Overhead Dumbbell Press

Action

The seated overhead dumbbell press may require the assistance of a spotter to help in getting the dumbbells positioned. Dumbbells may be preferred over a barbell when performing an overhead press because of the additional range of motion they offer. Select the dumbbells of appropriate resistance. Typically, a greater resistance may be selected than the amount associated with the standing barbell or dumbbell overhead press activities. To perform the seated overhead dumbbell press, assume a sitting position on an inclined bench. Fix the back support of the bench in a vertical position. Precaution should be taken to keep the back, shoulders, head, and hips in contact with the back support during the lifting movements. Lightly grasp the dumbbells using a pronated grip and position the dumbbells directly overhead with the arms fully extended. The wrists should be fixed and extended above the elbows. During the upward or concentric phase, press the dumbbells directly overhead to a point where the arms are fully extended. Do not lock the elbows out during extension. The downward or eccentric phase requires the elbows to be flexed, lowering the dumbbells toward the chest. Stop the downward movement when the dumbbells are even with the clavicles. Proper breath control is strongly recommended. Inhale during the eccentric phase of the lift and exhale during the concentric phase. The action of the seated overhead dumbbell press is shown in Figure 7.52.

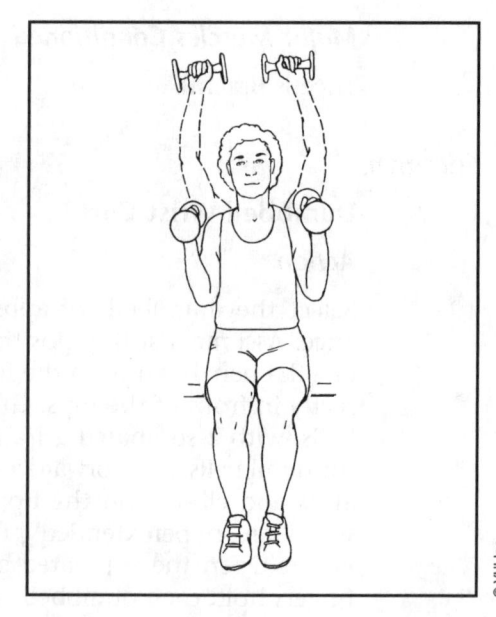

Figure 7.52 ■ Free Weight Dumbbell - Seated Overhead Dumbbell Press

Major Muscles Conditioned

Deltoid (anterior, medial)

Standing Dumbbell Lateral Row

Action

Select the dumbbells of appropriate resistance. It should be noted that because of the extreme leverage associated with the fully extended arms, the dumbbell lateral row will normally require very light dumbbells. Grasp the dumbbell with a pronated grip. Assume a standing position and allow the dumbbells to rest comfortably on the thigh. In order to provide a more stable stance, position the feet slightly outside the shoulders and turn the toes slightly out. During the concentric or upward phase, lift or abduct the dumbbells directly upward, away from the sides, until the dumbbells are approximately on the level with the clavicles or parallel to the floor. During the lifting motion, keep the arms extended with a slight bend in the elbows. Precaution should be taken to keep the back straight and the head up during the lifting motion. During the downward or eccentric phase adduct the upper arms toward the sides lowering the dumbbells back to their original position. Proper breath control is strongly recommended. Inhale during the eccentric phase of the lift and exhale during the concentric phase. The action of the standing dumbbell lateral row is shown in Figure 7.53.

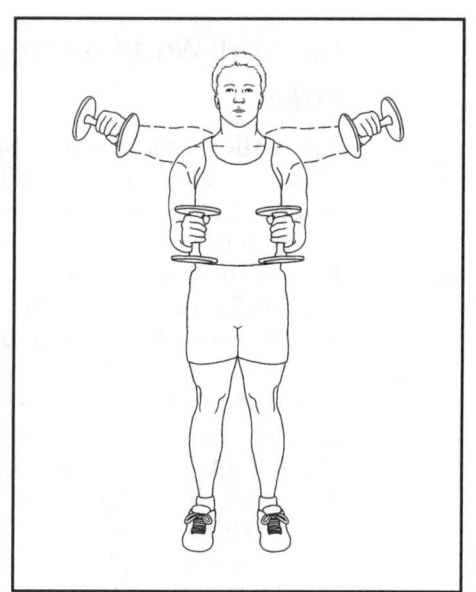

Figure 7.53 ■ Free Weight Dumbbell - Standing Dumbbell Lateral Row

Major Muscles Conditioned

Deltoids (anterior, middle, posterior), Trapezius (upper)

Standing Dumbbell Upright Row

Action

Select the dumbbells of appropriate resistance. Grasp the barbell with a pronated grip. Assume a standing position and allow the dumbbells to rest comfortably on the thigh. In order to provide a more stable stance, position the feet slightly outside the shoulders and turn the toes slightly out. During the concentric or upward phase, pull or lift the dumbbells directly upward against the abdomen and chest toward the chin until the dumbbells are approximately on the level with the clavicles. During the lifting motion, keep the elbows high. Precaution should be taken to keep the back straight and the head up during the lifting motion. During the downward or eccentric phase extend the elbows and adduct the upper arms toward the side lowering the dumbbells back to their original position. Proper breath control is strongly recommended. Inhale during the eccentric phase of the lift and exhale during the concentric phase. The action of the standing dumbbell upright row is shown in Figure 7.54.

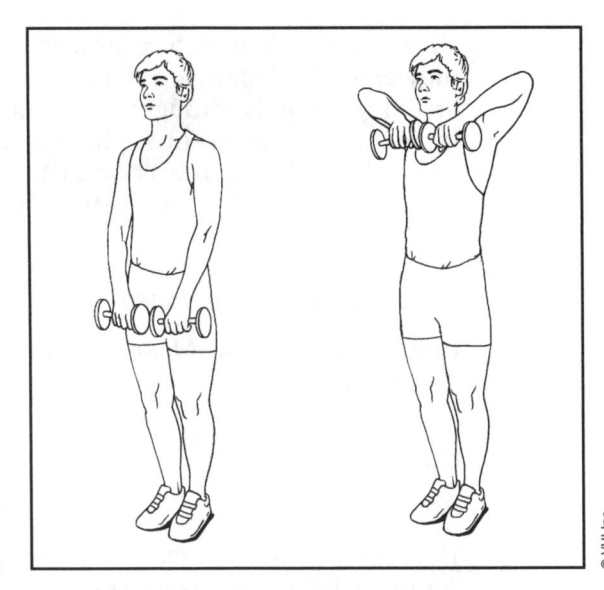

Figure 7.54 ■ Free Weight Dumbbell - Standing Dumbbell Upright Row

Major Muscles Conditioned

Deltoids (anterior, middle, posterior), Trapezius (upper)

Upper Back

Dumbbell Bent Over Row

Action

The dumbbell bent over row is often preferred over the barbell bent over row. There are several reasons for this preference. First, the dumbbells offer a greater range of motion during the lift. Second, the barbell bent over row is an unsupported activity. The dumbbell row offers the participant the option of stabilizing and supporting the upper body. Finally, the dumbbell bent over row offers the option of working each arm individually. To perform the dumbbell bent over row, select the dumbbells of the appropriate resistance. Assume a standing position so the dumbbells are just outside the feet. The feet should be placed approximately shoulder width apart with the toes turned slightly outward. Squat down, keeping the hips slightly lower than the shoulders, and grasp a dumbbell with a pronated grip. Precaution should be taken to keep the back flat and the head up with the eyes focused ahead. Do not tuck the head and look downward. Keeping the back flat, lift the dumbbells slightly off the floor by slightly extending the hips and knees. Do not stand erect. Extend the passive arm and rest it on the top of a flat bench. This arm should be used to support the upper body. The active arm should remain extended and hang straight down. The action of the dumbbell bent over row is similar to the barbell bent over row. The concentric phase of the dumbbell bent over row is to pull the dumbbell up toward the lower chest and upper abdominal area of the trunk. Keep the elbows high during this movement. The back should continue to remain flat with little or no movement occurring outside the area of the shoulder and shoulder girdle. During the downward or eccentric phase, slowly extend the active arm at the elbow and allow the shoulder to flex until the arm is fully extended below the shoulders. Proper breath control is strongly recommended. Inhale during the eccentric phase of the lift and exhale during the concentric phase. The action of the dumbbell bent over row is shown in Figure 7.55

Major Muscles Conditioned

Latissimus Dorsi, Teres Major, Trapezius (middle), Rhomboids

Dumbbell Pull-Over

Action

The action of the dumbbell pull-over is similar to the barbell pull-over. The primary difference is that typically the arms are fully extended when performing the dumbbell pull-over. Because of this difference, the dumbbell weight is significantly lower than the weight used when performing a barbell pull-over. To perform the dumbbell pull-over, select a dumbbell of appropriate resistance. Assume a supine position on a flat bench with the head, shoulders, back, and hips resting on the bench. The feet should be placed flat on the floor with the knees bent to approximately 90-degree angles. Grasp the end of the dumbbell with both hands. In the original position the dumbbell is held directly over the chest with the arms fully extended. The first action of the dumbbell pull-over is the eccentric phase. During the eccentric phase, carefully lower the dumbbell behind the head, toward the floor. Precaution should be taken to slowly lower the dumbbell. This will help in controlling how far the musculature is stretched. During the concentric phase, the dumbbell is pulled back up and over the face until it is returned to its original position. Proper breath control is strongly recommended. Inhale during the eccentric phase of the lift and exhale during the concentric phase. The action of the dumbbell pull-over is shown in Figure 7.56.

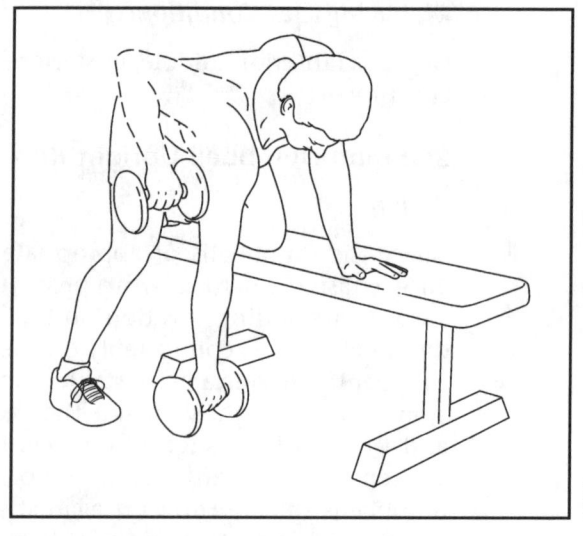

Figure 7.55 ■ Free Weight Dumbbell - Dumbbell Bent Over Row

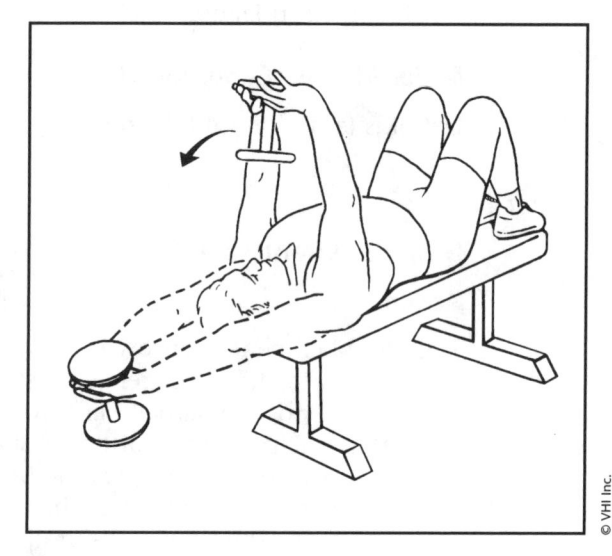

Figure 7.56 ■ Free Weight Dumbbell - Dumbbell Pull-Over

Major Muscles Conditioned

Lattissimus Dorsi, Deltoid (posterior)

Lower Legs – Posterior

Standing Dumbbell Heel Raise

Action

The standing heel raise can be performed with dumbbells. Because of the large load required, some may find the standing barbell heel raise a more appropriate activity. To perform the standing dumbbell heel raise, select the dumbbells of appropriate resistance. Grasp the dumbbells using a neutral grip and allow them to hang, and rest on the outside of the thigh. Assuming a standing position, place the toes and balls of the foot on an elevated platform or board.

Platform height should not exceed more than a couple of inches. The heels of the foot should rest comfortably on the ground when the toes are elevated. The concentric phase of the standing dumbbell heel raise is the first action. During the concentric phase, plantar flex the toes and lift the heels off the ground. To complete the eccentric phase, return the heels back to ground. Proper breath control is strongly recommended. Inhale during the eccentric phase of the lift and exhale during the concentric phase. The action of the standing dumbbell heel raise is shown in Figure 7.57.

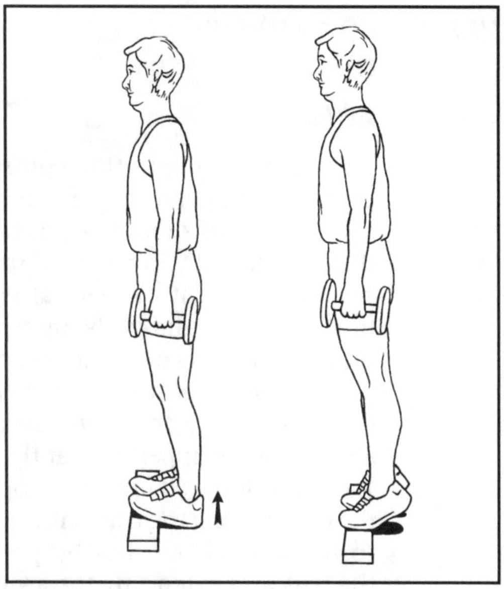

Major Muscles Conditioned

Soleus, Gastrocnemius

Resistance Training without Free Weights or Resistance Machines

Figure 7.57 ■ Free Weight Dumbbell - Standing Dumbbell Heel Raise

There are many appropriate resistance training activities that can be recommended that do not require the use of free weights or resistance machines. These activities rely solely on gravitational pull on the body or selected body segments for resistance. As a result, they are referred to as gravitational activities. If properly incorporated into a regular muscular strength and endurance training program, each would allow for positive gains in both muscular strength and muscular endurance. To illustrate and describe such a large number of procedures is beyond the scope of this manuscript. As a result, examples of the more common procedures have been provided. For reader ease, procedures have been grouped by body segment.

Upper Arms – Anterior

Reversed, Closed Grip Pull-Up

The reversed, closed grip pull-up requires enough strength to lift your own body weight. This may limit the usefulness of this activity for some. If, however, additional resistance is needed, weights can be easily suspended from the waist. The action of a reversed, closed grip pull-up is similar to a machine lat pull-down. To perform a reversed, closed grip pull-up, position yourself under a secure bar positioned at a height that will allow you to hang freely when your arms are fully extended. Jump up and grasp the bar using either a pronated grip (hands facing toward you). The concentric phase of the reversed, closed grip pull-up is the first action. During the concentric phase, pull yourself up until your face and chin pass the bar. During the eccentric phase, slowly lower yourself back to the suspended position. The action of the reversed, closed grip pull-up is shown in Figure 7.58.

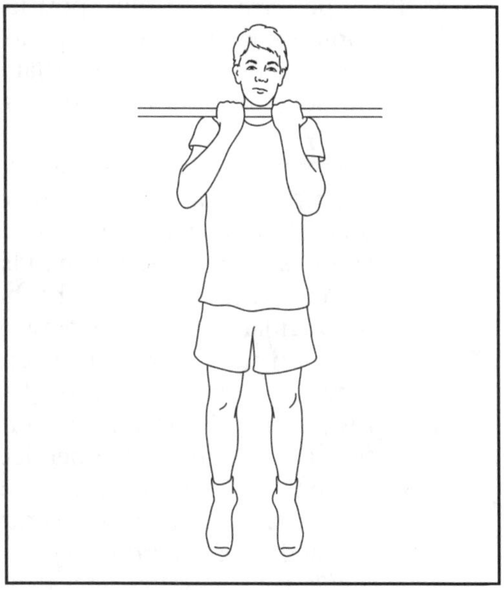

Figure 7.58 ■ Resistance Training - Reversed, Closed Grip Pull-Up

Major Muscles Conditioned

Latissimus Dorsi, Teres Major, Trapezius (middle), Rhomboids, Deltoid (posterior), Biceps

Upper Arms – Posterior

Dips

Action

To perform dips, position yourself between two support bars that are approximately shoulder width apart. The bars should be positioned at about shoulder level. Initially, you should suspend yourself grasping each bar with a neutral grip and jumping up until the arms and body are fully extended. Do not lock your elbows out. The eccentric phase is the first action. To perform the eccentric phase, lower your body by flexing the lower arms at the elbows and abducting the upper arms at the shoulders. The body should be lowered until the upper chest is even with the bars. During the concentric phase, return the body to its original position by pressing downward on the bars and extending the arms. Precaution should be taken to keep the body erect. The body should not be allowed to swing. Proper breath control is strongly recommended. Inhale during the eccentric phase of the lift and exhale during the concentric phase. The action of dips is shown in Figure 7.59.

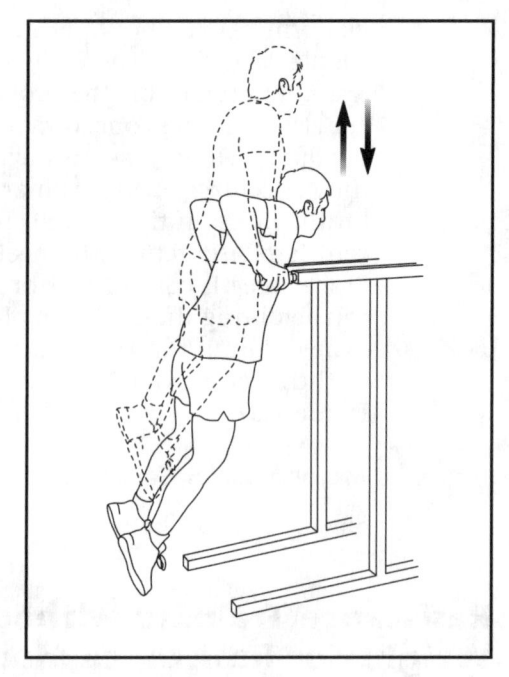

Figure 7.59 ■ Resistance Training - Dips

Major Muscles Conditioned

Pectoralis Major, Triceps, Deltoid (anterior), Latissimus Dorsi

Chair Dips

Action

To perform chair dips, position yourself between two stable chairs that are approximately shoulder width apart. Suspend yourself, facing away from the chairs, by placing your hands under your shoulders and flat on the chair bottoms. The arms should be fully extended. Do not lock the elbows out during extension. The legs should be fully extended in front of you as if you were attempting to sit on air. The eccentric phase is the first action. To perform the eccentric phase, lower your body by flexing the lower arms at the elbows and abducting the upper arms at the shoulders. The body should be lowered until the upper chest is even with the hands. During the concentric phase, return the body to its original position by pressing downward on the chairs and extending the arms. Precaution should be taken to keep the lower body erect. Proper breath control is strongly recommended. Inhale during the eccentric phase of the lift and exhale during the concentric phase. The action of chair dips is shown in Figure 7.60.

Major Muscles Conditioned

Pectoralis Major, Triceps, Deltoid (anterior), Latissimus Dorsi

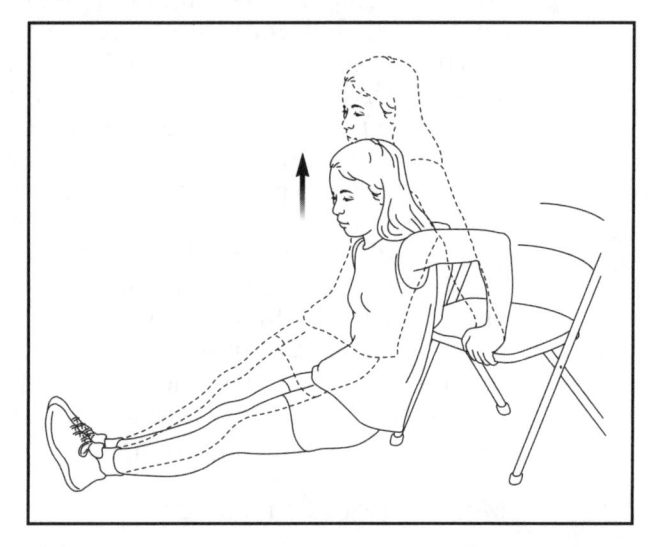

Figure 7.60 ■ Resistance Training - Chair Dips

Push-Up

Action

...ing the upward phase or concentric phase, push down on the floor and lift the body upward until the arms are fully extended. The arms should be externally rotated so the elbows are positioned or pointed outward. In the up position, the only points of contact should be the hands and toes. During the downward or eccentric phase, lower the body until the chest is just off the ground. During the action of the arms, precaution should be taken to keep the body rigid. Arching or swaying of the back should be avoided. Proper breath control is strongly recommended. Inhale during the eccentric phase of the lift and exhale during the concentric phase. It should be noted that for those with limited strength, the knees can serve as the support point instead of the toes. This change will lower the resistance and make it easier to elevate the upper body. Again, even when using the knees as the support point, it is important to keep the back straight and the body rigid. The action of a push-up is shown in Figure 7.61.

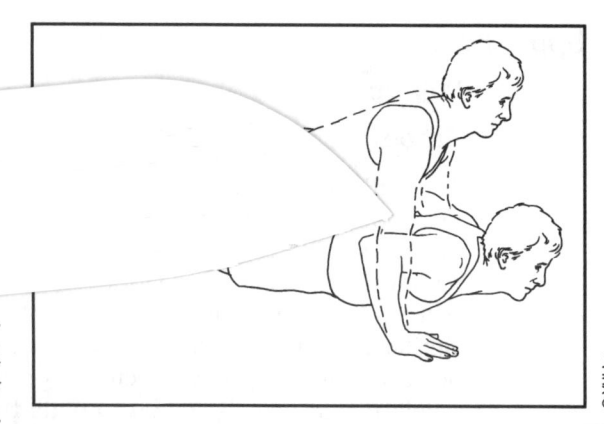

Figure 7.61 ■ Resistance Training - Push-Up

Major Muscles Conditioned

Pectoralis Major, Triceps

Closed Hand Push-Up

Action

The action of the closed hand push-up is similar to the push-up. The primary difference is the location of the hands. By placing the hands closer together, greater emphasis is placed in the triceps musculature. To perform a closed hand push-up, assume a prone position with the hands placed flat on the floor, just under the chest. The distance between the hands should be minimal. The fingertips should be pointed toward the head. Dorsi flex the feet so the toes serve as a support point. During the upward phase or concentric phase, push down on the floor and lift the body upward until the arms are fully extended. The arms should be externally rotated so that the elbows are positioned or pointed outward. In the up position, the only points of contact should be the hands and toes. During the downward or eccentric phase, lower the body until the chest is just off the ground. During the action of the arms, precaution should be taken to keep the body rigid. Arching or swaying of the back should be avoided. Proper breath control is strongly recommended. Inhale during the eccentric phase of the lift and exhale during the concentric phase. It should be noted that for those with limited strength the knees can serve as the support point instead of the toes. This change will lower the resistance and make it easier to elevate the upper body. Again, even when using the knees as the support point, it is important to keep the back straight and the body rigid. The action of the closed hand push-up is shown in Figure 7.62.

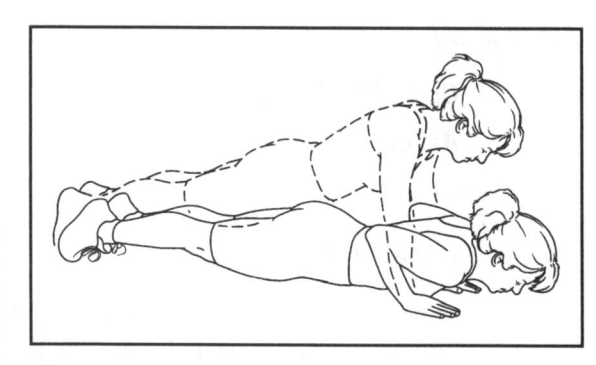

Figure 7.62 ■ Resistance Training - Closed Hand Push-Up

Major Muscles Conditioned

Pectoralis Major, Triceps

Upper Back

Pull-Up

Action

The pull-up requires enough strength to lift your own body weight. This may limit the usefulness of this activity for some. If, however, additional resistance is needed, weights can be easily suspended from the waist. The action of a pull-up is similar to a lat pull down. To perform a pull-up, position yourself under a secure bar positioned at a height that will allow you to hang freely when your arms are fully extended. Jump up and grasp the bar using either a pronated grip (hands facing away). The concentric phase of the pull-up is the first action. During the concentric phase, pull yourself up until your face and chin pass the bar. During the eccentric phase, slowly lower yourself back to the suspended position. The action of the pull-up is shown in Figure 7.63.

Figure 7.63 ■ Resistance Training - Pull-Up

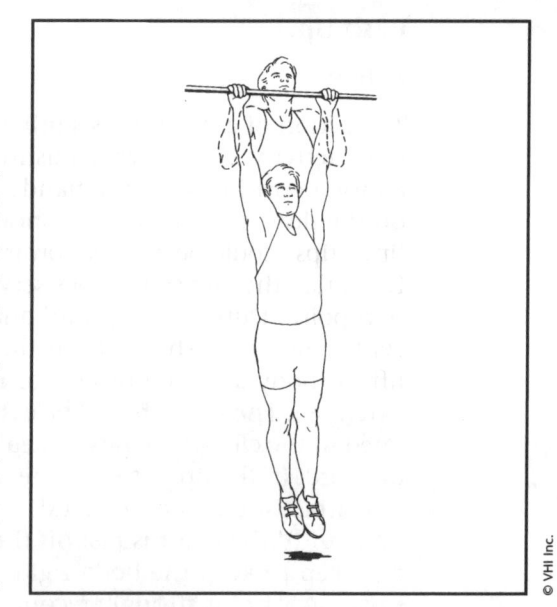

Major Muscles Conditioned

Latissimus Dorsi, Teres Major, Trapezius (middle), Rhomboids, Deltoid (posterior), Biceps

Abdominals

Crunches (Curl-Ups)

Action

Crunches are also commonly referred to as curl-ups. To perform the curl-up the subject is placed, in a supine position, on his/her back with their arms and hands extended until the hands are touching his/her thighs. The legs should be bent at the knees so his/her heels are 12–8 inches from the buttocks or his/her knees are bent at 90 degrees. An assistant may hold the ankles to keep the feet firmly on the ground and to provide support. A correct curl-up is performed when a subject curls-up, lifting his/her shoulder blades off the mat, while sliding his/her hands up his/her thighs until the hands touch the kneecap. The lower back, buttocks, and feet should remain in contact with the mat. The trunk should be at approximately a 30-degree angle to the mat. To complete the curl-up, the subject returns to the mat and makes full contact with the back and shoulders. The subject's lower back should be fully flattened before he/she begins another curl-up. The subject should not hold his/her breath during the activity, but should breathe freely with each repetition. The action of crunches (curl-ups) is shown in Figure 7.64.

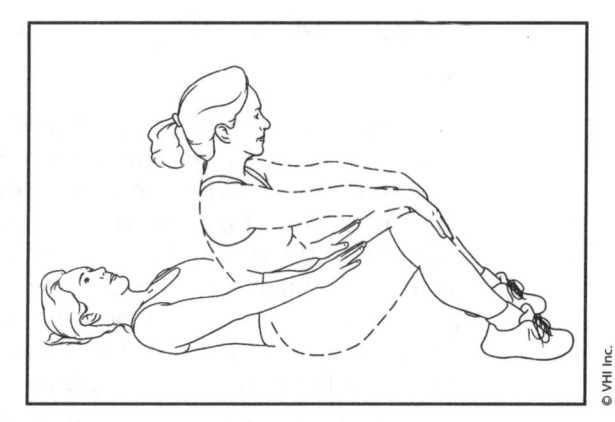

Figure 7.64 ■ Resistance Training - Crunches (Curl-Ups)

Major Muscles Conditioned

Rectus Abdominis

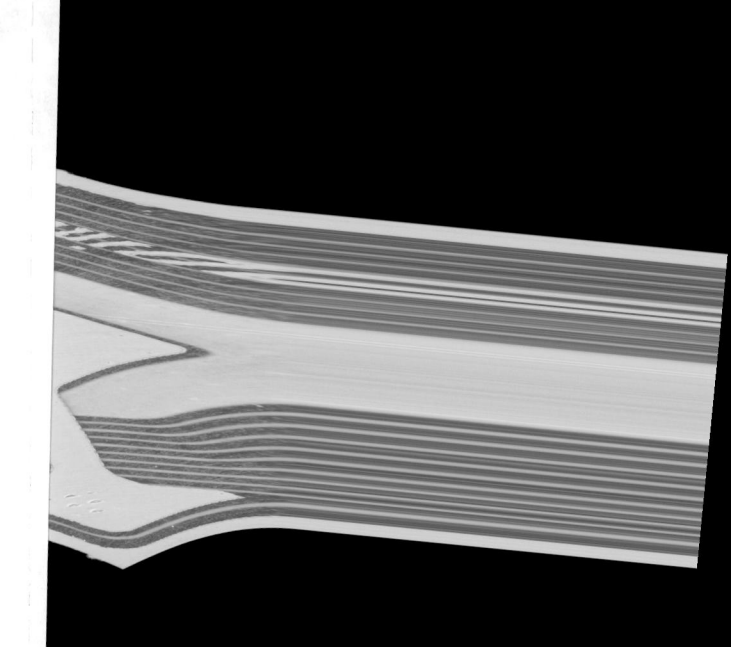

Inclined Bent Knee Sit Ups

Action

The action of the inclined bent knee sit-up is similar to the curl-up. The primary difference is that an inclined board is used. By varying the height of the board, greater or lesser resistance is offered. In simple, the higher the board, the more difficult the bent knee sit-up. The subject assumes a supine position on his/her back with hands interlocked over the chest touching the shoulders. The legs should be bent at the knees so the heels are 12–8 inches from the buttocks. The feet are held in place by hooking the toes under the roller pad on the end of the incline board. A correct sit-up is performed when a subject curls his/her torso up while keeping his/her feet, buttocks, and lower back flat on the inclined board. The hands/arms remain in contact with his/her chest and shoulders during the curl-up. To complete the sit-up, the subject must return to the inclined board and make full contact with the back and shoulders. The subject should not hold his/her breath during the sit-up, but should breathe freely with each repetition. The action of inclined bent knee sit-ups is shown in Figure 7.65.

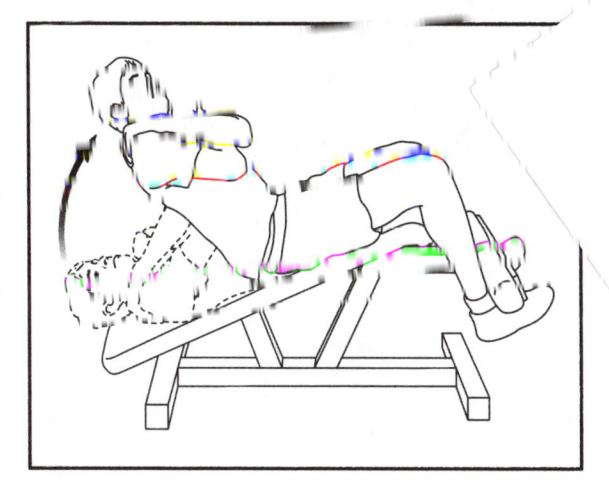

Figure 7.65 ■ Resistance Training - Inclined Bent Knee Sit-Ups

Major Muscles Conditioned

Rectus Abdominis, External Abdominal Oblique, Internal Abdominal Oblique

8

Principles of Flexibility

*Two-thirds of people with diabetes mellitus
die of some form of heart or blood vessel disease*
American Heart Association

*People with diabetes are two to four times more likely to have
heart disease or stroke than people without diabetes*
Center for Disease Control and Prevention

■ Chapter Outline ■

What Is Flexibility?
    Active Flexibility
    Passive Flexibility
Benefits of Flexibility
Factors that Influence Flexibility
    Muscle Spindles
    Golgi Tendon Organs
    Joint Structure
    Soft Body Tissue
    Age

Gender
Muscle Temperature
Pregnancy
Principles and Procedures of Flexibility Training
    or Stretching
    How Can Range of Motion Be Improved?
    Static Stretching
    Dynamic or Ballistic Stretching
    Proprioceptive Neuromuscular Facilitation
        (PNF)

■ Learning Objectives ■

The student should be able to:

- Define flexibility (range of motion).
- Distinguish the difference between active and passive flexibility.
- Identify the benefits and importance of good joint flexibility.
- Describe the relationship between the principle of overload and the development of flexibility.
- Describe the relationship between the principle of specificity and the development of flexibility.

- Identify biomechanical and physiological factors that influence joint flexibility.
- Describe techniques, procedures and exercises for developing joint flexibility using dynamic, static, and proprioceptive neuromuscular facilitation stretching protocols.
- Describe the advantages and disadvantages of dynamic, static, and proprioceptive neuromuscular facilitation stretching protocols.
- Describe the stretch-reflex mechanism as it relates to muscle lengthening and contraction.

Keywords

- Active flexibility
- Agonistic contraction
- Autogenic inhibition
- Ballistic/dynamic stretching
- Contract-relax
- Elastic elongation
- Flexibility
- Golgi tendon organs
- Hold-relax
- Muscle spindles
- Passive flexibility
- Plasticity
- Plastic elongation
- Principle of overload
- Principle of specificity
- Proprioceptive neuromuscular facilitation Stretching (PNF)
- Range of motion (ROM)
- Reciprocal inhibition
- Static stretching
- Stretch-reflex mechanism

What Is Flexibility?

Flexibility is defined and is also referred to as the **range of motion (ROM)** of a single joint (i.e., knee) or a series of joints (i.e., spine). It is specific to each joint. Gaining flexibility in one joint does not result in a gain in another joint. In other words, increasing flexibility in the right shoulder has no effect on the range of motion of the left shoulder. Similarly, to have good flexibility in a particular joint does not mean that you will have good flexibility throughout the body. It is possible to have good range of motion in the upper body and limited range of motion in the lower body. Flexibility is often subdivided as to whether it is active or passive.

Active Flexibility

Active flexibility is referred to as dynamic flexibility. By definition, it is *the degree to which the force of a muscle contraction can move a joint.* Active stretches occur when the individual stretching provides the muscular force needed to stretch the muscle tissue. Active stretching requires a greater degree of energy expenditure as compared to passive stretching. In cases of rapid movement, active flexibility may elicit a stretch-reflex.

Passive Flexibility

Passive flexibility is referred to as static flexibility. It may be defined as *the ROM a joint may passively be moved.* It involves no muscle contraction, but rather relies on some external force to generate the movement. Typically, the ROM associated with passive flexibility is greater than active flexibility. Passive stretches occur when a partner or external apparatus such as a stretching machine provides the force needed for the stretch.

Benefits of Flexibility

Flexibility is an important component of health-related fitness and should be considered essential for establishing and maintaining mobility. Good overall flexibility is directly related to daily living activities. It has been shown to:

- Reduce muscle soreness
- Reduce muscle tension
- Reduce risk of low back pain
- Improve muscle performance
- Improve posture
- Improve muscle coordination

From a physical performance perspective, it assists in reducing risk of injury, reducing the severity and frequency of injuries, assists in the treatment of musculoskeletal injuries, and improves performance. Psychologically, it has been shown to relieve stress and tension (Alter, 1988) and improve and/or developed an enhanced sense of body awareness.

Factors That Influence Flexibility

The range of motion of a joint(s) is influenced by both biomechanical and physiological properties. Biomechanical factors include the joint structure and related connective tissues. Physiological factors are related to the muscle tissue, including the muscle spindles and golgi tendon bodies. These are described under separate subheaders below.

Which factors limit the range of motion of a joint are joint specific. For example, the hip and shoulder are limited by connective tissues. A joint such as the elbow is more structurally limited.

Muscle Spindles

Muscle spindles are proprioceptors located within the muscle fibers that monitor and detect changes in muscle length. They are particularly sensitive to *rapid changes* in muscle length and when activated induce stretch-reflex, a phenomenon which should be avoided when stretching.

Golgi Tendon Organs

Golgi tendon organs are mechanoreceptors located in the region of the musculotendinous junction. They are particularly sensitive to *muscle tension* and when activated cause the contracting muscle (agonist) to relax and the antagonistic muscles to become excited. This action serves as a protective mechanism by preventing muscle injury that results when excessive force or muscle tension is generated during skeletal muscle contraction.

Joint Structure

The human body is composed of a variety of joints. These joints vary in structure and design. The range of motion associated with each joint may vary. Synarthrodial joints (i.e., sutures of the scull) present little or no movements. Diarthrodial joints (i.e., shoulder) allow for extensive range of motion. The specific movement patterns that occur at each joint are directly related to: (1) the articular joint structure, and (2) the connective and muscle tissues associated with the joint (see Soft Body Tissue).

Soft Body Tissue

Several soft body tissues influence the range of motion of a joint. These include:

- Muscle tissue
- Connective tissue, including the muscle tendons and joint capsule ligaments
- Skin
- Scar tissue
- Adipose tissue

Precaution must be taken when developing stretching programs to avoid altering the plasticity of the nonelastic properties of these tissues, particularly the capsular ligaments. The plasticity of a tissue is the tendency or ability of the tissue to adapt to or assume a new and greater length after stretching. Tissues such as capsular ligaments are particularly important in providing joint stability and should not be altered. Gains in range of motion should result from plastic elongation of the elastic connective tissues surrounding the muscle. It should be noted that injuries that lead to tearing or scarring of connective tissue may lead to reduced ROM.

Age

In general, aging is negatively related to flexibility. In simple, as we grow older we lose flexibility. There are several possible explanations for this finding. Perhaps, the most probable explanation lies in the sedentary nature that we adopt as we grow older. Some of the loss can be attributed to physical changes including the chemical structure of the tissues, loss of fluids in the tissues, increased amounts of calcium deposits, and the replacement of the muscle fibers with collagenous fibers (Alter, 1988). Collagenous tissues typically are nonelastic and provide strength and rigidity to the joint. Additionally, older individuals tend to become susceptible to a process known as fibrosis. Fibrosis occurs when fibrous connective tissue replaces degenerating muscle fibers.

Gender

Are men less flexible than women? Clearly, this is a common perception. While gender differences do exist (Corbin, 1984; Surburg, 1995), the differences appear to be joint specific and do not always favor women. Additionally, some of the differences that have been reported appear to be related to male joint asymmetry (ACSM, 1993). In other words, some men present less range of motion on their dominant side than on their nondominant side.

Muscle Temperature

Increases in muscle temperature are related to changes in muscle tissue flexibility and joint range of motion. These changes appear to result from changes in tissue viscosity. For optimal muscle tissue elongation to occur, muscle tissue should be raised to between 102 and 110 degree Fahrenheit (Johnson & Nelson, 1986). As muscle tissue temperature rises, connective tissue and collagen become softer, allowing for more plastic elongation to occur. These findings suggest a need to warmup the body before stretching. Light calisthenics, walking/jogging or other activities which raise core body temperature should occur **before** stretching activity. This is contrary to the usual practice of relying on stretching activities to warmup the body.

Pregnancy

During pregnancy the hormone relaxin is released. It causes a change in the elastic properties of ligaments and connective tissues, and subsequently, improves muscle and joint flexibility (Robergs and Roberts, 1997).

Principles and Procedures of Flexibility Training or Stretching

How Can Range of Motion Be Improved?

There are three common procedures that can improve joint range of motion. These include ballistic, static, and proprioceptive neuromuscular facilitation. Each is described under separate headers below. General guidelines for flexibility training based on these procedures are summarized in Table 8-1. Before discussing each procedure, it is important to understand how soft tissue can allow for increased range of motion.

When attempting a stretching exercise, two types of elongation are involved, these being elastic and plastic. **Elastic elongation** is a temporary increase in the soft tissue length resulting from agonistic muscle force or some external force, depending on whether the flexibility activity is active or passive. **Plastic elongation** is a long-term tissue adaptation resulting in a permanent lengthening of the soft tissue. It does not result in a change in the elastic properties of the connective, ligamentous, or capsular tissues. Because joint capsules, ligaments, and cartilage provide stability to a joint, it is recommended that plastic elongation of these tissues be avoided (Komi, 1986).

The principles of overload and specificity apply when developing programs for increasing flexibility. Flexibility is very joint and soft tissue specific. As a result, the **principle of specificity** would suggest that any flexibility program include all joints. Any area that is not directly trained will not be affected.

The **principle of overload** implies that plastic elongation will occur over time if repeated bouts of tension are applied to the soft tissues. It has been reported that the time required for increasing flexibility is inversely related to the force used (Sapega, Quedenfeld, Moyer, & Butler, 1981). It should be stressed that increases in the amount of force used when stretching is related to increased tissue damage and injury. It is recommended that lower force be used and

Table 8-1 ■ Recommended Guidelines for Static, PNF, and Ballistic Flexibility Training

Component	Static	PNF	Ballistic/Dynamic
Frequency	4 Repetitions minimum per stretching activity	4 Repetitions minimum per stretching activity	Not Recommended
Duration	10–30 seconds per stretching activity	6-second isometric contraction followed by a 10–30-second passive stretch at mid discomfort at end range of motion	Not Recommended
Intensity	Point of mild discomfort at end range of motion	Point of mild discomfort at end range of motion; submaximal isometric contraction	Not Recommended
Progression	3–5 times per week	3–5 times per week	Not Recommended

a long-term program adopted. When beginning a flexibility program, allow 4 to 6 weeks minimum for tissue adaptations to occur.

Static Stretching

When **static stretching**, a muscle or selected musculature is isolated and **slowly stretched** or elongated until slight tension or discomfort is experienced. If done properly, static stretching **will not** induce the muscle stretch-reflex or stretch-shortening cycle.

Opinions vary as to the length of time the stretched position should be held. Currently, ACSM (2001) recommends holding each stretch for 10 to 30 seconds, relaxing, and then repeating the stretch, for each muscle group, at least four times. Flexibility exercise sessions should occur a minimum of two to three days per week to develop or maintain flexibility. Three to five days per week are appropriate. Precaution should be taken to gradually (slowly) stretch the tissue to avoid muscle spindle activity and elicit reciprocal inhibition or inverse stretch-reflex. Limited evidence would suggest improved gains when holding stretches longer than 30 seconds.

Static stretching is the most common and recommended stretching procedure. When done properly, it is easy to learn, safe, and allows for the development and retention of muscular flexibility. It is not associated with the development of muscle soreness and, in fact, may reduce muscle soreness.

Dynamic or Ballistic Stretching

Ballistic stretching is the most dangerous of the stretching procedures. It involves the use of movement or bouncing to elongate the isolated muscle or group of muscles. The stretched or end position may or may not be held. Generally, ballistic stretching is not a recommended procedure. It may lead to muscle soreness and muscle injury if the extensibility limits of the muscle are exceeded (Bandy & Irion, 1994) or the stretch-reflex is induced (Smith, 1994; Surburg, 1995). It must be emphasized that **ballistic stretching typically induces stretch-reflex**. As a result, most consider the disadvantages of ballistic stretching to outweigh its advantages. Clearly, when compared to static stretching, static stretching is safer, requires less energy expenditure, and is associated with far less muscle soreness and muscle injury.

As previously mentioned, the **stretch-reflex** is a protective mechanism related to the muscle spindles of the body. Muscle spindles are muscle proprioceptors found in most skeletal muscles. They monitor the magnitude and rate of length change of the muscle. Sudden, forceful movements, which occur in ballistic stretches, may excite muscle spindle activity and induce the stretch-reflex phenomenon leading to intrafusal muscle contraction. As a result, the very muscle or muscles being forcefully *lengthened* by the ballistic stretching movement are also being *shortened* by the intrafusal muscle contraction. This action of the muscle tissue being pulled into two opposite directions can of course lead to tissue tearing and damage.

Dynamic stretching is similar to ballistic stretching in that it relies on controlled body movements to stretch the muscle tissue. Dynamic stretching activities do, however, try to avoid bouncing or violently stretching the muscle tissue. They do, this by mimicking and exaggerating sport or movement specific patterns in a way that actively stretches the tissue, but at the same time, avoids the high speed of movement associated with a bouncing activity. Dynamic stretching activities are commonly used during a sport-specific warm-up. While somewhat safer than ballistic stretching, dynamic stretching activities still present an unnecessarily high level of risk of injury for the average individual and are not recommended for these types of individuals.

Proprioceptive Neuromuscular Facilitation (PNF)

There are two types of proprioceptive neuromuscular facilitation (PNF) procedures. These include: (1) Hold-Relax, also referred to as Contract-Relax, and (2) Hold-Relax with agonist contraction, which is also referred to as Contract-Relax with agonist contraction (ACSM, 2001; Nieman, 1995). While procedural differences exist between the two types, both are designed to increase flexibility by facilitating muscular inhibition. For example, the Contract-Relax procedure calls for an isometric contraction of the muscle group prior to static stretching of the muscle group. In comparison, the Contract-Relax with agonist contraction procedure requires the same steps as the Contract-Relax procedure, except that during the period of static or passive stretching the agonist muscle group is submaximally contracted. Those promoting this procedure believe that the agonistic contraction may help to better relax the stretched muscles.

The underlying premise of proprioceptive neuromuscular facilitation can be presented by discussing the two separate and distinct phases or actions. Before beginning either phase, the muscle or muscle group should be positioned and held at a point of full range of motion (see Figure 8.1). After an assistant fixes the muscles in their initial stretched position, proprioceptive neuromuscular facilitation stretching procedures call for the prestretched muscle or group of muscles to contract for approximately six seconds. This contraction is isometric in nature since the muscle position remains fixed or held constant (by the assistant) during contraction. The six-second contraction is considered phase one. Immediately following the completing of the six-second isometric contraction, the active muscles should be passively stretched (see Figure 8.2).

The process of actively contracting a muscle or muscles before they are passively stretched helps the stretched muscle(s) to experience **autogenic inhibition.** Autogenic inhibition is a reflex muscle relaxation that occurs in the contracting muscle(s) as a result of the Golgi ten-

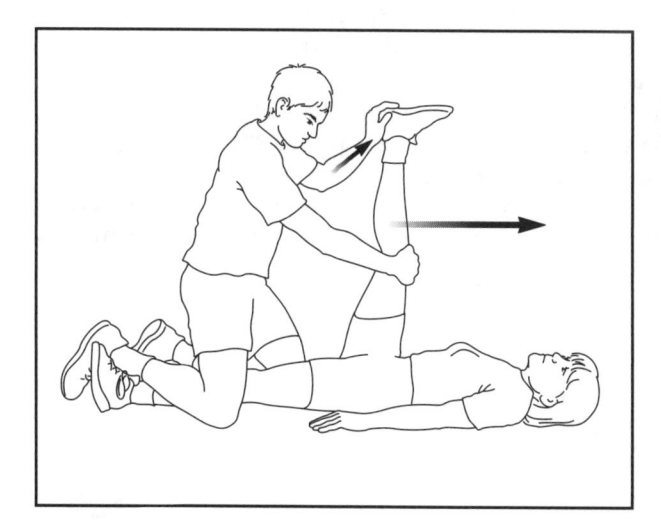

Figure 8.1 ■ PNF - Initial Position

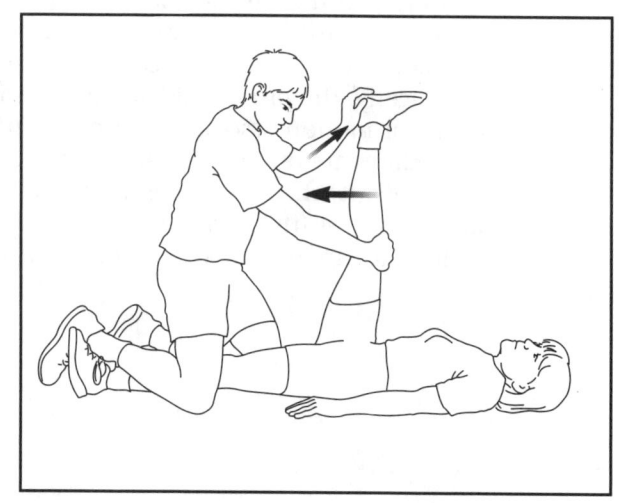

Figure 8.2 ■ PNF - Isometric Contraction

don organs being stimulated during concentric contraction or tension build up. The isometric action of the stretched muscle is referred to as *hold*, while the concentric contraction of the stretched muscle is referred to as *contract*. This duel referencing contributes to the multiple methods, and often confusing methods, of referring to this phase of the PNF procedure.

Following the six-second isometric contraction, the muscle is passively elongated (see Figure 8.3). Passive elongation is considered the second phase of the PNF procedure. Passive elongations require the assistance of a partner, who applies a slow, constant pressure or force directed in such a manner as to statically stretch the muscle tissue. This process is referred to as the *Relax* Phase of the PNF procedure.

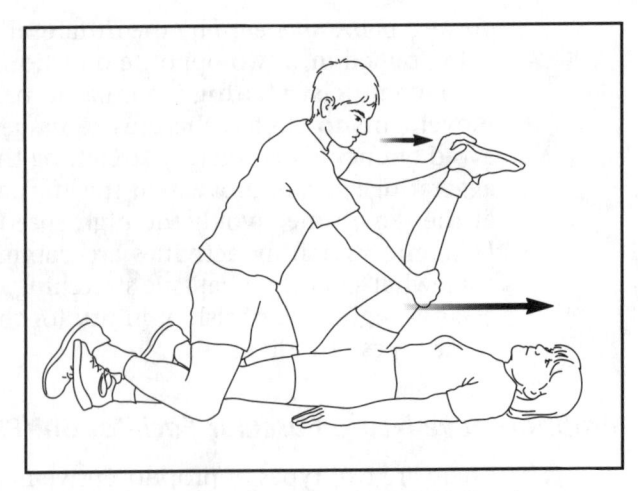

Figure 8.3 ■ PNF - Passive Stretch Following Contraction

The partner-assisted passive stretching occurring during the *Relax* phase may also be accompanied by agonistic muscle contraction by the subject. Contracting the agonist muscle group leads to an active elongation, by the subject, of the stretched tissue. It is believed that the agonistic contraction will help elicit **reciprocal inhibition** in the antagonist muscle(s) or, in this situation, the muscles being passively stretched. Reciprocal inhibition may be defined as a muscle relaxation that occurs in the muscle or muscles that act in opposition to the muscle(s) experiencing increased tension or contraction. In less scientific parlance, reciprocal inhibition helps relax the muscle(s) being passively stretched by contracting the muscle that normally acts in opposition to them. During the *Relax* phase of PNF, the muscle tissue being passively stretched should remain elongated or stretched for 10 to 30 seconds following isometric contraction.

PNF is an effective method of increasing flexibility. While opinions vary as to whether it is superior to static or ballistic stretching protocols, most would suggest it is a superior procedure for developing flexibility (ACSM, 2001; Holcomb, 2000).

PNF is associated with increased muscle soreness and injury (ACSM, 2000). The soreness may be associated, in part, with the eccentric or isometric contraction phase of the procedure. At one time, maximal contraction at end-ROM was recommended and may have contributed to the majority of the muscular soreness. Current practice is to restrict maximal isometric contractions during the contraction phase of the procedure, especially at end range of motion. Like static stretching, a PNF protocol should include at least four repetitions for each stretch, three to five times per week, for each muscle group.

Clearly, the primary advantage of the PNF stretching procedure is the increased gains in range of motion associated with it. Unfortunately, there are numerous disadvantages. PNF procedures are often difficult to teach and, in most cases, require the assistance of a partner. Additionally, the procedures are associated with more personal discomfort, muscle soreness, and muscle stiffness than that associated with static stretching. Finally, PNF stretching procedures are more time-consuming than static stretching methods.

Laboratory Activities

CHAPTER 8

Name: _____ Class Time/Day: _____ Score: _____

LABORATORY 8-A

Flexibility: Shoulder and Wrist Elevation

- **Purpose:** This test measures shoulder and wrist flexibility.

- **Precautions:** Individuals with shoulder joint or shoulder girdle limitations should consult with the instructor before participating. Individuals should warmup properly before participating.

- **Equipment:** Yardstick and cloth tape measure.

- **Procedure:** Place the subject in a prone position, face down with his/her arms extended. The subject should grasp the yardstick, shoulder width apart. Then the subject should raise the yardstick upward as high as possible, keeping the elbows extended and his/her chin on the floor. When the subject reaches his/her highest point, the assistant, using the tape measure, measures the distance from the bottom of the yardstick to the floor (see Figure 8.4). Finally, the assistant should measure the subject's arm length as it hangs naturally down by the subject's side. The arm measurement should be recorded from the acromion process of the shoulder to the tip of the middle finger. All measurements should be made to the nearest quarter-inch.

- **Scoring:** The subject's score represents the best of the three shoulder elevation measurements subtracted from the arm length. The closer to zero, the better the score. Determine the normative rating by using Table 8-2.

- **Data/Calculations:**

Name: _____   Date: __/__/__

Gender: _____ Age: _____ Height: _____ Weight: _____

Trial	Arm Length*		Shoulder Elevation	Score
1.		—		
2.		—		
3.		—		

*Arm length is measured (in inches) from acromion process to tip of middle finger.

Best score: _____   Rating: _____

Table 8-2 ■ Normative Values by Gender for Shoulder and Wrist Elevation

Rating	Shoulder and Wrist Elevation
	Men
Excellent	6–0
Good	8¼–6¼
Average	11½–8½
Fair	12½–11¾
Poor	12¾ and above
	Women
Excellent	5½–0
Good	7½–5¾
Average	10¾–7¾
Fair	11¾–11
Poor	12 and above

From Johnson & Nelson *Practical Measurements for Evaluation in Physical Education.* Copyright © 1986 by Allyn and Bacon.

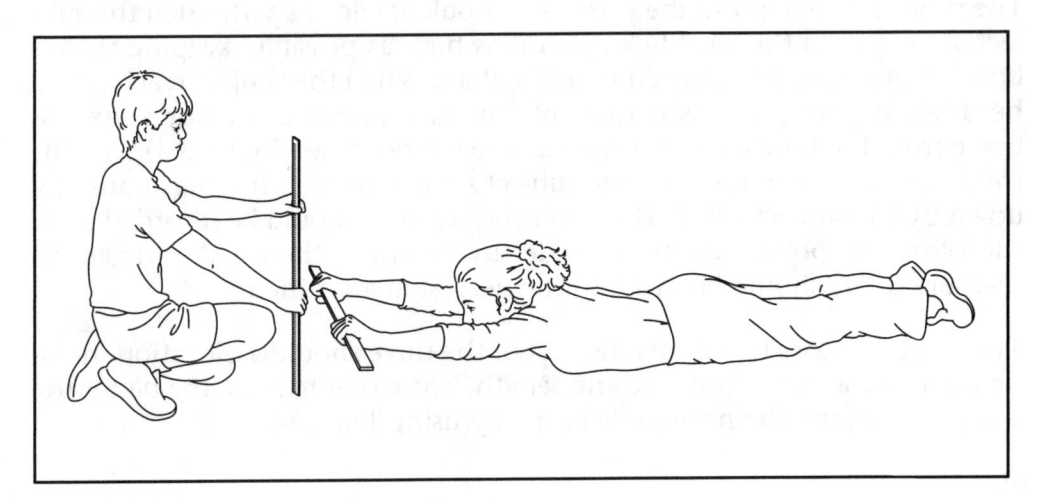

Figure 8.4 ■ Shoulder and Wrist Elevation

Name: _____ Class Time/Day: _____ Score: _____

LABORATORY 8-B

Flexibility: Trunk and Neck Extension

- **Purpose:** This test measures an individual's ability to extend the trunk and neck.

- **Precautions:** Individuals with trunk and neck limitations should consult with the class instructor before participating. Individuals should warmup properly before participating.

- **Equipment:** Yardstick or cloth measuring tape.

- **Procedure:** Two measurements are needed. The first measure represents the trunk extension score. To determine this measure, place the subject prone position, face down on the mat with your hands resting in the small of the back. The subject should raise his/her trunk upward as high as possible from the floor while keeping the hips stationary to the floor. The assistant should measure the vertical distance between the mat and the tip of the nose (see Figure 8.5). A second measurement of the subject's trunk and neck length must be determined. Position the subject in a chair or on the floor with legs fully extended. Precaution should be taken to keep the back straight and eyes looking directly forward. Measure from the tip of the nose to the seat of the chair (or floor). All measurements should be made to the nearest quarter-inch.

- **Scoring:** The best of the three trunk extension scores subtracted from the trunk and neck length represents the subject's score. The closer to zero, the better the score. Determine the normative rating by using Table 8-3.

- **Data/Calculation:**

Name: Date: /   /

Gender: Age: Height: Weight:

Trial	Trunk and Neck Length*		Trunk Extension	Score
1.		—		
2.		—		
3.		—		

*Trunk and Neck length (Torso) is measured from the tip of the nose to the seat bottom.

Best score: _____   Rating: _____

Table 8-3 ■ Normative Values by Gender for Trunk and Neck Extension

Rating	Trunk and Neck Extension
	Men
Excellent	3–0
Good	6–3¼
Average	8–6¼
Fair	10–8¼
Poor	10¼ and above
	Women
Excellent	2–0
Good	5¾–2¼
Average	7¾–6
Fair	9¾–8
Poor	10 and above

From Johnson & Nelson *Practical Measurements for Evaluation in Physical Education.* Copyright © 1986 by Allyn and Bacon.

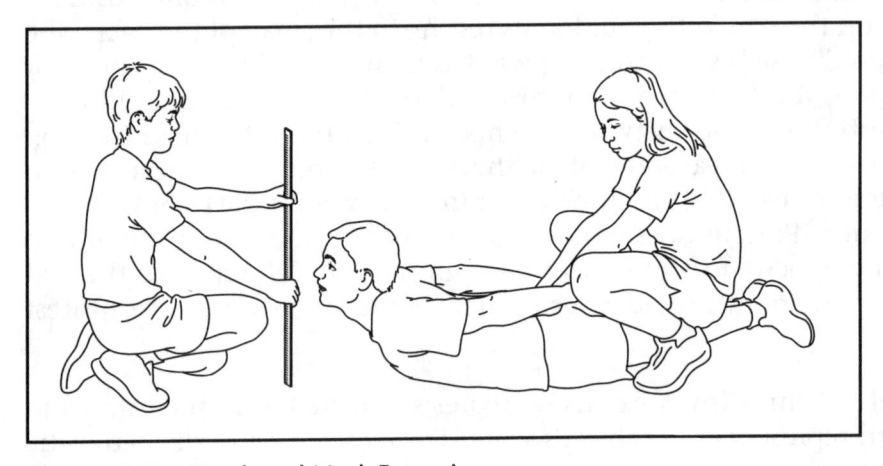

Figure 8.5 ■ Trunk and Neck Extension

Name: _____ Class Time/Day: _____ Score: _____

LABORATORY 8-C

Flexibility: Ankle Plantar Flexion

- **Purpose:** This test measures ankle extension or plantar flexion.

- **Precautions:** Individuals with a history of ankle injuries or limitations should consult with the class instructor before participating. Individuals should warmup properly before participating.

- **Equipment:** Yardstick or cloth tape measure.

- **Procedure:** The subject should remove his/her shoes and take a seated position on the floor with one leg extended straight out. Two measurements should be made. All measurements are made to the nearest quarter-inch. The first measurement is made from the floor to the lowest point of the tibia (shin bone). The second measurement is made from the floor to the highest point of the foot (toes or arch of the instep) while the foot if fully plantar flexed (see Figure 8.6). Repeat the procedure on the other leg.

- **Scoring:** The difference between the foot and shin measurements for each leg should be determined. These scores are referred to as the average difference right foot score and average difference left foot scores, respectively. Average the right foot difference score with the left foot difference score. This value represents the subject's final plantar flexion score. Determine the normative rating by using Table 8-4.

- **Data/Calculations:**

Name: _____   Date: / /

Gender: _____ Age: _____ Height: _____ Weight: _____

Right leg

Trial	Highest (Foot) Measure		Lowest (Shin) Measure	Right Foot Score
1.		—		
2.		—		

Average Difference (Right Foot) Score = (Right Foot Score (trial 1) + Right Foot Score (trial 2)) / 2

Average Difference (Right Foot) Score = (_____ + _____) / 2

Average Difference (Right Foot) Score: _____

Left leg

Trial	Highest (Foot) Measure	Lowest (Shin) Measure	Right Foot Score
1.		—	
2.		—	

Average Difference (Left Foot) Score = (Left Foot Score (trial 1) + Left Foot Score (trial 2)) / 2

Average Difference (Left Foot) Score = (_____ + _____) / 2

Average Difference (Left Foot) Score: _____

****

Final Plantar Flexion Score = [Average Difference (Right Foot) + Average Difference (Left Foot)] / 2

Final Plantar Flexion Score = (_____ + _____) / 2

Final Score: _____

Normative Rating: _____

Table 8-4 ■ Normative Values by Gender for Ankle Plantar Flexion

Rating	Ankle Plantar Flexion
Men	
Excellent	¾ and below
Good	1½–1
Average	2–1¾
Fair	3–2¼
Poor	3¼ and above
Women	
Excellent	½ and below
Good	1¼–1½
Average	1¾–1½
Fair	2¼–2
Poor	2½ and above

From Johnson, B. & Nelson, J. *Practical Measurements for Evaluation in Physical Education.* Copyright © 1986 by Allyn and Bacon.

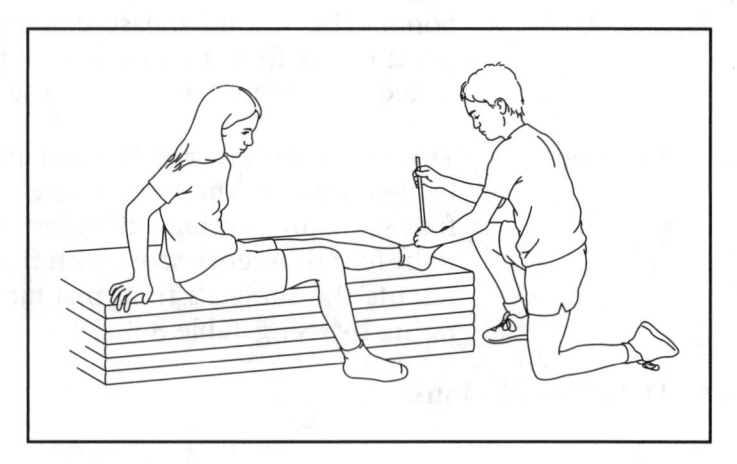

Figure 8.6 ■ Ankle Plantar Flexion

Name: _____ Class Time/Day: _____ Score: _____

LABORATORY 8-D

Flexibility: Ankle Dorsi Flexion

- **Purpose:** This test measures ankle flexion or dorsiflexion.

- **Precautions:** Individuals with a history of ankle injuries or limitations should consult with the class instructor before participating. Individuals should warmup properly before participating.

- **Equipment:** Yardstick or cloth measuring tape.

- **Procedure:** Two measurements should be made. First, standing height is determined by measuring from the chin to the floor with the subject standing erect looking forward. The second measure, the leaning measurement, is the maximum distance taken from the toe line to the wall. This measure is taken with the subject standing as far back from the wall as possible, keeping the heels on the floor, while leaning into the wall, touching the wall with hands, chin, and chest (see Figure 8.7). Precaution should be taken to keep the body and legs straight and the heels flat on the floor. Three leaning measurements should be taken. All measurements should be taken to the nearest quarter-inch.

- **Scoring:** The best leaning measure subtracted from the standing height represents the subject's score. Determine the normative rating by using Table 8-5.

- **Data/Calculations:**

Name: _____   Date: __/__/__

Gender: _____ Age: _____ Height: _____ Weight: _____

Standing Height (inches): _____

Best Lean Measurement (inches): _____

Trial	Lean Measure
1.	
2.	
3.	

Ankle Dorsiflexion Score = Standing height (inches) − best lean measure (inches)

Ankle Dorsiflexion Score = _____ − _____

Ankle Dorsiflexion Score: _____

Normative Rating: _____

Table 8-5 ■ Normative Values by Gender for Ankle Dorsi Flexion

Rating	Ankle Dorsi Flexion
Men	
Excellent	26½ and below
Good	29½–26¾
Average	32½–29¾
Fair	35¼–32¾
Poor	35½ and above
Women	
Excellent	24¼ and below
Good	26½–24½
Average	30¼–26¾
Fair	31¾–30½
Poor	32 and above

Source: Modified from Johnson, B. and Nelson, J. (1986). *Practical Measurements for Evaluation in Physical Education.* Minneapolis: Burgess Publishing.

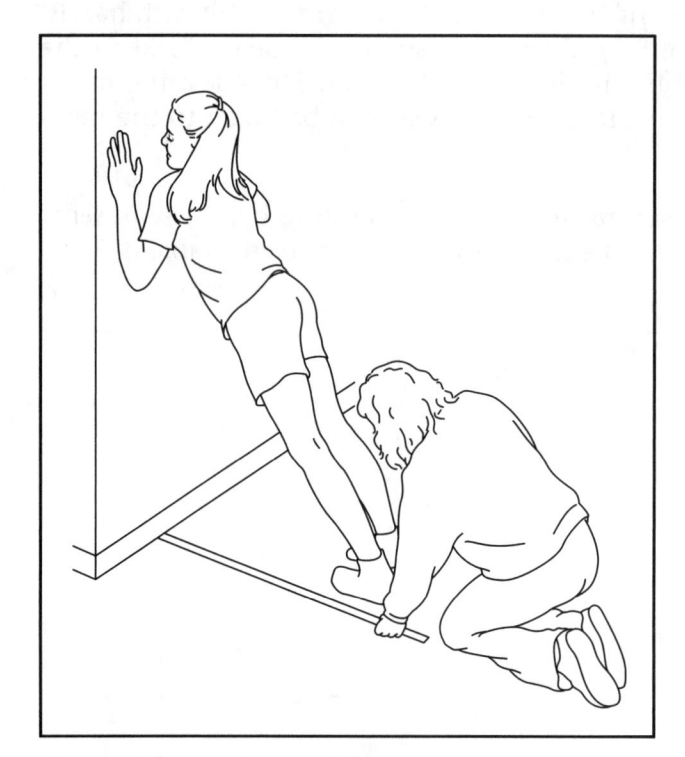

Figure 8.7 ■ Ankle Doral Flexion

Name: _____ Class Time/Day: _____ Score: _____

LABORATORY 8-E

Flexibility: Modified (Accuflex) Sit And Reach

- **Purpose:** This test measures hip and back flexion, as well as extension of the hamstring muscles of the legs. This test is designed to see how far an individual can extend the fingertips beyond the foot line with legs extended.

- **Precautions:** Individuals with trunk limitations should consult with the class instructor before participating. Individuals should warm up properly before participating.

- **Equipment:** Accuflex sit and reach box.

- **Procedure:** Secure the slide bar on the Accuflex sit and reach box with the pin provided. The subject sits on the floor, with his/her shoes removed, and his/her legs extended straight against the Accuflex sit and reach box. His/her back should be placed straight against the wall. The subject places the index finger of both hands together and slowly reaches forward, as far as possible, on the box while holding his/her position on the wall. An assistant should slide the reach indicator along the top of the box until it touches the subject's fingers. Allowing the head and back to move off the wall, the subject should gradually stretch forward as far a possible (see Figure 8.8). The final stretch should be held for several seconds. The tip of the fingers should be measured as the position is held. The knees must be straight and the legs and hips must remain in contact with the floor at all times.

- **Scoring:** The average of two trials, measured to the nearest quarter-inch or cm, represents the subject's score. Use scale C to measure in inches and scale E to measure in centimeters. Determine the normative rating by using Table 8-6 for measurements taken in inches, and Table 8-7 for measurements take in cm.

- **Data/Calculations:**

Name: _____   Date: / /

Gender: _____   Age: _____   Height: _____   Weight: _____

Trial	Distance
1.	
2.	

Average score/ reach: _____   Rating: _____

213

Fitness Classification: _____

Flexibility Percentile Score: _____

Table 8-6 ■ Normative Values by Age and Gender for Sit and Reach Box (Inches*)

Classification	Percentile	18–25	26–35	Age 36–45	46–55	56–65	> 65
				Men			
Excellent	90	22	21	21	19	17	17
	80	20	19	19	17	15	15
Above Average	70	19	17	17	15	13	13
	60	18	17	16	14	13	12
Average	50	17	15	15	13	11	10
	40	15	14	13	11	9	9
Below Average	30	14	13	13	10	9	8
	20	13	11	11	9	7	7
Poor	10	11	9	7	6	5	4
				Women			
Excellent	90	24	23	22	21	20	20
	80	22	21	21	20	19	18
Above Average	70	21	20	19	18	17	17
	60	20	20	18	17	16	17
Average	50	19	19	17	16	15	15
	40	18	17	16	14	14	14
Below Average	30	17	16	15	14	13	13
	20	16	15	14	12	11	11
Poor	10	14	13	12	10	9	9

*Use scale C on the Accuflex sit and reach box to measure in inches.

From: *ACSM's Guidelines For Exercise Testing and Prescription,* 6th Edition. 2000. Philadelphia: Lippincott, Williams, & Wilkins.

Table 8-7 ■ Normative Values by Age and Gender for Sit and Reach Box (cm*)

Classification	Percentile	Age 20–29	30–39	40–49	50–59	60–69
Men						
Excellent	90	42	40	37	38	35
	80	38	37	34	32	30
Above Average	70	36	34	30	29	26
	60	33	32	28	27	24
Average	50	31	29	25	25	22
	40	29	27	23	22	18
Below Average	30	26	24	20	18	16
	20	23	21	16	15	14
Poor	10	18	17	12	12	11
Women						
Excellent	90	43	42	40	40	37
	80	40	39	37	37	34
Above Average	70	28	37	35	35	31
	60	26	35	33	32	30
Average	50	34	33	31	30	28
	40	32	31	29	29	26
Below Average	30	29	28	26	26	24
	20	26	25	24	23	23
Poor	10	22	21	19	19	18

*Use scale E on the Accuflex sit and reach box to measure in cm.

From: *ACSM's Guidelines For Exercise Testing and Prescription*, 6th Edition. 2000. Philadelphia: Lippincott, Williams, & Wilkins.

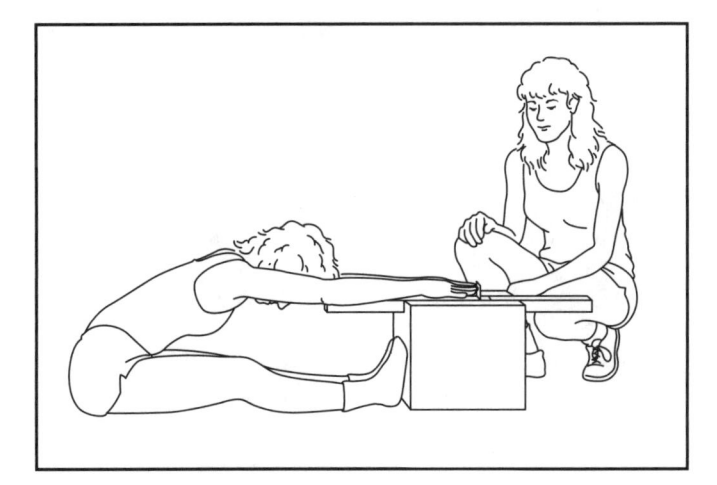

Figure 8.8 ■ Modified (Accuflex) Sit and Reach

9

Flexibility Activities

People who are sedentary have twice the risk of heart disease of those who are physically active.
Center for Disease Control and Prevention

■ Chapter Outline ■

Stretching Protocols: General Guidelines
    Static Stretching Activities
        Contraindicated Static Stretching
            Activities
                Plough
                Hurdler's Stretch
                Full or Deep Knee Squats or
                    Lunges
                Standing Straight Legged Toe
                    Touch
                Standing Straight Legged
                    Straddle Toe Touch
                Full Neck Rolls
                Waist Circles
                Back Bends (Bridges)
        Recommended Static Stretching
            Activities
                Feet
                    Plantar Arch
                    Anterior Foot and Toes
                Lower Legs
                    Anterior Lower Leg
                    Lateral Lower Leg
                    Posterior Lower Leg
                Upper Legs
                    Anterior Upper Leg
                    Posterior Upper Leg
                    Adductors
                Hips

                Back and Trunk
                    Supine Single Leg Trunk
                      Rotation
                    Supine Double Leg Hip
                      Rotation
                    Cat Stretch
                    Double Leg Hip Flexion
                    Single Leg Hip Flexion
                Neck
                    Anterior
                    Lateral
                    Posterior
                Chest
                Shoulders
                    Anterior
                    Posterior
                Arms
                    Anterior (Biceps)
                    Posterior (Triceps)
    Ballistic Stretching Activities
    Proprioceptive Neuromuscular
        Facilitation Stretching Activities
            Upper Leg
                Anterior
                Posterior
            Lower Back
            Chest
            Shoulders
            Adductors

Learning Objectives

The student should be able to:

- Identify three common procedures of flexibility training.
- Identify selected variables that influence flexibility.
- Identify general guidelines that need to be incorporated into any flexibility training program.
- Identify static stretching activities for each major muscle group.
- Identify contraindicated static stretching activities and describe their potential risk.
- Identify proprioceptive neuromuscular facilitation (PNF) stretching activities for selected major muscle groups.

Keywords

Ballistic stretching

Proprioceptive neuromuscular facilitation stretching

Static stretching

Stretching Protocols: General Guidelines

Static Stretching Activities

Recall, there are three common procedures of flexibility training. These include ballistic, static, and proprioceptive neuromuscular facilitation. Specific guidelines to each procedure have been described in Chapter 8. For reader ease, the recommended flexibility activities have been grouped according to specific flexibility training procedure.

It is important to emphasize that these activities are recommendations only. Individual differences in factors such as age, existing joint range of motion, disabilities, and muscular strength and endurance may influence the appropriateness of the activities. Activities that present greater risk of injury have been identified. These activities should be avoided (see Contraindicated Static Stretching Activities).

Individuals presenting recent soft tissue injuries to either the musculotendinous unit (strain) or ligaments (sprains) should avoid participation. Those presenting joint inflammation resulting from infections, known or suspected osteoporosis, unusual or unexplained tissue discomfort during elongation or other types of medical complications should limit flexibility training until they have established medical clearance.

To allow for maximal benefit and minimal risk of injury, several general guidelines should be followed. These guidelines may be fitted to any of the procedures or recommended flexibility activities.

As may be expected, first and foremost, is to establish medical clearance before beginning any flexibility training program. Any limitations and/or precautions should be clearly identified and understood by the participant and the exercise leader (if appropriate).

Warmup before any stretching activities. Warm-up activities, such as light calisthenics and walking/jogging are appropriate. The critical issue is to raise core body temperature. The exact time and nature of required warm-up activities may vary. When possible, identify the muscle groups you intend to include in flexibility training. Be sure these muscle groups are adequately warmed up **before** stretching activities are performed.

Wear clothes that are non-restrictive. All joint structures should be able to move through a full range of motion. Avoid footwear and exercise mats that allow skidding. Unwanted slipping of body parts such as feet or hands may result in injury.

Perform all stretching routines in a controlled, slow, and non-jerky manner. Never bounce or force a muscle through a range of motion. Focus your mind on the muscles involved. Try to relax the active tissue. Avoid rapid movements that may induce the stretch-reflex mechanism. Return from stretched positions slowly and carefully. Always determine the appropriate postural position to be used before beginning any stretching activity. Table 9.1 summarizes the sequence of action for static stretching activities.

Avoid breath holding. Normal, free breathing patterns should be included in flexibility training. It may be beneficial to control breathing. Many find it beneficial and relaxing to sequence a deep exhalation with the more extreme ranges of motion.

Finally, remember to use caution when relaxing a muscle from a stretched position. Always return a muscle slowly and carefully to its natural resting length. As in the case when stretching a muscle, avoid rapid and jerky movements.

Table 9-1: Sequence of Action for Static Stretching Activities

Step	Action
1	Assume the recommended body position and slowly stretch the selected muscle tissue to a point of end range of motion.
2	Slowly apply mild tension to passively stretch the selected muscle tissue to a point of mild discomfort. Slowly exhale during the stretch.
3	Hold the passive stretched position for 10–30 seconds.
4	Relax the tissue by slowly returning the selected muscle tissue to normal resting length.
5	Repeat steps 1–4 a minimum of 4 times per stretching activity.

Contraindicated Static Stretching Activities

Individual differences in variables such as age, soft tissue characteristics, muscular strength and endurance, disabilities and fitness levels may predetermine the appropriateness of some flexibility training activities. The exercises described below should be considered **inappropriate for general use.** Simply stated, they offer too much risk of injury for the general public.

That is not to say that some, if not all, of these flexibility training activities are not used by highly trained and fit individuals. This of course leads to much of the confusion surrounding these activities.

Individuals who regularly train or participate in activities such as dance, gymnastics, martial arts, wrestling, and yoga may find these higher risk training procedures present less risk of injury. This, of course, is a direct result of the advanced levels of flexibility training required for these activities. It must be emphasized; this finding is true for only those participants who have an established, advanced levels of flexibility. Participants new to these types of activities should use caution and train using the flexibility activities recommended for the general public.

Plough

Potential Risk: The plough flexibility training procedure places unwanted and unnecessarily high levels of strain on the cervical ligaments of the lower back (see Figure 9.1). Additionally, increased and potentially excessive pressure is placed on the cervical discs. The plough procedure should be considered extremely dangerous for individuals presenting a history of low back complications.

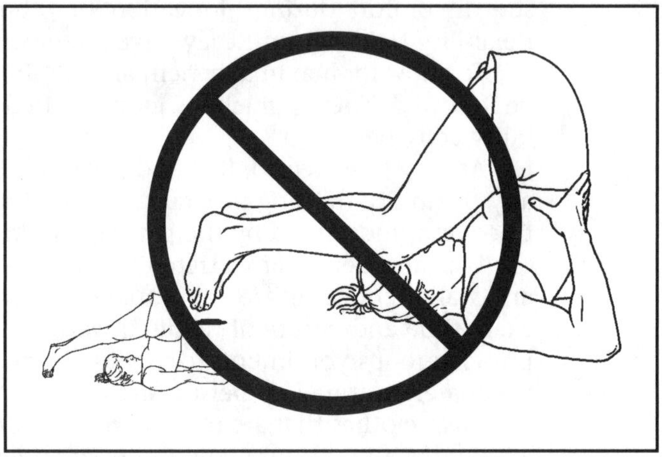

Figure 9.1 ■ Plough

Hurdler's Stretch

Potential Risk: The single or double legged hurdler's stretch (see Figure 9.2) places unwanted and unnecessarily high levels of strain on the medial collateral ligament of the knee. Additionally, increased and potentially excessive pressure is placed on the meniscus of the knee. This pressure leads to increased risk of meniscal tears. The hurdler's stretch should be considered extremely dangerous for individuals presenting a history of knee joint complications. This is particularly true for those with a history of ligamental and/or menisci trauma or tears.

Full or Deep Knee Squats or Lunges

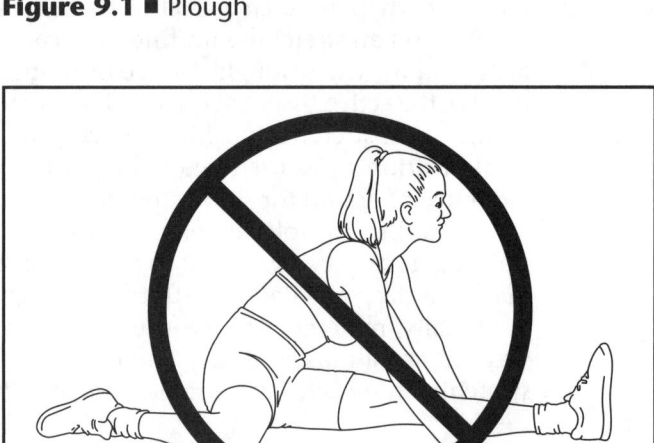

Figure 9.2 ■ Hurdlers Stretch

Potential Risk: Full or deep knee squats or lunges are defined as squatting or lunging movements that allow for knee flexion of 90 degree or greater (see Figure 9.3). A practical, easily observable criteria to prevent excessive knee flexion would be to limit movements that allow for the knee to be moved or positioned over the ankle. Full or deep knee squats or lunges place unwanted and unnecessarily high levels of strain on the lateral ligaments of the knee. Additionally, increased and potentially excessive

Figure 9.3 ■ Full or Deep Knee Squats or Lunges

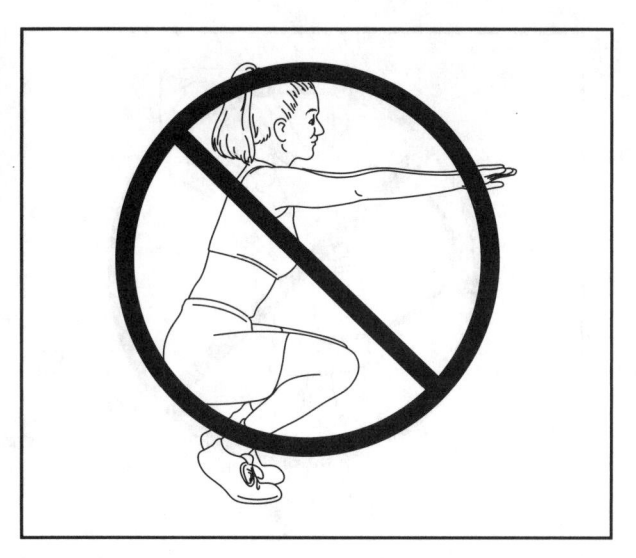

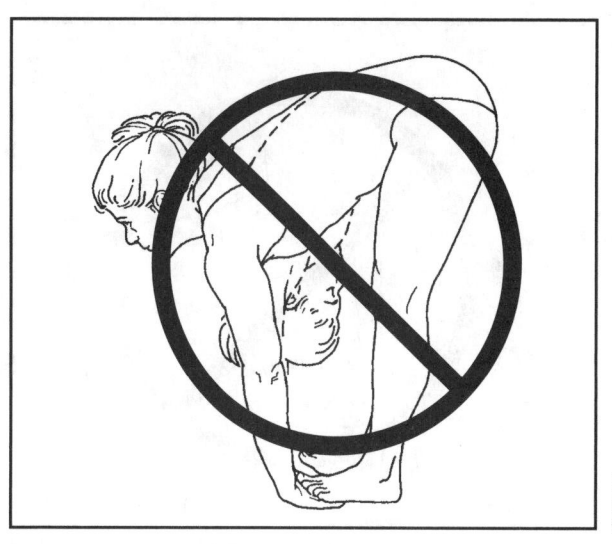

Figure 9.4 ■ Standing Straight Legged Toe Touch

patellar tendon forces, occurring during knee flexion, compress the patella (kneecap). This pressure leads to increased risk of chrondomalacia and/or meniscal tears. Full or deep knee squats or lunges should be considered extremely dangerous for individuals presenting a history of knee joint complications. This is particularly true for those with a history of ligamental and/or menisci trauma or tears.

Standing Straight Legged Toe Touch

Potential Risk: The standing straight legged toe touch flexibility procedure places unwanted and unnecessarily high levels of strain on the lumbar ligaments (see Figure 9.4). Additionally, increased and potentially excessive pressure is placed on the lumbar (lower vertebrae of the back) discs. The standing straight legged toe touch procedure should be considered extremely dangerous for individuals presenting a history of low back complications.

Standing Straight Legged Straddle Toe Touch

Potential Risk: Similar to the standing straight legged toe touch, the standing straight legged straddle toe touch flexibility procedure places unwanted and unnecessarily high levels of strain on the lumbar ligaments (see Figure 9.5). Additionally, increased and potentially excessive pressure is placed on the lumbar (lower vertebrae of the back) discs. If flexion occurs with rotation, such as in the case of moving the head toward one leg, shear or torsion forces are also placed on spinal disc. Lastly, the straddle position places unnecessarily high levels of strain on the medial collateral ligaments of the knees. The standing straight legged straddle toe touch procedure should be considered extremely dangerous for individuals presenting a history of low back and knee joint complications.

Full Neck Rolls

Potential Risks: Full neck rolls place unwanted and unnecessarily high levels of strain on the cervical ligaments (see Figure 9.6). Additionally, increased and potentially excessive pressure is placed on the cervical discs. Lastly, a

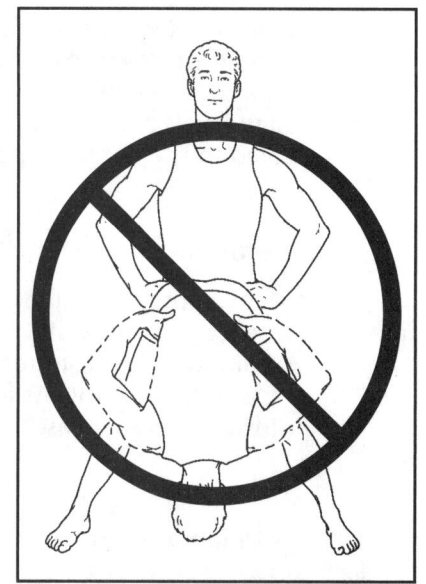

Figure 9.5 ■ Standing Straight Legged Straddle Toe Touch

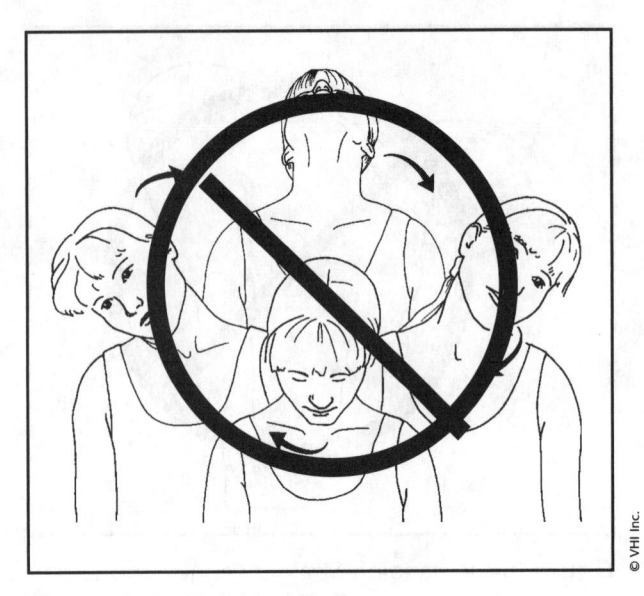

Figure 9.6 ■ Full Neck Rolls

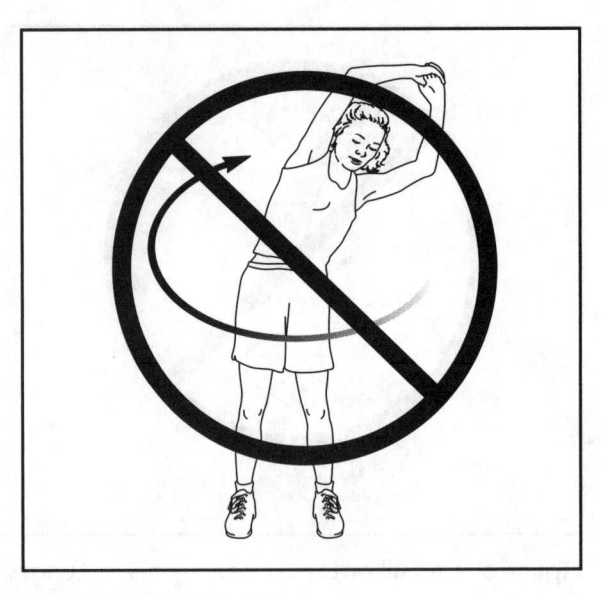

Figure 9.7 ■ Waist Circles

potential for arterial impingement may occur resulting in restricted blood flow and dizziness or syncope (temporary loss of consciousness).

Waist Circles

Potential Risks: Waist circles place unwanted and unnecessarily high levels of strain on the lower back musculature (see Figure 9.7). Additionally, increased and potentially excessive pressure is placed on the lumbar vertebrae of the lower back.

Back Bends (Bridges)

Potential Risks: Back bends (Bridges) hyperextend the lower back (see Figure 9.8). This action places unwanted and unnecessarily high levels of stress on the vertebral disc located in the lumbar region of the spine.

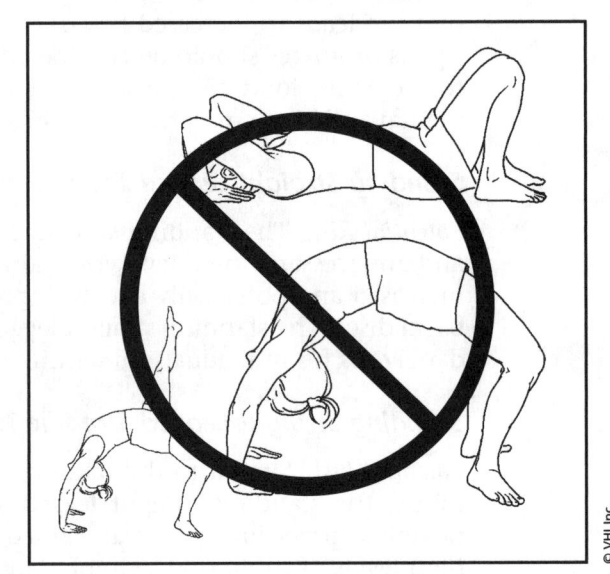

Figure 9.8 ■ Back Bends (Bridges)

Recommended Static Stretching Activities

Many appropriate static stretching activities could be recommended. If properly incorporated into a regular flexibility training program, each would allow for positive gains in joint range of motion. To illustrate and describe such a large number of procedures is beyond the scope of this manuscript. As a result, a sampling of the more common procedures has been provided. For reader ease, procedures have been grouped by body segment.

Feet

Plantar Arch

Procedure: Assume a standing position facing a wall. Stand approximately two feet away from the wall. Place your hands on the wall, at approximately chest level, in front of you for balance. While bending one leg, extend the other leg straight backward keeping the foot flat and pointed directly toward the wall. To stretch the plantar arch, raise the heel of the extended foot, bending the toes at the ball of the foot. Carefully shift more of your body weight onto the ball of this foot while pressing downward on the toes (see Figure 9.9). You should be able to control the tension of the stretch by how you shift your weight. Hold the stretch for approximately 10–30 seconds and then relax by shifting your weight off the extended leg to the nondominant foot. Repeat a minimum of four repetitions. Switch foot positions and repeat the procedure.

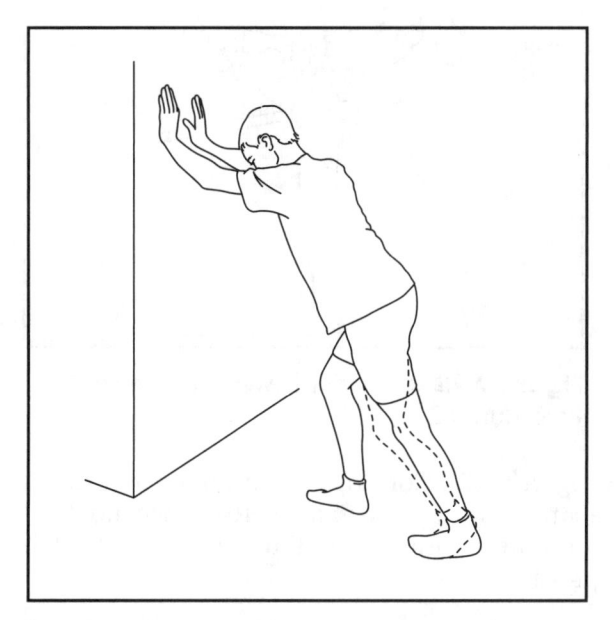

Figure 9.9 ■ Plantar Arch Stretch

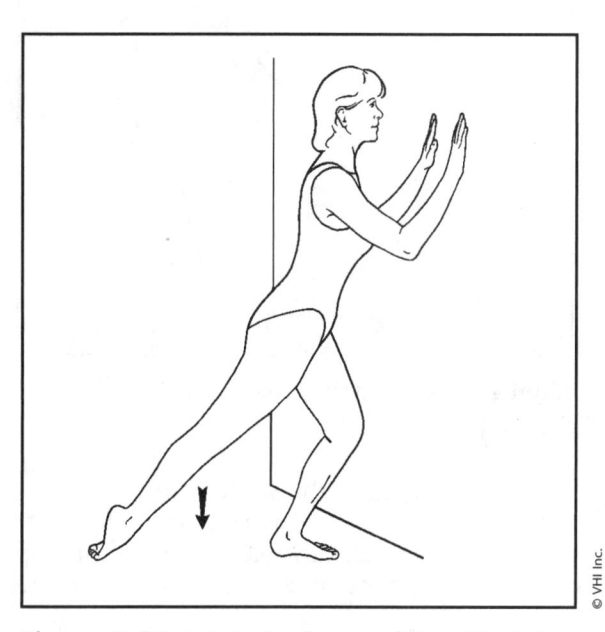

Figure 9.10 ■ Anterior Foot and Toes Stretch

Anterior Foot and Toes

Procedure: Assume a standing position with your body weight resting on a support leg. Position the other leg so the anterior foot and toes of the foot are plantar flexed or pointed and resting on the ground. Turn the toes of the foot under so the pressure can be felt on the top of the curled toes on the active leg. To stretch the anterior foot and toes, carefully shift your body weight onto the active leg, pressing downward on the top of the toes until tension is felt (see Figure 9.10). Hold the stretch for approximately 10–30 seconds and then relax by shifting your weight back to the support leg. Repeat a minimum of four repetitions. Switch foot positions and repeat the procedure.

Lower Legs

Anterior Lower Leg

Procedure #1: One of the more common methods of stretching the anterior aspect of the lower leg is to simply assume a kneeling position and then sit back on your heels while your feet are plantar flexed (see Figure 9.11). The feet may be placed directly on the floor or on a flat cushion or other soft surface. Shifting body weight on or off the heels controls the tension of the stretch. Hold the stretch for approximately 10–30 seconds and then relax by leaning forward and shifting body weight onto the knees. Repeat a minimum of four repetitions. **This activity should be considered contraindicated and avoided for individuals presenting knee limitations.**

Procedure #2: An alternative method of stretching the anterior aspect of the lower leg for individuals with knee limitations is to assume a sitting position in a chair or bench of normal height. Cross one leg and rest the ankle of this leg on the knee of the support leg. Plantar flex the foot of this leg. Grasp the toes of the foot on the crossed leg with one hand and the ankle with the other. Slowly pull the toes of the foot toward your body while stabilizing

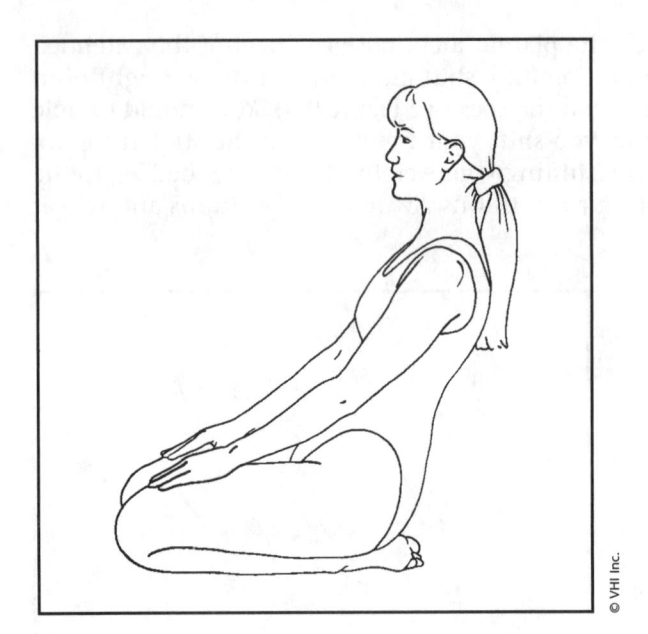

Figure 9.11 ■ Anterior Lower Leg Stretch Procedure #1

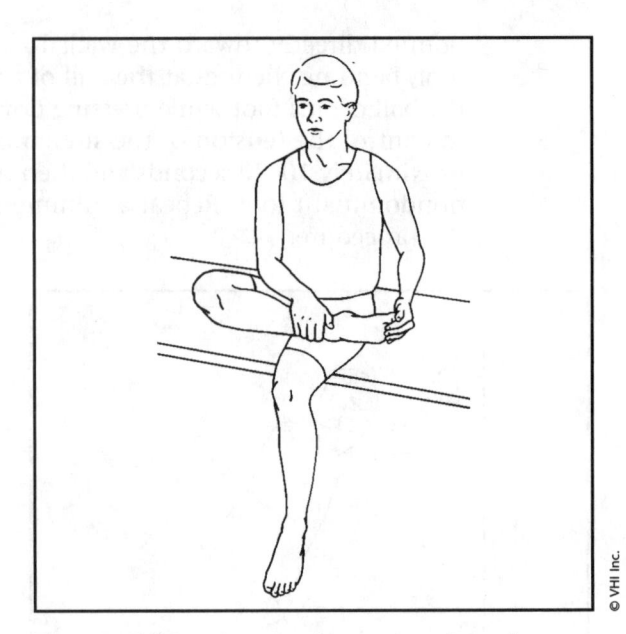

Figure 9.12 ■ Anterior Lower Leg Stretch Procedure #2

the leg at the ankle with the other hand (see Figure 9.12). Control the tension of the stretch by how hard you pull on the foot. Hold the stretch for approximately 10–30 seconds and then relax by releasing the pull. Repeat the procedure a minimum of four repetitions. Switch leg, foot, and hand positions and repeat the procedure.

Lateral Lower Leg

Procedure: To stretch the lateral (outside) aspect of the lower leg, assume a sitting position in a chair or bench of normal height. Cross one leg and rest the ankle of this leg on the knee of the support leg. Grasp the toes and outside portion of the foot on the crossed leg with one hand and the ankle with the other. Slowly invert the foot toward your body while stabilizing the leg at the ankle with the other hand (see Figure 9.13). Control the tension of the stretch by how hard you pull and lift the foot during inversion. Hold the stretch for approximately 10–30 seconds and then relax by releasing the pull. Repeat the procedure a minimum of four repetitions. Switch leg, foot, and hand positions and repeat the procedure.

Posterior Lower Leg

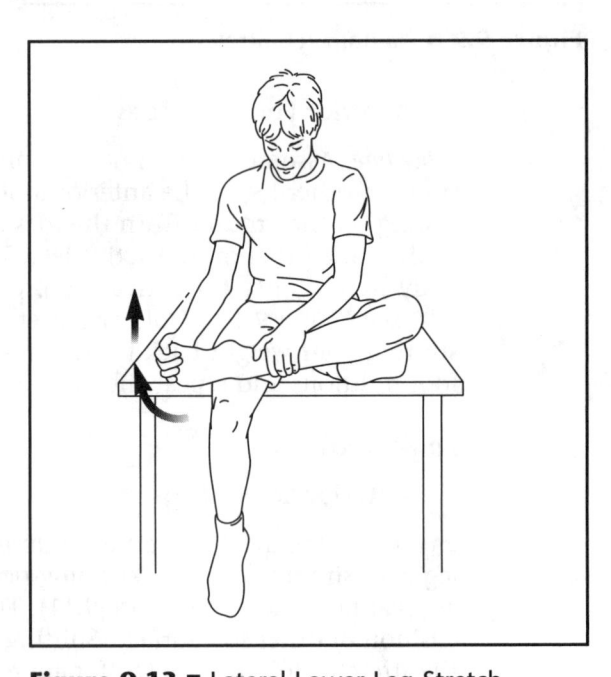

Figure 9.13 ■ Lateral Lower Leg Stretch

Procedure: Assume a standing position facing a wall. Stand several feet away from the wall. Place your hands on the wall, at approximately chest level, in front of you for balance. While bending one leg, fully extend the other leg straight backward keeping the foot flat and pointed directly toward the wall until your body is linearly extended from head to foot. To stretch the posterior lower leg, carefully shift your body weight forward while keeping the foot of the extended leg flat on the floor (see Figure 9.14). You should be able to control the tension of the stretch by how you shift your weight. Hold the stretch for approximately 10–30 seconds and then relax by shifting your weight off the extended leg to the nondominant foot. Repeat a minimum of four repetitions.

Switch foot positions and repeat the procedure. **Individuals presenting physical limitations with their knees should avoid locking out the knee on the extended leg.**

Upper Legs

Anterior Upper Leg

Procedure: Assume a standing position facing a wall. Stand approximately two feet from the wall. Extend one arm, at approximately chest level, in front of you for balance. Shift your body weight to the nonactive leg or the leg opposite of the extended arm. Bend your knee and raise the heel of the active leg toward your buttocks. Reach behind your hip with the same side arm as the active leg and grasp the raised foot of the active leg. To stretch the anterior upper leg muscles, collectively referred to as the quadriceps, lift or pull up on the heel bringing it toward your buttocks (see Figure 9.15). **Individuals presenting physical limitations with their knees should avoid fixing the active leg against the support leg during stretching.** To help eliminate risk of injury to the active knee, allow the knee of the active leg to drift backwards, hyperextending the active upper leg at the hip. Control the tension of the stretch by controlling the magnitude of the lifting force. Hold each stretch for approximately 10–30 seconds and then relax by releasing and lowering the heel of the active foot. Repeat a minimum of four repetitions. Switch foot and hand positions and repeat the procedure.

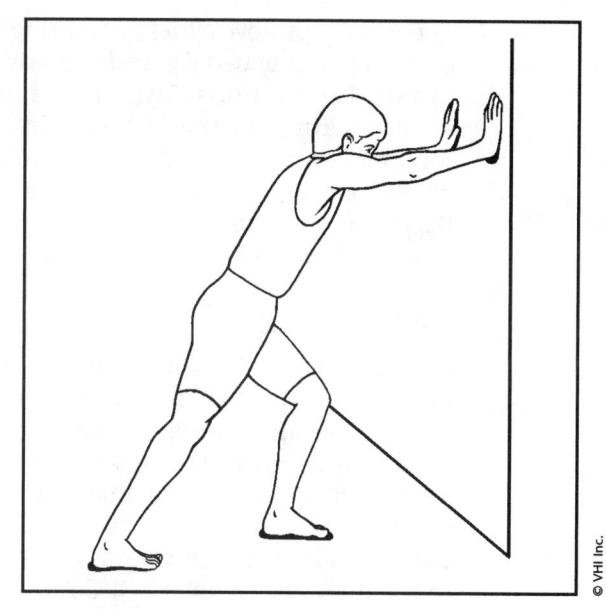

Figure 9.14 ■ Posterior Lower Leg Stretch

Posterior Upper Leg

Procedure: Assume a standing position facing a bench or chair of standard height. Shift your body weight to your support leg and raise the active leg and rest the heel of the foot of this leg on the surface of the chair or bench. To stretch the posterior upper leg muscles, collectively referred to as the hamstrings, keep both legs straight and bend forward at the waist, lowering your head and upper body to the raised leg. Precaution should be taken to keep your back straight (see Figure 9.16). Control the tension of the stretch by how far you lower your

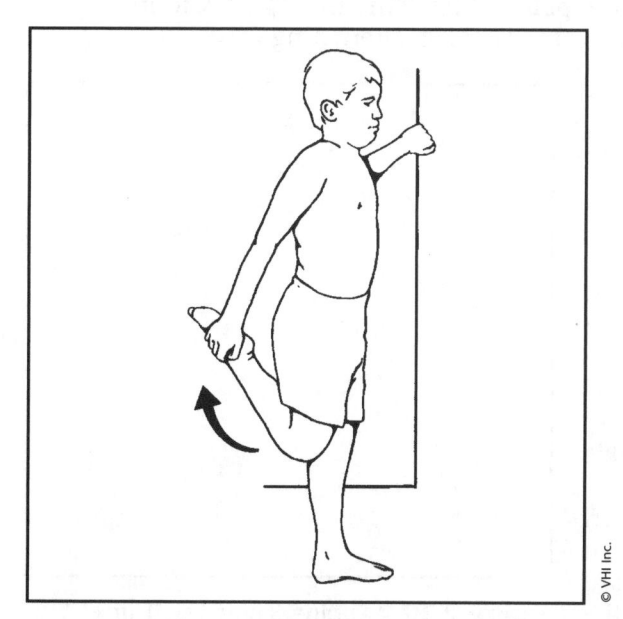

Figure 9.15 ■ Anterior Upper Leg Stretch

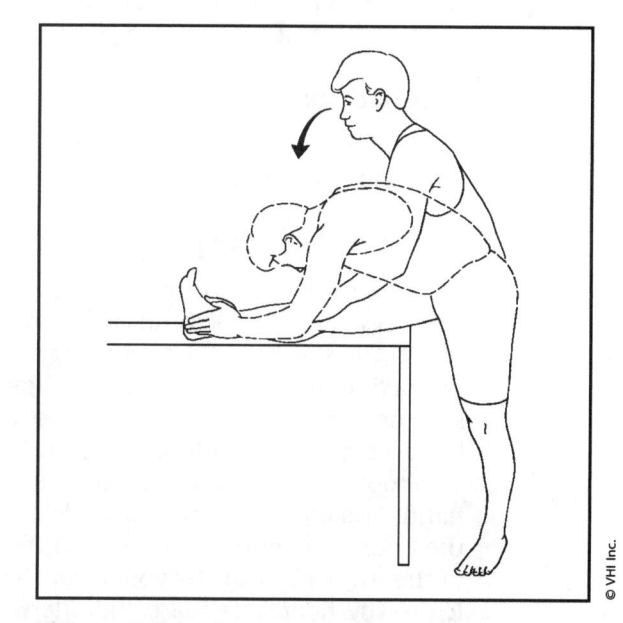

Figure 9.16 ■ Posterior Upper Leg Stretch

upper body or how closely you bring your upper body to the extended leg. **Individuals presenting physical limitations with their knees should avoid locking out the knees.** Hold each stretch for approximately 10–30 seconds and then relax by lifting your upper body and standing back up. Repeat a minimum of four repetitions. Switch foot and leg positions and repeat the procedure.

Adductors

Procedure: Assume a sitting position on the floor. Bring the soles of both feet together by flexing both knees and pulling the heels of the feet toward your crotch and buttocks. Keeping your back fully extended, place your elbows and lower arms on the same side knee. To stretch the adductors, use your elbows and lower arms to press your knees to the floor (see Figure 9.17). Control the tension of the stretch by how much pressure you place

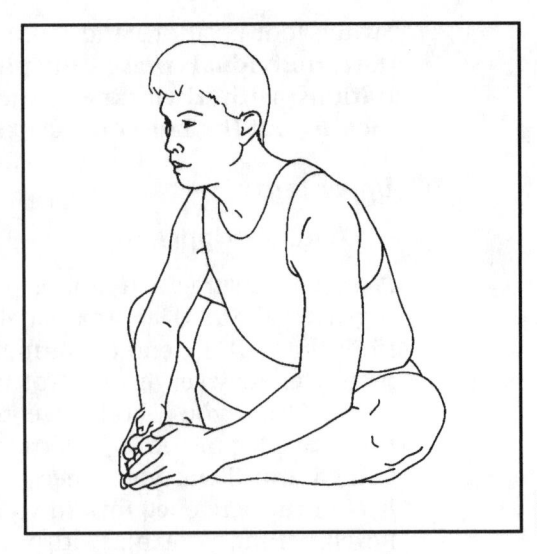

Figure 9.17 ■ Adductor Stretch

on the knees and how much you lower the knees toward the floor. Hold each stretch for approximately 10–30 seconds and then relax by releasing pressure and raising your knees. Repeat a minimum of four repetitions.

Hips

Procedure: Assume a supine position on your back with both legs fully extended. To stretch the hip, flex one leg at the hip until the knee is directly over the hip. Grasp the flexed leg at the knee and ankle and slowly externally rotate the knee outward while simultaneously pulling the ankle to the opposite shoulder until the lower leg is held at approximately 90-degrees. Keep the head and

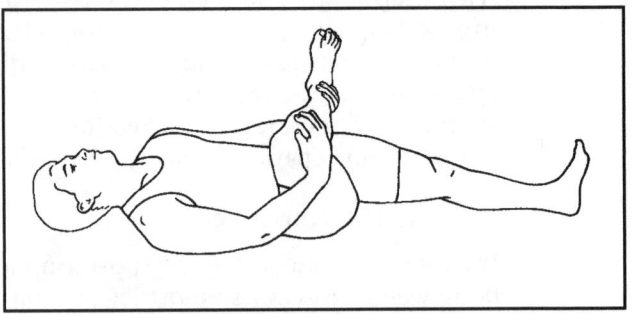

Figure 9.18 ■ Hip Stretch

shoulders flat on the floor at all times (see Figure 9.18). Hold each stretch for approximately 10–30 seconds and then relax by releasing the pull and lowering the leg back to its original position. Repeat a minimum of four repetitions for each leg, alternating legs.

Back and Trunk

The following procedures describe those recommended in Chapter 12—Low Back Pain.

Supine Single Leg Trunk Rotation

Assume a supine position on your back with both legs fully extended and each arm abducted out to the side, to a 90-degree angle from the long axis of the body. To stretch the lower back, keep one leg fully extended and cross the other leg over it at the hip level bringing the ankle and foot of the crossed leg to the extended hand. The hip of the crossed leg will rotate off the floor (see Figure 9.19). Control the tension of the stretch by how far you lower the crossed leg to the floor. The head, shoulders, and the

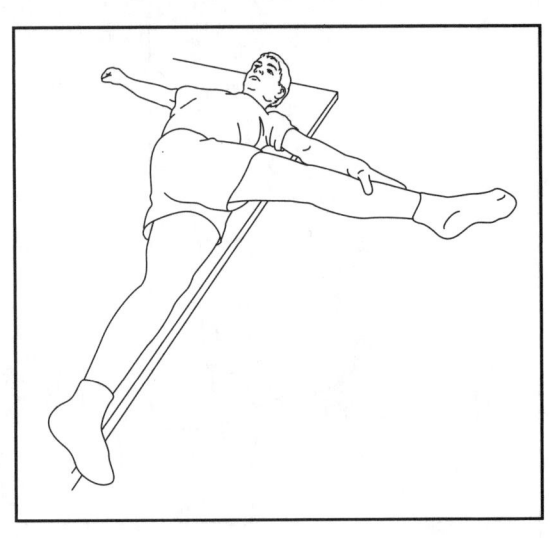

Figure 9.19 ■ Supine Single Leg Trunk Rotation

fully extended leg should remain flat on the floor during the stretch. Hold each stretch for approximately 10–30 seconds and then relax by lowering the crossed leg and rotating the hips until both gluteal masses are back in contact with the floor. Repeat a minimum of four repetitions and then switch legs.

Supine Double Leg Hip Rotation

Assume a supine position on your back with your knees bent to approximately a 90-degree angle. Each arm should be abducted out to the side approximately 90 degrees from the long axis of the body. To stretch the lower back, slowly rotate both legs to the floor on one side of the body keeping the head, shoulders, and arms flat on the floor (see Figure 9.20). Control the tension of the stretch by controlling how far you lower your knees to the floor. Hold each stretch for approximately 10–30 seconds and then relax by rotating both legs back up to their original position. Repeat a minimum of four repetitions to each side, alternating sides.

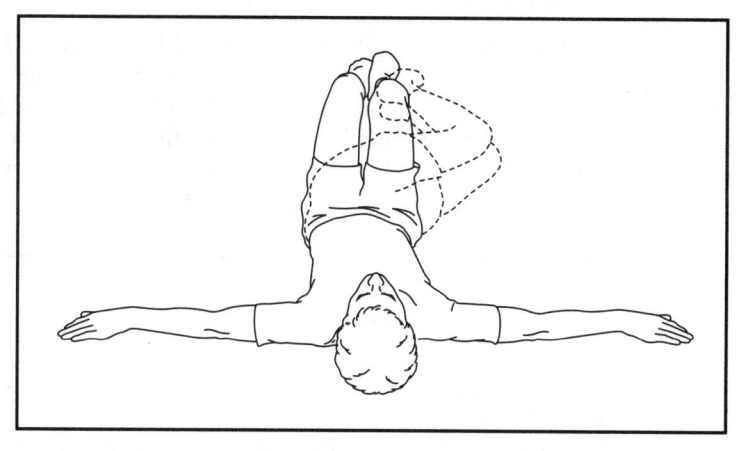

Figure 9.20 ■ Supine Double Leg Hip Rotation

Cat Stretch

Assume a kneeling position. Position your hips directly over your knees and place your hands directly under your shoulders. Fully extend both arms. To stretch your lower back, slowly lower your head between your extended arms and fully round your lower back by contracting your abdominal musculature (see Figure 9.21). Control the tension of the stretch by how much you round your lower back. Hold each stretch for approximately 10–30 seconds and then relax by lifting your head and flattening your back. Repeat a minimum of four repetitions.

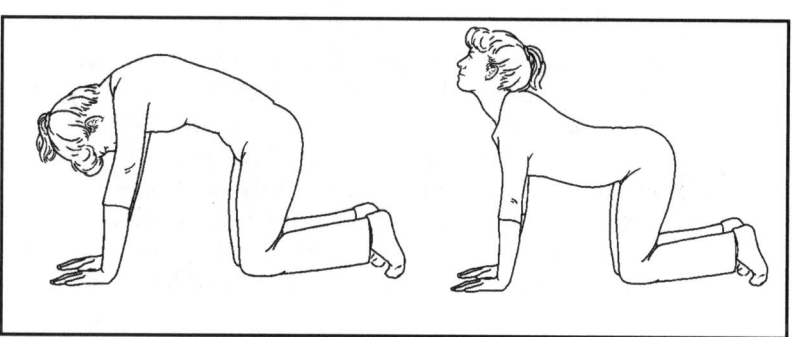

Figure 9.21 ■ Cat Stretch

Double Leg Hip Flexion

Assume a supine position on your back with both knees bent to approximately a 90-degree angle. To stretch your lower back, grasp behind each knee and pull both knees simultaneously toward your chest, rotating the hips off the floor (see Figure 9.22). Control the tension of the stretch by how far you pull the

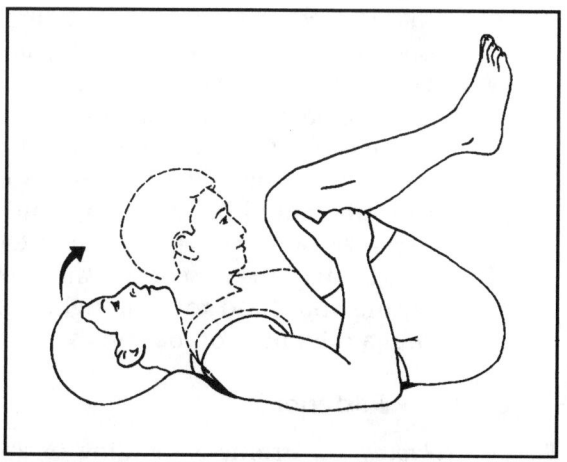

Figure 9.22 ■ Double Leg Hip Flexion

knees toward your chest. You may elect to keep your head and shoulders flat on the floor at all times. Hold each stretch for approximately 10–30 seconds and then relax by lowering your legs and rotating the hips back to their original position. Repeat a minimum of four times.

Single Leg Hip Flexion

Assume a supine position on your back with both knees bent to approximately a 90-degree angle. To stretch your lower back, grasp one knee with both hands and slowly pull it toward your chest. Keep your head and shoulders flat on the floor at all times (see Figure 9.23). Control the tension of the stretch by how far you pull the knee toward the chest. Hold each stretch for approximately 10–30 seconds and then relax by lowering the leg to its original position. Repeat a minimum of four times for each leg, alternating legs.

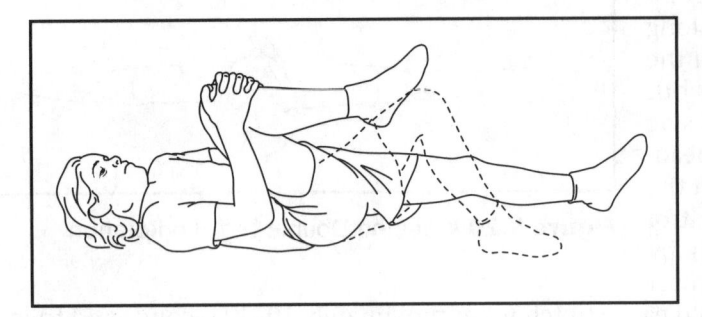

Figure 9.23 ■ Single Leg Hip Flexion

Neck

Anterior

Procedure: Assume a standing or an upright sitting position. To stretch the anterior aspect of the neck, place both hands on the top, front of the head (forehead) and slowly press backward (see Figure 9.24). Control the tension of the stretch by how hard and far you push the head backward. **Precaution should be taken to avoid excessive pressure or force.** Hold each stretch for approximately 10–30 seconds and then relax by raising your head to an upright position. Repeat a minimum of four times.

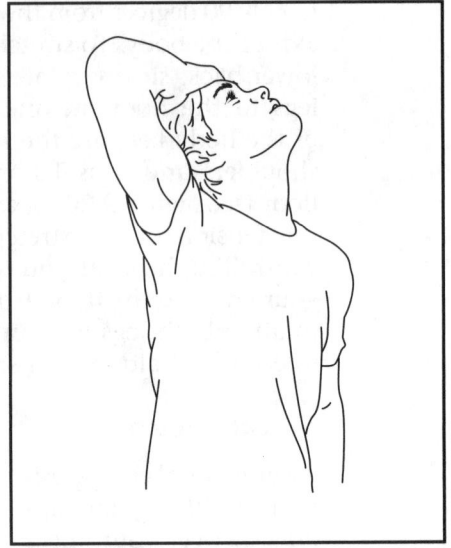

Figure 9.24 ■ Anterior Neck Stretch

Lateral

Procedure: Assume a standing or an upright sitting position. To stretch the lateral aspect of the neck reach over your head and grasp the opposite side of your head with your hand (see Figure 9.25). Slowly pull your head towards the shoulder of the reaching hand. Control the tension of the stretch by how hard and far you pull the head towards the shoulder. **Precaution should be taken to avoid excessive pressure or force.** Hold each stretch for approximately 10–30 seconds and then relax by raising your head to an upright position. Repeat a minimum of four times.

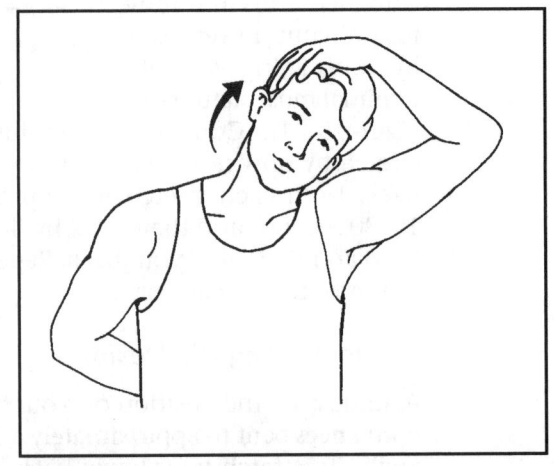

Figure 9.25 ■ Lateral Neck Stretch

Posterior

Procedure: Assume a standing or an upright sitting position. To stretch the posterior neck grasp the top, back aspect of your head with both hands and slowly pull your head down so that your chin rests against your chest (see Figure 9.26). Control the tension of the stretch by how hard and far downward you pull your head. **Precaution should be taken to avoid excessive pressure or force.** Hold each stretch for approximately 10–30 seconds and then relax by raising your head to an upright position. Repeat a minimum of four times.

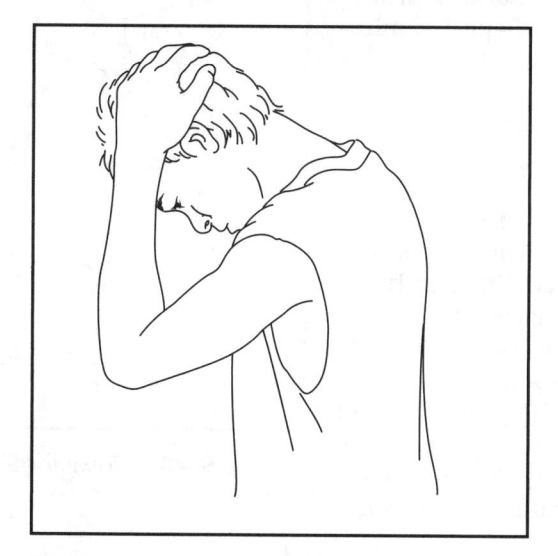

Figure 9.26 ■ Posterior Neck Stretch

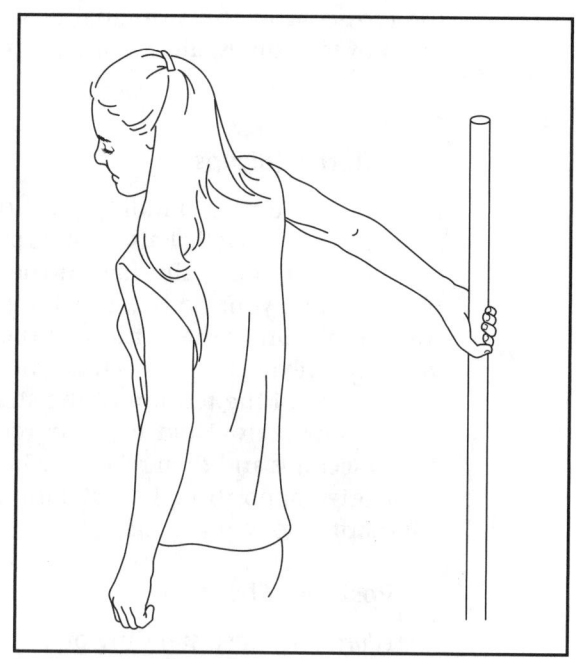

Figure 9.27 ■ Chest Stretch

Chest

Procedure: Assume a standing position, facing perpendicular next to a wall. Raise one arm to chest level and place or affix your palm flat on the wall. To stretch the chest, rotate your body on its long axis away from the wall. To maximize the tension on the chest muscles, maintain a linear line from the midline of the body to the hand (see Figure 9.27). Control the tension of the stretch by how far you rotate your body. Hold each stretch for approximately 10–30 seconds and then relax by rotating your body back to its original position. Repeat a minimum of four times, alternating body positions and arms.

Shoulders

Anterior

Procedure: Assume a sitting position with your hands placed at shoulder width behind your hips. To stretch the anterior aspect of the shoulder, keeping your hands flat and pointed backwards, slide the hips forward (see Figure 9.28). Control the tension of the stretch by how far you slide your hips forward. Hold each stretch for approximately 10–30 seconds and then relax by shifting your hips back, decreasing the distance between your hips and hands. Repeat a minimum of four times.

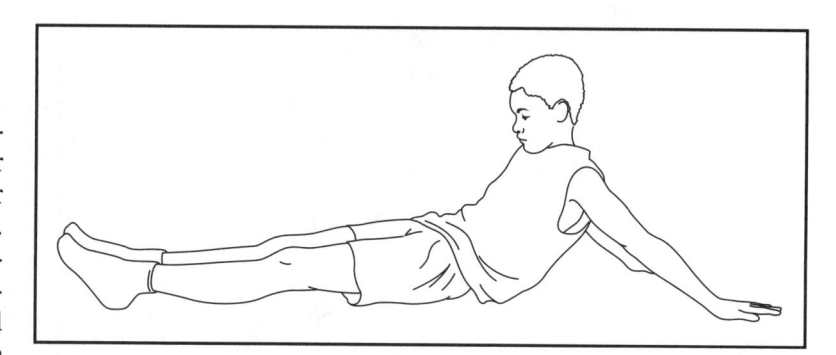

Figure 9.28 ■ Anterior Shoulder Stretch

Posterior

Procedure: Assume a standing or an upright sitting position. To stretch the posterior aspect of the shoulder, raise one arm to shoulder level and reach across your chest (see Figure 9.29).

Using your other hand, grasp the elbow of the crossed arm and pull the elbow toward your chest. Control the tension of the stretch by how hard you pull the crossed arm toward your chest. Hold each stretch for approximately 10–30 seconds and then relax by lowering and returning the crossed arm to its original position. Repeat a minimum of four times, alternating arms.

Arms

Anterior (Biceps)

Procedure: Assume a standing position, facing perpendicular next to a wall. Raise one arm to chest level and place or affix your palm flat on the wall. To stretch the biceps, rotate your body on its long axis away from the wall. To maximize the tension on the biceps, allow transverse hyperextension to occur at the shoulder (see Figure 9.30). Control the tension of the stretch by how far you rotate your body. Hold each stretch for approximately 10–30 seconds and then relax by rotating your body back to its original position. Repeat a minimum of four times, alternating body positions.

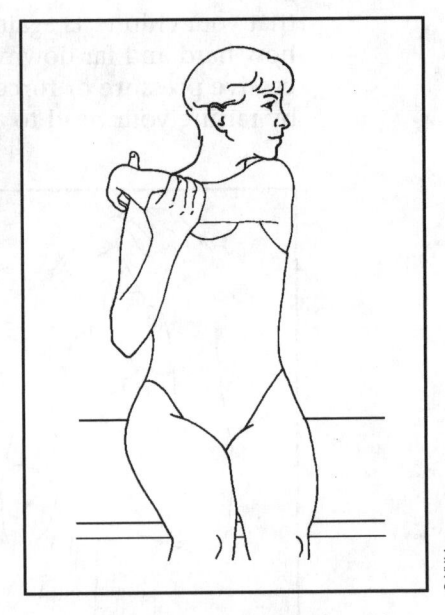

Figure 9.29 ■ Posterior Shoulder Stretch

Posterior (Triceps)

Procedure: Assume a standing or an upright sitting position. Both arms should be relaxed and hanging naturally at the sides. Reach behind your head with one hand as if to scratch the middle of your back. To stretch the triceps, grasp the elbow of the reaching arm and hand, with the opposite hand, and press the elbow behind the head (see Figure 9.31). Control the tension of the stretch by how hard you press the elbow behind the head. Hold each stretch for approximately 10–30 seconds and then relax by lowering both arms to their original position. Repeat a minimum of four times, alternating arms.

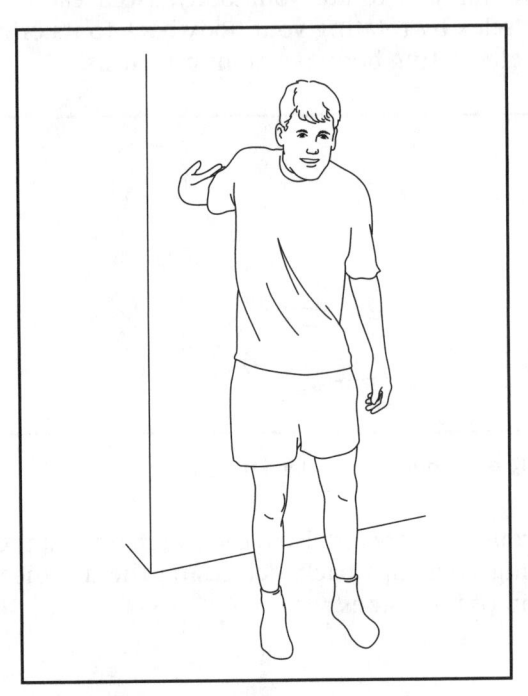

Figure 9.30 ■ Anterior Upper Arm (Biceps) Stretch

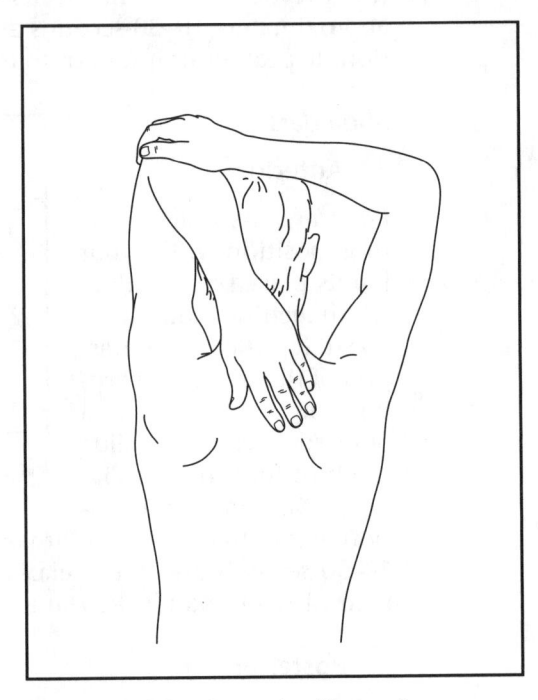

Figure 9.31 ■ Posterior Upper Arm (Triceps) Stretch

Ballistic Stretching Activities

Because of the inherent danger associated with ballistic stretching, no ballistic stretching activities are recommended.

Proprioceptive Neuromuscular Facilitation Stretching Activities

There are many appropriate proprioceptive neuromuscular facilitation stretching activities that could be recommended. If properly incorporated into a regular flexibility training program each would allow for positive gains in joint range of motion. To illustrate and describe such a large number of procedures is beyond the scope of this manuscript. As a result, a sampling of the more common procedures has been provided. For reader ease, procedures have been grouped by body segment. To control page space, fewer activities, as compared to static stretches, are offered. Table 9.2 offers an overall step sequence used in all PNF activities. Step 1 is illustrated in Figure 9.32. Steps 2 & 3 are illustrated in Figure 9.33. Steps 4–6 are illustrated in Figure 9.34.

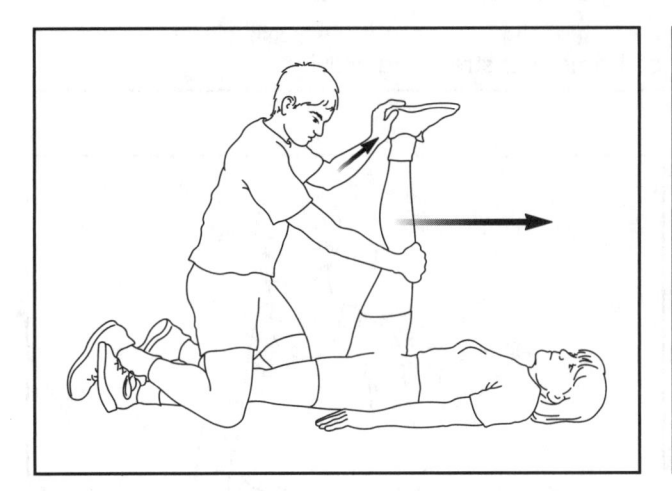

Figure 9.32 ■ Sequence of Action PNF Stretching - Step 1

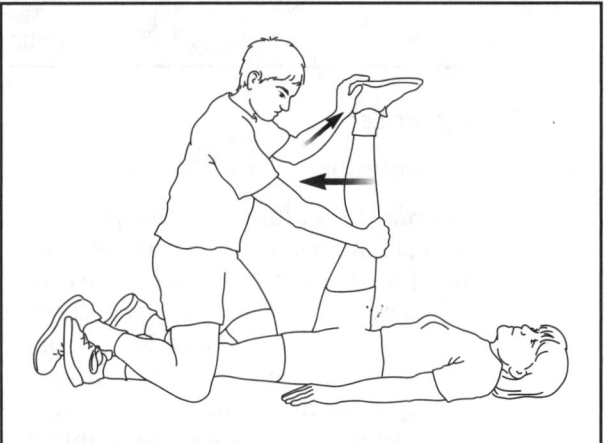

Figure 9.33 ■ Sequence of Action PNF Stretching - Steps 2 and 3

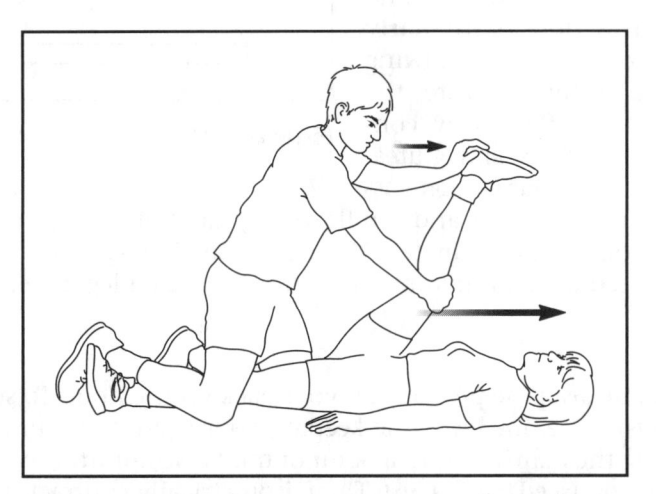

Figure 9.34 ■ Sequence of Action PNF Stretching - Steps 4–6

Table 9.2 ■ Sequence of Action for Proprioceptive Neuromuscular Facilitation Stretching Activities

Step	Action
1	Assume the recommended body position and slowly stretch the selected muscle tissue to a point of end range of motion.
2	Have a partner or use an external apparatus to stabilize the body segment at the point of end range of motion.
3	Submaximally isometrically contract the selected muscle tissue for 6 seconds while the body segment is being stabilized.
4	Following the isometric contraction, have a partner slowly apply mild force in a direction to passively stretch the selected muscle tissue.
5	Hold the passive stretched for 10–30 seconds.
6 (Optional)	Subject may contract agonist muscle group at the same time the partner is passively stretching the selected muscle tissue.
7	Relax the tissue by slowly returning the selected muscle tissue to normal resting length.
8	Repeat steps 1–7 a minimum of 4 times per stretching activity.

Upper Leg

Anterior

Procedure: Assume a supine position on your stomach. To stretch the anterior leg (quadriceps) and hip flexors, raise one leg while keeping your chest, arms, head, and opposite leg in contact with the floor. Stretch the quadriceps and hip flexors to a point of mild discomfort. Have a partner stabilize the raised leg in this position (see Figure 9.35). Then, isometrically contract the quadriceps and hip flexors for approximately six seconds. **Precaution should be taken to avoid maximal isometric contraction particularly at end range of motion.** Following contraction, actively elongate the quadriceps and hip flexors by contracting the hamstrings and gluteal musculature, or have your partner passively stretch the quadriceps and hip flexors by carefully and slowly lifting up on the knee. Hold this position for approximately 10–30 seconds. To relax, slowly lower the leg to the floor. Repeat this procedure a minimum of four times for each leg, alternating legs.

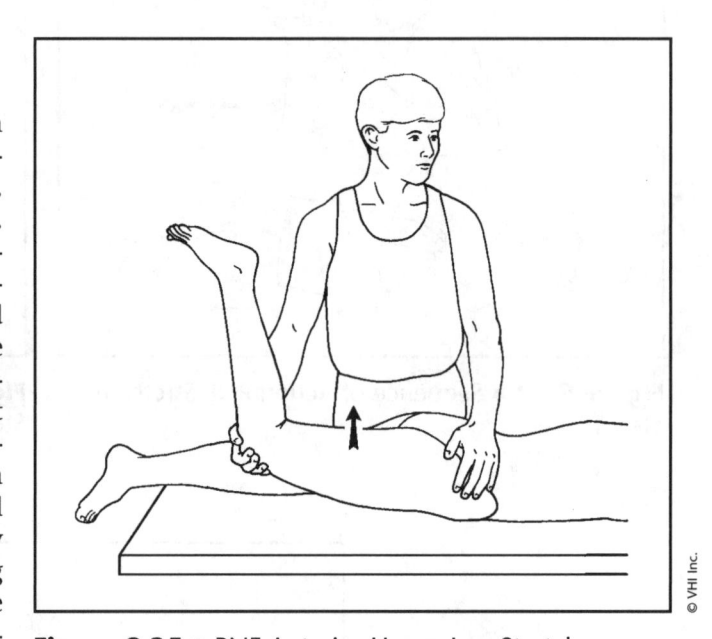

Figure 9.35 ■ PNF Anterior Upper Leg Stretch

Posterior

Procedure: Assume a supine position on your back on the floor. To stretch the posterior upper leg (hamstrings), raise one leg while keeping your head, hips, and back in contact with the floor, stretching the hamstrings to a point of mild discomfort. Have your partner stabilize the leg in this position (see Figure 9.36). Then, isometrically contract the hamstring musculature for approximately six seconds. **Precaution should be taken to avoid maximal isometric contraction particularly at end range of motion.** Following contraction, actively elongate the hamstrings by contracting the iliopsoas musculature (hip flexors), or have your partner passively stretch the hamstrings by carefully and slowly pushing your heel toward your head. Hold this position for approximately 10–30 seconds. To relax, slowly lower the leg to the floor. Repeat this procedure a minimum of four times for each leg, alternating legs.

Lower Back

Procedure: Assume a sitting position on the floor with your legs fully extended in front of you. Do not lock the knees out. To stretch the lower back, gradually lean forward, as if attempting to touch your toes, stretching the musculature of the lower back to a point of mild discomfort. Have your partner stabilize the back in this position (see Figure 9.37). Then, isometrically contract the low back musculature for approximately six seconds. **Precaution should be taken to avoid maximal isometric contraction particularly at end range of motion.** Following contraction, actively elongate the low back musculature by contracting the abdominal musculature, or have your partner passively stretch the low back by pressing on your shoulders for approximately 10–30 seconds. To relax, slowly sit back up. Repeat this procedure a minimum of four times.

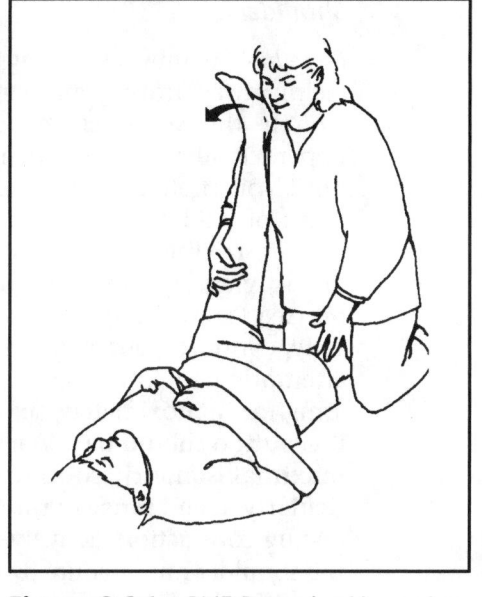

Figure 9.36 ■ PNF Posterior Upper Leg Stretch

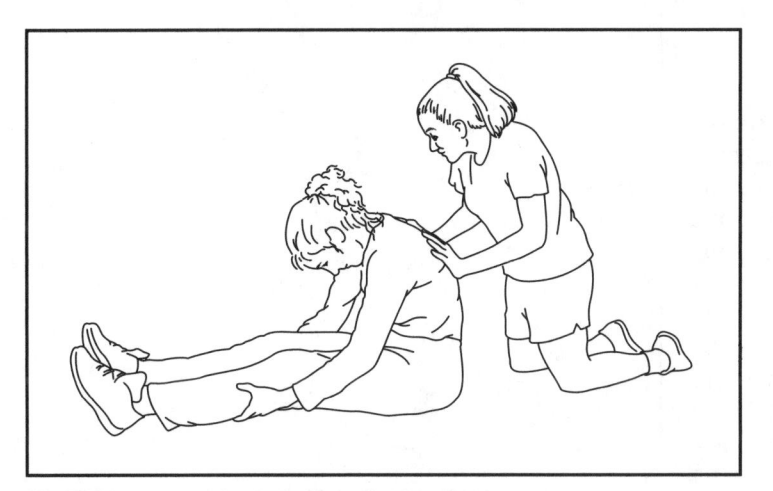

Figure 9.37 ■ PNF Low Back and Hamstring Stretch

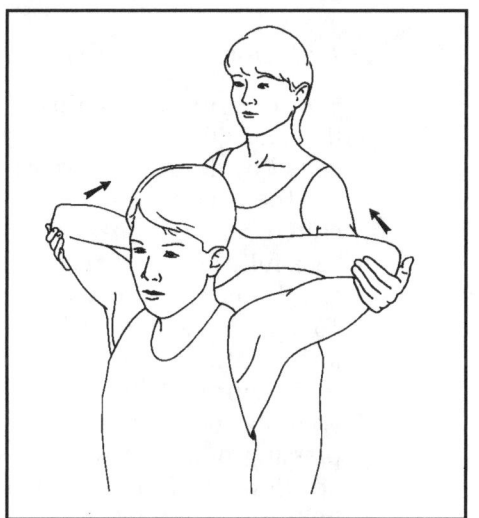

Figure 9.38 ■ PNF Chest Stretch

Chest

Procedure: Assume a sitting position on the floor with your hands placed behind your head. To stretch the chest draw your elbows back behind your head until you stretch the musculature of the chest to a point of mild discomfort. Have your partner stabilize your arms, by grasping your elbows, in this position (see Figure 9.38). Then, isometrically contract the chest musculature for approximately six seconds. **Precaution should be taken to avoid maximal isometric contraction particularly at end range of motion.** Following contraction, actively elongate the chest musculature by contracting the rhomboids, posterior deltoids and back (trapezius) musculature, or have your partner passively stretch the chest by pulling on your arms for approximately 10–30 seconds. To relax, slowly allow the elbows to move forward. Repeat this procedure a minimum of four times.

Shoulders

Procedure: Assume a standing position facing away from your partner. To stretch the shoulder musculature, hyperextend your arms behind you until you stretch the shoulders to a point of mild discomfort. Have your partner stabilize your arms in this position by grasping your wrists and lifting up (see Figure 9.39). Then, isometrically contract your shoulders while attempting to lower your stabilized arms for approximately six seconds. **Precaution should be taken to avoid maximal isometric contraction particularly at end range of motion.** Following contraction, actively elongate the shoulder musculature by attempting to further raise your arms behind you or by having your partner passively stretch the shoulders by lifting up on your arms for approximately 10–30 seconds. To relax, slowly lower your arms to your sides. Repeat this procedure a minimum of four times.

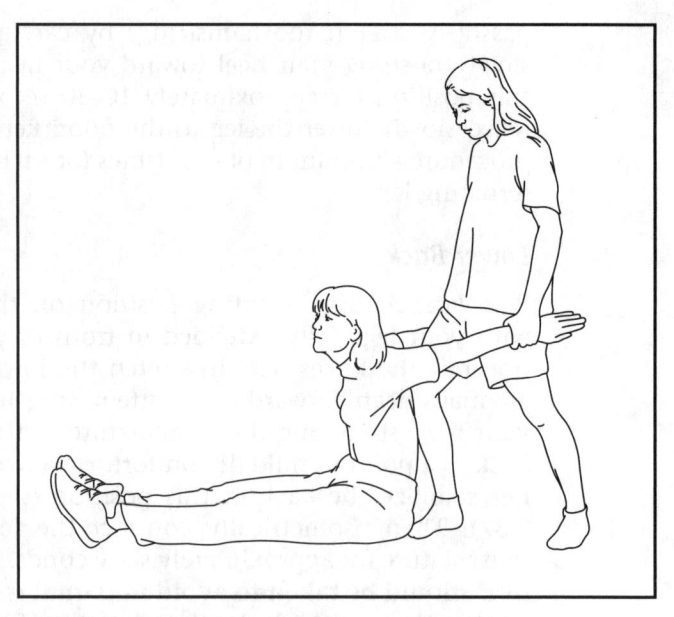

Figure 9.39 ■ PNF Anterior Shoulder Stretch

Adductors

Procedure: Assume a sitting position on the floor. Bring the soles of both feet together by flexing both knees and pulling the heels of the feet toward your crotch and buttocks. Keeping your back fully extended, relax your elbows and lower arms on your flexed legs. To stretch the adductors, lower your knees until you stretch the adductors to a point of mild discomfort. Have your partner stabilize your legs, by pressing down on the knees, in this position (see Figure 9.40). Then, isometrically contract the adductors for approximately six seconds. **Precaution should be taken to avoid maximal isometric contraction particularly at end range of motion.** Following contraction, actively elongate the adductors by contracting the leg abductors, or have your partner passively stretch the adductors by pressing down on your knees for approximately 10–30 seconds. To relax, slowly raise your knees. Repeat this procedure a minimum of four times.

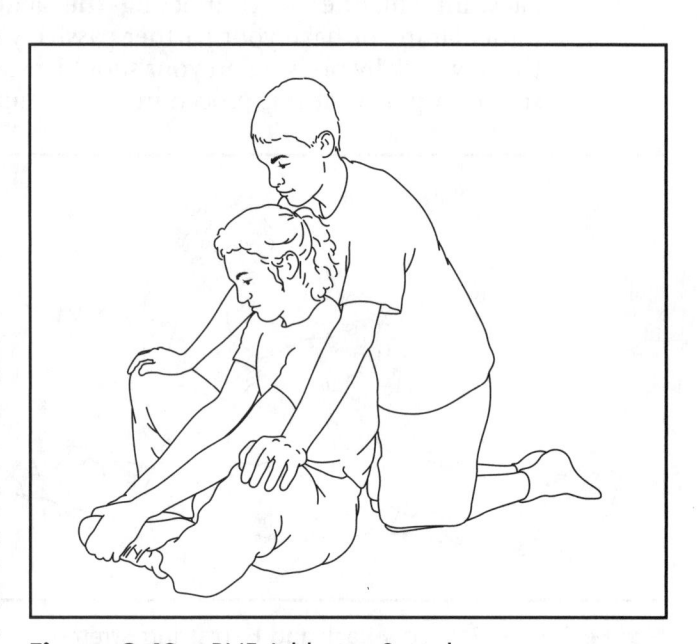

Figure 9.40 ■ PNF Adductor Stretch

10

Principles of Nutrition

300,000 deaths annually are related to poor diet and physical inactivity.
Center for Disease Control and Prevention

Only 18% of women and 20% of men report eating five servings of fruits and vegetables each day.
Center for Disease Control and Prevention

■ Chapter Outline ■

Nutrition
High Nutrient Density
Exploring the Essential Nutrients
    Carbohydrates
        Simple Carbohydrates
        Complex Carbohydrates
        Fiber
            Soluble Fiber
            Insoluble Fiber
    Fats
        Saturated Fat
            Hydrogenation and Trans Fatty Acids
        Unsaturated Fat
            Monounsaturated Fat
            Polyunsaturated Fat
                Omega-3 Fatty Acids
                Omega-6 Fatty Acids
            Olestra (Olean)
    Proteins
        Amino Acid Supplementation
            Creatine
    Vitamins
        Fat Soluble Vitamins
        Water Soluble Vitamins
        Antioxidant Vitamins
    Minerals
        Sodium and Potassium
        Iron
        Calcium
    Water
Nutrient Recommendation
Understanding the MyPyramid Food System
Supplements
Herbal Supplements
Food for Performance
    How Soon Can I Exercise after I Eat?
    Dietary Needs for the Physically Active
        Carbohydrate Intake
        Carbohydrate Loading
        Fat Intake
        Protein Intake
        Sodium Replacement
        Fluid Replacement
        Vitamin and Mineral Supplementation
Caffeine
Understanding the New Food Label
    % Daily Values
    Health Claims
    Nutrient Content Descriptors

Learning Objectives

The student should be able to:

- Define nutrition.
- Demonstrate an understanding of the differences between essential and non-essential nutrients.
- Demonstrate an understanding of high nutrient density.
- Identify and demonstrate understanding of the six classifications of essential nutrients.
- Demonstrate an understanding of the differences and characteristics of soluble and unsoluble fiber.
- Demonstrate an understanding of the differences and characteristics of saturated fat, monounsaturated fat, polyunsaturated fat, omega-3 fatty acids, and olean.
- Demonstrate an understanding of the dietary needs of the physically active.
- Demonstrate an understanding of supplementation and an understanding of specific supplements such as amino acids, creatine, herbs, and vitamins.
- Demonstrate an understanding of antioxidants.
- Demonstrate an understanding of minerals; more specifically, minerals associated with muscular contraction and physical activity.
- Demonstrate an understanding of the Food Label, including the term % Daily Value.
- Identify and demonstrate understanding of the 10 Health Claims that may be used on a Food Label.
- Identify and demonstrate understanding of the 12 Nutrient Content Descriptors that may be used when describing food products.

Keywords

Amino acids	Fuel nutrients	Omega-3 fatty acid
Amino acid supplementation	Glycogen supercompensation	Percent (%) daily values
Antioxidants	Health claims	Polysaccharides
Calcium	Herbal supplements	Polyunsaturated fat
Carbohydrates	High density lipoproteins (HDL)	Potassium
Carbohydrate loading	High nutrient density	Protein
Cholesterol	Hydrogenation	Refined grains
Complete protein	Hyponatremia	Saturated fat
Complex carbohydrates	Incomplete protein	Simple carbohydrates
Creatine	Iron	Simple sugar
Dehydration	Low density lipoprotein (LDL)	Sodium
Dissacharides	Low nutrient density	Soluble fiber
Empty calorie	Minerals	Supplements
Essential amino acids	Monosaccharides	Trans fatty acid
Essential nutrient	Monounsaturated fat	Unrefined grains
Fat	Non-essential nutrient	Unsaturated fat
Fat soluble vitamins	Nutrient claims	Unsoluble fiber
Fiber	Nutrition	Vitamin
Fluid replacement	Olestra (Olean)	Water soluble vitamins

Nutrition

Proper nutrition is scientifically linked to overall good health and well-being, as well as to athletic performance. Proper nutrition means that a diet includes sufficient amounts of nutrients to carry out normal tissue growth, repair, and maintenance of the body. Approximately forty-five to fifty nutrients are needed for these functions. Typically, these nutrients are categorized as carbohydrates, fats, proteins, vitamins, minerals and water. They also are classified as either essential or non-essential. Essential nutrients are those that may only be obtained from foods eaten, while non-essential nutrients are those produced within the body.

High Nutrient Density

It is important to understand that nutrient density and calorie content of foods *are not related*. High nutrient density refers to foods that are rich in nutrients relative to their energy content. That is, they are foods having a low or moderate amount of calories but are packed with nutrients. One should always try to choose foods high in nutrient density. The more a food resembles the original, farm-grown product, the more nutrient dense it is likely to be. For example, an orange would be more nutritious than orange juice, and orange juice is more nutrient dense than "orange drink."

Individuals eating a low-calorie diet should pay particular attention to the nutrient density of the foods they consume. There is no perfect food that contains all nutrients. Therefore, a variety of foods must be consumed to ensure proper nutrient intake. If, however, low nutrient density foods are consumed, the consumer will get proportionally limited nutrients for the calories consumed. If higher nutrient density foods are consumed, less food, and less calories will need to be consumed before appropriate levels of nutrients are taken in.

Exploring the Essential Nutrients

There are six classifications of essential nutrients: Carbohydrates, fats, proteins, minerals, vitamins, and water. These are often subdivided as macronutrients and micronutrients. The macronutrients are consumed daily in much larger volume than the micronutrients. Macronutrients include carbohydrates, fats, proteins, and water.

Three of the macronutrients, carbohydrates, fats, and proteins are also referred to as **fuel nutrients.** In other words, they are the source of calories for our body. Carbohydrates and fats are used primarily as sources of energy for physical activity; carbohydrates being the "high octane" fuel for activity. While protein is a source of energy, the body relies on proteins as a last resort for fuel. Table 10-1 provides recommended daily intake for fat, protein and carbohydrates based on low, average, and high levels of caloric intake. The fuel nutrients are discussed in detail under separate header below.

The micronutrients are minerals and vitamins. Much smaller levels of consumption of these nutrients are required. The micronutrients are discussed under separate headers below.

Carbohydrates

Plants are the source for carbohydrates. Carbohydrates are the primary providers of energy for the body, and may be identified as simple or complex. When carbohydrates are metabolized or transformed into energy for the body, they produce glucose or blood sugar. The cells then make this "sugar" or glucose available for use.

Carbohydrates supply the body with *4 calories per gram* of food weight. Fifty-five **(55)** to sixty **(60)** percent of an individual's total daily caloric intake should be comprised of carbohydrates, mostly complex carbohydrates. It is recommended that 6 to 11 servings of carbohydrates should be consumed daily. Active individuals may need even higher levels of carbohydrate intake (70% of total calories consumed). Unfortunately, in the typical American diet only 40 to 45% of calories come from carbohydrate intake.

Table 10-1 ■ Recommended Daily Intake for Fat, Protein, and Carbohydrate Based on Low, Average, and High Levels of Caloric Intake

Nutrient (Energy/Gram)	Percent of Total Calories	Low: 1600 Caloric (Grams) Intake	Average: 2200 Caloric (Grams) Intake	High: 2800 Caloric (Grams) Intake
Total Fat (9 calories/gram)	30% or less	480 Calories (53 grams)	660 Calories (73 grams)	840 Calories (93 grams)
Saturated Fat (9 calories/gram)	7% or less	112 Calories (12 grams)	154 Calories (17 grams)	196 Calories (22 grams)
Monounsaturated Fat (9 calories/gram)	20% or less	320 Calories (35 grams)	440 Calories (49 grams)	560 Calories (62 grams)
Polyunsaturated Fat (9 calories/gram)	10% or less	160 Calories (18 grams)	220 Calories (24 grams)	280 Calories (31 grams)
Protein (4 calories/gram)	15%	240 Calories (60 grams)	330 Calories (83 grams)	420 Calories (105 grams)
Total Carbohydrate (4 calories/gram)	55–60%	880 Calories (220 grams)	1210 Calories (303 grams)	1540 Calories (385 grams)
Simple (4 calories/gram)	15% or less	240 Calories (60 grams)	330 Calories (83 grams)	420 Calories (105 grams)
Complex (4 calories/gram)	40% or greater	640 Calories (160 grams)	880 Calories (220 grams)	1120 Calories (280 grams)

Source: Modified from Insel, P. and Roth, W. (2002). *Core Concepts in Health,* 9th ed. Boston, MA: McGraw-Hill.

Simple Carbohydrates

Simple carbohydrates contain one or two sugars in each molecule. Specifically, they can be subdivided into monosaccharides and disaccharides. **Monosaccharides** are the simplest sugars and contain only one sugar. They include: glucose (natural sugar), fructose (fruit sugar), and galactose. **Disaccharides** contain two sugar units in each molecule. They include: sucrose or simple table sugar (glucose + fructose), lactose (glucose + galactose), and maltose (glucose + glucose).

Cakes, cookies, and candies are typically thought to contain simple carbohydrates. In general, they provide us with calories, but very little in the way of vitamins and minerals or fiber (due to excessive processing). Simply stated, simple carbohydrates are low in nutrient density. As a result, the calories associated with simple sugars are often referred to as **"empty calories,"** meaning they offer little or no nutritional value. Unfortunately, and wrongfully, many interpret the term "empty calorie" to mean there are no calories associated with simple sugars.

Most Americans consume far too many simple sugars. As a general rule, simple carbohydrate intake should be limited to 15% or less of total calories consumed.

Although fruits are single sugars, the body responds to them as though they were complex carbohydrates. They do not cause spikes in blood sugar, as simple carbohydrates do, so they are often thought of as complex carbohydrates. Currently 2–4 servings of fruit are recommended daily.

Complex Carbohydrates

These carbohydrates are referred to as "complex" due to the nature of their molecular make-up. **Complex carbohydrates** are also known as **polysaccharides** and consist of chains of united simple sugars. Common complex carbohydrates are starches, dextrins, and glycogen. Complex carbohydrates are found in foods such as rice, cereals, breads, potatoes, beans, and vegetables. Most of one's diet should come from these food sources. Significant amounts of vitamins, minerals, and fiber are found in these foods.

Grains, such as rice, barley, oats, wheat, millet, and rye, represent an excellent food source for complex carbohydrates. They are often categorized as either *refined* or *unrefined*. Refined grains are simply processed or milled whole grains. In the process of refinement, the inner germ layer and the outer bran layer are removed, leaving only the starchy middle layer known as the endosperm. Unfortunately, refined grains maintain most of their caloric value even though they are lower in fiber, and are less nutrient dense than whole, unrefined grains. Sources of refined grains include, but are not limited to, wheat flour, unbleached flour, enriched flour, wheat germ, wheat bran, and degerminated corn meal.

Whole grains are unrefined grains and consist of the entire, edible portion of the grain. This includes the germ, endosperm, and bran. Whole grains are far more nutrient dense than their refined counterparts. Whole grains are slower to digest and, because of their high fiber content, have been linked to disease risk reduction including, but not limited to, heart disease, diabetes, hypertension, stroke, and colon and rectal cancer. Whole grains are the preferred dietary grain and should be incorporated into the diet whenever possible. Sources of whole grain include, but are not limited to, whole wheat, whole rye, whole oats, oatmeal, popcorn, brown rice, and barley.

Fiber

Fiber is the indigestible portion of the fruits, vegetables and grains we eat (i.e., seeds, skins). Even though some nutritionists consider it a seventh nutrient, fiber is simply a form of a complex carbohydrate. Animal sources do not contain fiber; complex carbohydrates do. Fiber may be classified as soluble or insoluble.

It is estimated that most Americans consume 10 to 15 grams of fiber per day. Recommended amounts, for adults, are 20 to 35 grams per day. In simple, "an apple a day does not provide enough fiber to keep the doctor away."

Simple dietary behaviors can be employed to help increase fiber intake. For example, when selecting foods for purchase and later consumption, choose whole-grain breads instead of white bread, or brown rice instead of white rice. Take the time to read the food label. Look for breads and crackers that list a whole grain first in the ingredient list. Try to avoid foods made from processed grains. Eat whole fruits rather than drinking only juice. Include beans in soups and salads, and use beans as a base for dip rather than cheese.

Soluble Fiber

Soluble fiber dissolves in water and is broken down by bacteria in the large intestine. Sources of soluble fiber include, but are not limited to, fruits, legumes, oats, and barley. When soluble fiber breaks down it is capable of binding with fat and can contribute to increased fat excretion from the body. This is considered a positive characteristic. Diets high in soluble fiber intake have been linked to decreased levels of blood cholesterol and blood sugar.

Insoluble Fiber

Insoluble fiber does not dissolve in water or break down in the intestine. Sources of insoluble fiber include, but are not limited to, wheat, wheat bran, cereals, and vegetables. Insoluble fiber increases bulk in the stools because it binds water. This helps create a softer, bulkier stool that is more easily and more rapidly passed. This is an extremely critical feature. Moving the stool more quickly through the intestine has been shown to lower colon cancer risk because the colon is less exposed to cancer-causing agents.

Other health problems have been associated with high fiber intake. In addition to colon and rectal cancer risk reduction, disease risk reductions with high fiber intake have been linked to constipation, hemorrhoids, and diverticulitis. Diverticulitis is an inflammation in the diverticulum, where abnormal pouches or sacs are formed or open in the intestine.

Fats

Excessive consumption of fats pose major health problems in our country such as cardiovascular diseases and colon cancer. Sources of fats are vegetable oils, animal oils, butter, and cheese. *One gram of fat contains 9 calories,* the highest concentration of energy in all the nutrients.

Fats are essential for many body processes, especially for the absorption of the fat-soluble vitamins: A, D, K, and E. These vitamins bind to sites on fat molecules enabling the vitamins to be absorbed in the small intestine. Fat is also necessary for cushioning organs.

Only about **30%** of daily caloric intake should come from fats, with less than 10% coming from saturated fat. If lowering cholesterol and/or body weight are of concern, one should lower his/her fat percentage to 20% of his/her daily caloric intake.

Insel and Roth (2002) cite the findings of a 2001 report by the National Cholesterol Education Program (NCEP). In this report the NCEP recommends a total fat intake of 25–35%. Additionally, it suggests that less than 7% should come from saturated fat intake, up to 10% from polyunsaturated fat, and up to 20% from monounsaturated fat. Lastly, the NCEP recommends limited trans fatty acid consumption.

Fats are typically subdivided by hydrogen saturation level. Included are saturated and unsaturated fats. Unsaturated fats are further subdivided into monounsaturated fats and polyunsaturated fats. These subdivisions are discussed under separate headers below.

Saturated Fat

Sources of saturated fats include primarily animal products and by-products such as red meats, butter, whole milk, cream, and cheese. Saturated fats are typically solid at room temperature. Coconut and palm oils, while plant sources, are somewhat unusual in that they too are very high in saturated fat and should be avoided. Many commercially baked products and "movie popcorn" contain these oils. The skin and fat of poultry is also high in saturated fat.

Frequently, these products are and can be labelled as cholesterol free. This type of labelling is extremely misleading. The high levels of saturated fat prove to be extremely problematic by contributing to the production of serum cholesterol by the body. Therefore, though they are technically cholesterol free, the consumption of these products can and will lead to high total serum cholesterol levels.

While excessive fat consumption (no matter the source) will lead to obesity, saturated fats are a primary culprit in contributing to heart disease. Additionally, foods high in saturated fat frequently contain high levels of cholesterol. Some examples are chicken livers and other organ meats.

When saturated fat is consumed, the liver responds by using this saturated fat to produce increased amounts of cholesterol. Cholesterol plays an integral part in the formation of waxy, fatty, plaque deposits that build up in the arteries, especially in the coronary arteries that supply blood to the heart. This leads to a number of cardiovascular problems, especially coronary artery disease.

The amount of saturated fat in the diet should be limited to no more than **10%** of your total caloric intake. Because the body produces cholesterol, there is no need to consume additional amounts. In fact, every precaution should be taken to limit dietary consumption of cholesterol (250 to 300 milligrams per day). Table 10-2 provides a summary recommendation offered by the United States Department of Agriculture, of methods to lower total fat, saturated fat, and cholesterol intake.

In addition to increased risk of heart disease, excessive consumption of saturated fats has been linked to elevations in total serum cholesterol levels and LDL "bad" cholesterol levels. Finally, saturated fat consumption may increase risk of colon and prostate cancers.

Hydrogenation and Trans Fatty Acids

Unsaturated fats are sometimes put through a process that adds hydrogen to the fat. This increases the saturation of the liquid oils and turns them into a product that more closely resembles saturated fat. The term "hydrogenation," therefore, should communicate that a food item may be higher in saturated fat than previously thought. *Foods high in "trans fatty acids" have been linked with elevations in serum cholesterol levels.* Sources of food high in trans fatty acids include, but are not limited to, 1) hydrogenated vegetable oils such as hard or stick margarines and shortenings, 2) many commercially fried foods such as French fries and other deep-fried foods, 3) many commercially prepared bakery goods such as cookies and crackers, and 4) processed sweets and snacks.

The consumption of trans fatty acids has been shown to raise total serum and LDL (bad) cholesterol levels. Additionally, trans fatty acids have been shown to lower HDL (good) cholesterol levels. Finally, increased risk of heart disease and breast cancer have been linked to trans fatty acids.

Table 10-2 ■ Recommended Methods to Lower Total Fat, Saturated Fat, and Cholesterol Intake

Fats and Oils

- ♥ Choose vegetable oils rather than solid fats (meat and dairy fats, shortening).
- ♥ Decrease the amount of fat used in cooking and at the table.

Meat, Poultry, Fish, Shellfish, Eggs, Beans, and Nuts

- ♥ Choose 2 to 3 servings of fish, shellfish, lean poultry, other lean meats, beans, or nuts daily. Trim fat from meat and take skin off poultry. Choose dry beans, peas, or lentils often.
- ♥ Limit your intake of high-fat processed meats such as bacon, sausages, salami, bologna, and other cold cuts. Try the lower fat varieties.
- ♥ Limit your intake of liver and other organ meats. Use egg yolks and whole eggs in moderation. Use egg whites and egg substitutes freely when cooking since they contain no cholesterol and little or no fat.

Dairy Products

- ♥ Choose fat-free or low-fat milk, fat-free or low-fat yogurt, and low-fat cheese most often. Try switching from whole to fat-free or low-fat milk. This decreases the saturated fat and calories but keeps all other nutrients the same.
- ♥ Prepared Foods
- ♥ Check the Nutrition Facts Label to see how much saturated fat and cholesterol are in a serving of prepared food. Choose foods lower in saturated fat and cholesterol.

Foods at Restaurants or Other Eating Establishments

- ♥ Choose fish or lean meats. Limit ground meat and fatty processed meats, marbled steaks, and cheese.
- ♥ Limit your intake of foods with creamy sauces, and add little or no butter to your food.
- ♥ Choose fruits as desserts most often.

Source: U.S. Department of Agriculture, *Dietary Guidelines for Americans, 2000*, Home and Garden Bulletin No. 232.

Unsaturated Fat

Unsaturated fat sources are primarily vegetable oils, and are normally "soft or liquid" at room temperature. Unsaturated fats are sub-classified as monounsaturated or polyunsaturated and are discussed below under separate subheaders.

Monounsaturated Fat

Sources of monounsaturated fats include canola, peanut, safflower, and olive oil, avocados, olives, and tub margarine. Other sources include peanut butter, almonds, cashews, pecans, and pistachios. Monounsaturated fats are more desirable in the diet than polyunsaturated fats because they tend to lower only the "bad" cholesterol (LDL) and not the "good" cholesterol (HDL). This contributes to a more positive total cholesterol–HDL ratio. Therefore, these fats may protect against heart disease.

Additionally, monounsaturated fats are associated with reduced blood pressure, lower triglyceride levels, and reduced heart disease, stroke, and cancer risk. It is recommended that no more than 10% of total caloric intake should come from monounsaturated fats.

Polyunsaturated Fat

Sources of polyunsaturated fats include oils from corn, cottonseed, sunflower, and soybeans. It is thought that these fats lower both the "good" and the "bad" cholesterol. This will lead to a lower total cholesterol level, but will not alter the total cholesterol–HDL ratio. No more than 10% of total caloric intake should come from these fats.

Omega-3 Fatty Acids

Omega-3 fatty acids are found in cold-water fish such as salmon, herring, white albacore, mackerel, tuna, anchovies, and sardines, but are not found in canned fish. These fatty acids are affected during the canning process, reducing the positive effects otherwise gained. Additional sources include walnuts, flaxseed, canola, soybeans and the oils made from these products. Dark-green leafy vegetables also contain limited amounts of omega-3 fatty acids.

Research indicates that omega-3's are capable of reducing heart disease, fatal heart attacks, stroke, and hypertension (Hoeger and Hoeger, 1999). Fish oils appear to increase HDL levels, indirectly improving the total cholesterol–HDL ratio. Consumption of omega-3 fatty acids has been linked to reduced blood clotting, as well as assisting to inhibit abnormal heart rhythms.

Omega-6 Fatty Acids

Omega-6 fatty acids are found in corn, soybean, and cottonseed oils. All are frequently used in margarine, mayonnaise, and commercially produced salad dressings. These fatty acids have been linked with lower total and LDL (bad) cholesterol levels. They also may lower HDL (good) cholesterol levels, as well as reduce the risk of heart disease. A slight increase in cancer risk has been demonstrated if omega-6 fatty acids intake is high and omega-3 fatty acid intake is low.

Olestra (Olean)

Proctor & Gamble spent approximately 25 years and 250 million dollars developing the new fat substitute "olean" in which "WOW" potato chips are fried. The olean fat molecules, fortified in part with vitamins A, D, K, and E, are too large to be absorbed in the small bowel and pass right through the body.

While this may sound desirable, it really proves to be somewhat problematic as fat-soluble vitamins A, D, K, and E are absorbed into the body only after they bind to fat molecules. Negative side effects associated with olean include: potential vitamin deficiency, gastrointestinal problems such as diarrhea and cramping, and potentially cardiovascular problems.

Proteins

Proteins are essential for maintenance and repair of all body tissues (muscle, bone, cell membranes), enzymes, and some hormones. While proteins are an energy source for the body *(4 calories per gram),* they are not a preferred source of energy. Sources include meats, milk and milk by-products, eggs, and a variety of legumes (beans). Other common functions include, but are not limited to (Thompson, 1997):

- Carry oxygen (hemoglobin),
- Fight disease (antibodies),
- Catalyzes reactions (enzymes),
- Essential to movement (actin, myosin, troponin and tropomyosin),
- Acts as a connective tissue (collagen),
- Clots blood (prothrombin),
- Acts as a messenger (protein hormones such as growth hormone).

Proteins are composed of **amino acids.** Twenty common amino acids are found in food, nine of which are essential; that is, they can only be obtained from the foods we eat. Animal sources provide all of the essential amino acids and are therefore identified as high quality or **complete proteins.** Some foods, such as plant sources, do not provide enough of the essential amino acids. These are referred to as **incomplete proteins.** Some plant sources for incomplete proteins are beans, peas, and nuts.

It is possible to combine two incomplete protein sources to satisfy the body's need for amino acids. Red beans and rice, or beans and cornbread are examples. As long as these foods are eaten within the same day, they will sufficiently supply the body with essential amino acids. In this way, vegetarians are capable of consuming adequate amounts of amino acids or protein.

Twelve to fifteen percent of one's daily caloric intake should come from proteins. Excessive amounts of protein are, for the most part, non-problematic. It may, however, contribute fat to the diet because protein-rich foods are often fat-rich. For example, a fat marbled steak contains both fat and protein.

The amount of protein varies in both quantity and quality between food products. Animal sources are normally considered better sources of protein because they are complete proteins. Below is a list of selected foods to illustrate the range in quantity of protein in differing food items.

- 1 McDonald's quarter pounder has 23 grams of protein,
- 1 KFC chicken breast: 31 grams,
- 1/2 c. pinto beans: 6.5 grams,
- 1 c. skim milk: 9 grams,
- 1 c. of pasta: 4 grams.

In general, if a person consumes two to three servings of animal protein daily (depending on body weight), with each serving being about the size of a deck of cards, he/she will meet his/her protein requirement. To meet the RDA (Recommended Daily Allowance) these totals should be between 3 and 6 ounces.

The general rule for the average adult is to consume about .8 grams of protein for each kilogram of body weight (National Research Council, 1989). Younger individuals, and individuals involved in excessive amounts of exercise, may need more protein intake. For example, it has been suggested that an extremely active individual may require 1.2 to 2 grams of protein per kilogram of body weight. Most Americans, however, regardless of their exercise habits, consume more protein than is necessary.

Food labels do not give information concerning protein requirements. This is due to the fact that protein requirements, as previously mentioned, are individualized. Recall, the average adult should receive .8 grams of protein per kilogram of body weight. For example, consider a 150-pound man. To determine his daily protein requirement, first convert his body weight (150 pounds) to kilograms by dividing 150 by 2.2. In this case, this 150-pound individual weighs 68.2 kilograms. Next, multiply .8 by the determined body weight in kg (68.2). Based on this example, it would be recommended that this individual consume approximately 54–56 grams of protein daily.

Amino Acid Supplementation

Many athletes feel their bodies perform better when they supplement their diets with amino acids. Additionally, it is common for some body builders to declare amino acid supplementation is essential for muscle hypertrophy.

Given these feelings, amino acid supplementation is common. Precaution should be taken. Amino acid supplementation can be dangerous. High levels of some amino acids may prevent absorption of others. Additionally, consider this: a 3-ounce serving of meat or fish provides 20,000 mg of amino acids, as well as iron, niacin, and thiamine; while a 500 mg amino acid supplement provides only the amino acids listed and no additional nutrition. The cost per tablet is much greater than the cost of meat or fish. It should also be mentioned that the body absorbs nutrients from foods more completely and efficiently than it does from tablets. These findings suggest that proper diet should be considered more important than supplementation.

Creatine

Research has shown the amino acid, creatine, does help in increasing muscle mass and in the recovery of fatigued muscles. The long-term side effects, however, have not been determined and may prove to be harmful (Mihoces, 1997). It is therefore safest and best to increase muscle mass through physical training according to the "overload principle" rather than supplementation. Simply stated, if an individual eats properly, amino acid supplementation is not necessary.

Vitamins

There are thirteen vitamins, none of which can be manufactured by the body. They are the regulators of body processes. Vitamins have no caloric value and are destroyed by heat. They may be classified as fat-soluble or water-soluble, meaning they are absorbed in the small intestine when combined with either fat or water. Fat-soluble and water-soluble vitamins are discussed under separate subheader below.

Fat Soluble Vitamins

Fat-soluble vitamins are identified as: A (liver, milk, deep green and yellow fruits and vegetables), D (dairy products, eggs, fish oils, but primarily - exposure to sunlight), E (vegetable oils, some fruits and vegetables, and whole grains), and K (green leafy vegetables, and is also produced from normal bacteria in the intestines). These vitamins bind to fat molecules and are absorbed in the small intestine. This should point out the necessity for some consumption of fat in the diet. Excessive amounts of these vitamins can be toxic or poisonous since excessive amounts are stored in the body and not flushed out or removed. Because they are stored in the body, the risk for fat-soluble vitamin toxicity is greater than water-soluble vitamin toxicity (Sizer and Whitney, 1994).

Water Soluble Vitamins

Water-soluble vitamins include all of the B complex vitamins and vitamin C. They must be supplied daily as they cannot be stored in the body. Excessive amounts are excreted in the urine. In order to decrease vitamin losses during cooking, natural foods should be microwaved or steamed rather than boiled in water.

Antioxidant Vitamins

When oxygen is utilized during metabolism, a small amount ends up in an unstable form referred to as oxygen free radicals. Each free radical molecule steals an electron from another molecule in order to try to repair itself. In the process, it does not become repaired and turns the other molecule into a free radical. As the number of free radicals increases, so does the potential for increased damage to the body. Free radicals attack and damage proteins, cells, and DNA, thereby contributing to cardiovascular disease, cancer, emphysema, and other diseases.

Certain vitamins appear to play the role of antioxidants. It is thought that antioxidants (vitamin A, vitamin C, vitamin E, Beta-carotene (the precursor for vitamin A) and the mineral selenium) offer protection by absorbing free radicals before damage occurs. A well-balanced diet should provide all the antioxidants one needs. Because vitamin toxicity can occur from over intake of antioxidant, recommended levels of consumption are strongly encouraged. Recent research does support vitamin E supplementation, but not in excess of 600 international units per day (Hoeger and Hoeger, 1999). Excessive (> 800 IU/day) vitamin E intake has been linked to internal bleeding.

Antioxidants have been linked with reduced risk of certain types of cancer. Additionally, antioxidants are believed to lower diabetes risk for both men and women. Finally, antioxidants have been linked to reduced risk of heart attack, and they also appear to stop or blunt the progression of coronary artery narrowing (McArdle, Katch, and Katch, 2001).

Minerals

There are approximately 25 minerals, none of which contain calories, but all are essential to the body processes. Minerals are stored in the liver and bones, although an excess of minerals can pass out of the body through the digestive tract. Due to their relationship to muscular contraction and physical activity, a few minerals are discussed below.

Sodium and Potassium

Sodium and potassium are both important for physical activity, as they play a major role in the transmission of nerve impulses. Salt should be iodized to prevent goiters. Potassium additionally affects heart functioning. Good sources of potassium include baked white or sweet potatoes, spinach, winter squash, bananas, plantains, dried fruits such as apricots and prunes, and cooked dry beans and lentils.

Iron

Iron is the mineral most important in helping with oxygen transport. Iron helps form hemoglobin, the compound that transports oxygen in red blood cells. Insufficient iron consumption and absorption can lead to anemia, which is a condition where one's blood volume is below normal. When this occurs, an individual's body is receiving less oxygen than it should. Fatigue is a classic symptom of anemia. Normal daily functioning may be affected, as well as athletic performance. The best source of iron is red meats. Other sources include, but are not limited to, shellfish such as shrimp, clams, mussels, and oysters, cereals fortified with iron, dark turkey meat, sardines, spinach, dry beans, peas and lentils, and enriched whole grain breads. Only about 10% of the iron consumed is absorbed. Cooking in iron cookware will increase iron consumption. Eating foods that contain a significant source of iron is strongly advised.

Calcium

Calcium is the most abundant mineral in the body. It is necessary for the formation of bones and teeth, blood clotting, and muscular contraction. Milk products are the most reliable source of calcium. Other sources include spinach, tofu, dried beans, sardines, and broccoli. The body cannot manufacture calcium; therefore, sufficient amounts must be consumed in the diet. Average recommendations for calcium range from 1000 mg to 1500 mg daily. A cup of milk has slightly less than 300 mg. This helps to illustrate how difficult it is for most to consume the recommended amounts. Because of this, calcium supplementation is often recommended. If calcium intake is too low, the body will resorb calcium from the bones. This leads to the development of osteoporosis, a disease where bone mineral content or density decreases, leading to broken bones. Because 60% of postmenopausal women develop osteoporosis, awareness of calcium consumption is of critical importance. While calcium is important, weight-bearing activity and proper estrogen levels are important in preventing osteoporosis. Small-framed females are at highest risk of developing this disease. Men may develop osteoporosis as well, but usually not until approximately 70 years of age.

Water

Water is the most essential nutrient. The body is composed of approximately 70% water. Eight glasses of fluid are recommended daily. Because of the higher levels of perspiration associated with participation in vigorous activity and particular environments, this value may be higher for extremely active individuals or those that live in, or are exposed to, hotter climates.

Nutrient Recommendation

The nutrient requirement for any vitamin or mineral is the amount needed to prevent deficiency diseases. The RDA or recommended daily allowance is an amount greater than the nutrient requirement and includes a "margin of safety." If one consumes ⅔ of the RDA, that should be a sufficient amount to meet the body's needs. It should be remembered that exactly predicting the RDA for each individual is not possible due to physiological differences; however, the RDA is appropriate for the masses.

A new term, adequate intake (AI), has been coined by the FDA and may soon appear on nutritional charts and food labels. It represents the amount of vitamins and minerals needed for optimizing health.

Understanding the MyPyramid Food System

In 1992, the U. S. Department of Agriculture (USDA) adopted a new food group plan, commonly referred to as the Food Guide Pyramid. The pyramid replaced the more traditional, basic four food groups (i.e., Meats, Milk Products, Fruits and Vegetables, Breads and Cereals) with five groups or categories. The newer five food groups include: 1. Meats, Poultry, Fish, Dry Beans, Eggs and Nuts, 2. Milk, Yogurt, and Cheese, 3. Vegetables, 4. Fruits, and 5. Breads, Cereal, Rice and Pasta. While not considered a food group, fats, oils, and sweets were included in the Food Guide Pyramid. The USDA recommends limited intake and use of these products.

More recently, the USDA released the MyPyramid food guidance system and replaced the Food Guide Pyramid with a new MyPyramid symbol. This symbol is shown in Figure 1. While the Pyramid shape is still a part of the new MyPyramid symbol, the symbol has been revised. The revision is designed to reflect several different "consumer messages." These "consumer messages" stem from key recommendations found in the 2005 Dietary Guidelines for Americans (www.healthierus.gov/dietaryguidelines). Specifically, they are: physical activity, variety, proportionality, moderation, gradual improvement, and personalization. The underlying premise behind each part is described below.

- **Physical Activity** is illustrated by the individual climbing the steps. The premise of this particular part of the pyramid is to emphasize the importance of daily physical activity.
- **Variety** is illustrated by bands representing the five food groups and oils. Each individual food group band is systematically colorized. The premise of this particular part of the pyramid is to emphasize the importance and value in eating a large variety of foods from all food groups and subgroups.
- **Proportionality** is illustrated by the varying the widths of the food group bands. The basic premise of this particular part of the pyramid is to visually demonstrate how much food from each particular food group should be eaten when compared to the other food groups. This approach is quite different from the old Food Pyramid where being at the top or bottom of the Pyramid implied importance or greater value to a particular food group. The underlying tenet behind the shape of the Old Food Pyramid was to show that individuals should eat more servings from the food group at the base of the Pyramid and fewer servings from the groups placed higher in the Pyramid. For purposes of illustration, consider the top and bottom most aspects of the Old Food Pyramid, Fats, Oils, and Sweets and Bread, Cereal, Rice, and Pasta Group, respectively. The recommendation for intake of Fats, Oils, and Sweets was extremely limited. The Bread, Cereal, Rice and Pasta Group had the highest recommended servings of any of the food groups. While the new MyPyramid Food System continues to support this recommendation dietary recommendation it makes this recommendation visually quite differently.
- **Moderation** is illustrated by the narrowing of the food bands as they approach the top of the pyramid. The premise of this particular compoent is to suggest a need to eat more frequently the foods at the bottom of the pyramid. Foods at the bottom of the pyramid reflect those that are lower in solid fats such as fruits, vegetables, whole grains, and fat-free or low-fat milk and added sugars.

- **Gradual improvement** is illustrated by the slogan "Steps To a Healthier You" shown under the MyPryamid symbol. The basic premise of this particular aspect of the symbol is to suggest that small daily changes in diet and activity can lead to a healthier individual and life.
- **Personalization** is illustrated by the MyPyramid symbol in three different ways. First, is the symbolic representation of an individual climbing steps. Secondly, the slogan has been written to personalize the symbol. And lastly, the government website is particularly focused on helping each individual user establish personalized dietary and activity history. It is particular helpful in helping individuals to find the foods they need to eat, understand what they are currently eating and makes suggestions to help each person to make changes that will lead to a more healthy and positive lifestyle.

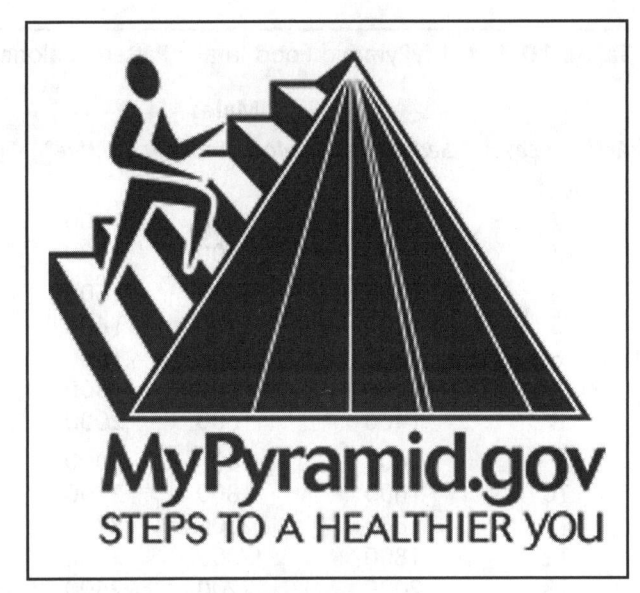

Figure 10.1 ■ The MyPyramid Symbol
Source: U.S. Department of Agriculture

Unlike the previous Food Pyramid and the Basic Four Group plans, the MyPyramid system offers a reasonably simple symbol design (described above) and relies on materials provided at MyPyramid.gov website to provide specific diet and physical activity guidance. The basic principle behind the MyPyramid system is to provide an individualized approach to healthy eating and physical activity. The system assigns each person, individually, to a specific caloric intake level based on their gender, age and current activity level. Activity levels are reflected in the following three categories: Sedentary, Moderately Active, and Active. Caloric intake levels are provided, by year, for individuals between the ages of 2 and 18 and by multi-year increments for adults for each activity category. Table 10.3 provides the recommended MyPyramid Food Intake Pattern Calorie Levels. There are a total of 12 levels shown. Activity levels are defined by the amount of time an individual spends physically active about normal daily living activity. Individuals are considered sedentary if they participate in less than 30 minutes of physical activity daily. Moderately active individuals participate in 30 to 60 minutes of physical activity a day. Active individuals are defined as those persons participating in more than 60 minutes of activity a day.

Specific food intake patterns for the twelve different caloric levels are shown in Table 10.5. The MyPyramid Food System offers a range of servings per group. This range is provided to correct for individual differences in caloric need. For example, a sedentary, 20 year old, female requires a daily caloric intake of approximately 2000 calories. Her recommended daily amount of food from each food group includes, 2 cups of fruits, 2.5 cups of vegetables, 6 ounces of grains, 5.5 ounces of meats and beans, 3 cups of milk and 27 grams or approximately 6 teaspoons of oil. By comparison, an active, 20 year old, male requires 3000 calories per day. His recommended food intake by food group would be 2.5 cups of fruit, 4 cups of vegetables, 10 ounces of grains, 7 ounces of meat and beans, 3 cups of milk and 44 grams or approximately 10 teaspoons of oils. For purposes of illustration, Table 10.4 presents serving size recommendations or equivalents for each food group.

Recall that no food item contains all food nutrients. In a similar vein, foods within a particular food group do not contain the same nutrient content. As a result, it is important to eat a variety of foods from each food group. This practice will help to ensure that adequate levels of all necessary nutrients are consumed. Individuals eating fewer calories or servings are encouraged to select foods in each group wisely. Foods that are more nutrient dense are recommended.

Table 10-3 ■ MyPyramid Food Intake Pattern Calorie Levels

	Males				Females		
Activity Level	Sedentary*	Mod. Active*	Active*	Activity Level	Sedentary*	Mod. Active*	Active*
AGE				AGE			
2	1000	1000	1000	2	1000	1000	1000
3	1000	1400	1400	3	1000	1200	1400
4	1200	1400	1600	4	1200	1400	1400
5	1200	1400	1600	5	1200	1400	1600
6	1400	1600	1800	6	1200	1400	1600
7	1400	1600	1800	7	1200	1600	1800
8	1400	1600	2000	8	1400	1600	1800
9	1600	1800	2000	9	1400	1600	1800
10	1600	1800	2200	10	1400	1800	2000
11	1800	2000	2200	11	1600	1800	2000
12	1800	2200	2400	12	1600	2000	2200
13	2000	2200	2600	13	1600	2000	2200
14	2000	2400	2800	14	1800	2000	2400
15	2200	2600	3000	15	1800	2000	2400
16	2400	2800	3200	16	1800	2000	2400
17	2400	2800	3200	17	1800	2000	2400
18	2400	2800	3200	18	1800	2000	2400
19–20	2600	2800	3000	19–20	2000	2200	2400
21–25	2400	2800	3000	21–25	2000	2200	2400
26–30	2400	2600	3000	26–30	1800	2000	2400
31–35	2400	2600	3000	31–35	1800	2000	2200
36–40	2400	2600	2800	36–40	1800	2000	2200
41–45	2200	2600	2800	41–45	1800	2000	2200
46–50	2200	2400	2800	46–50	1800	2000	2200
51–55	2200	2400	2800	51–55	1600	1800	2200
56–60	2200	2400	2600	56–60	1600	1800	2200
61–65	2000	2400	2600	61–65	1600	1800	2000
66–70	2000	2200	2600	66–70	1600	1800	2000
71–75	2000	2200	2600	71–75	1600	1800	2000
76 and up	2000	2200	2400	76 and up	1600	1800	2000

Key:
Sedentary = less than 30 minutes a day of moderate physical activity in addition to daily activities.
Moderately Active = at least 30 minutes up to 60 minutes a day of moderate physical activity in addition to daily activities.
Active = 60 or more minutes a day of moderate physical activity in addition to daily activities.

Source: US Department of Agriculture, Center for Nutrition Policy and Promotion, April 2005. http://www.mypyramid.gov

The consumer is often confused when it comes to the question of "how much food is the appropriate amount. In the case of a food label, the term "serving" represents the specific amount of the food described on the label that contains the exact amount of nutrients as described on the label. The serving size on the label *does not necessarily reflect* an appropriate amount of food based on the MyPyramid food system.

To further complicate the issue, consider the concept of "portion size." Portion size reflects the amount of food we choose to serve ourselves or the amount that is served in restaurants. Again, these portion sizes are not necessarily fitted to the MyPyramid food system recommendations. They may be bigger or smaller than the recommendations or the serving size as described by a particular food label. For example, consider our 20 year old, sedentary female again. She may order a 12-ounce steak, at her favorite restaurant, for dinner. This order represents one portion

Table 10-4 ■ What Counts?

Grains Group: Examples of 1 ounce equivalents of Bread, Cereal, Rice, and Pasta
- 1 slice of bread
- About 1 cup of ready-to-eat cereal
- ½ cup of cooked cereal, rice, or pasta

Vegetable Group: Examples of 1 cup equivalents
- 2 cup of raw leafy vegetables
- 1 cup of other vegetables—cooked or raw
- 1 cup of vegetable juice

Fruit Group: Examples of 1 cup equivalents
- 1 cup of fresh fruit
- 2 medium size fresh fruit (i.e. apple, banana, orange, pear)
- 1 cup of chopped, cooked, or canned fruit
- 1 cup of 100% fruit juice
- ½ cup of dried fruit

Milk Group: Examples of 1 cup equivalents of Milk, Yogurt, and Cheese
- 1 cup of milk or yogurt
- 1½ ounces of natural cheese
- 2 ounces of processed cheese

Meat and Beans Group: Examples of 1 ounce equivalents of Meat, Poultry, Fish, Dry Beans, Eggs, and Nuts
- 1 ounce of cooked lean meat, poultry, or fish
- ½ cup of cooked dry beans or ½ cup of tofu counts as 1 ounce of lean meat
- 1 egg counts as 1 ounce of lean meat
- ½ ounce of nuts or seeds
- 1 Tablespoon of peanut butter

Source: Modified from *Nutrition and Health: Dietary Guidelines for Americans, 2000.* Washington, DC: United States Department of Agriculture and Department of Health and Human Services, 2000 and *Dietary Guidelines for Americans, 2005* Washington, DC: United States Department of Agriculture and Department of Health and Human Services.

as defined and delivered by the restaurant. Yet, in terms of the MyPyramid recommendations, it represents more than twice her recommended daily intake of the meat and beans food group.

Supplements

For healthy people consuming a balanced diet, most supplements are not necessary. But for those who insist on taking supplements, the following information may prove helpful. The body processes foods much better than pills. The regular use of a one-a-day multivitamin and mineral supplement will not cause problems if it yields less than 2 times the RDA. Be concerned with the binding agents in supplements. If a tablet does not dissolve in an appropriate time or way, the product will be passed from the body without sufficiently being absorbed. Additionally, there is no evidence that vitamin C, taken in mega-doses is beneficial.

At present, there seems to be valid information supporting vitamin E supplementation. This is especially true for athletes and heavy exercisers. And, as mentioned, calcium supplementation is often recommended. Educate yourself before you use supplements, as they may become associated with some health problems. Be apprised that the information on supplementation is based on current knowledge in a field that is ever changing. As we expand our nutritional knowledge, we may find one day that some supplements (other than calcium) may be recommended.

Table 10-5 ■ Recommended Daily Food Intake for Each Food Group by Calorie Level

Daily Amount of Food From Each Group (vegetable subgroup amounts per week)

Calorie Level	1,000	1,200	1,400	1,600	1,800	2,000	2,200	2,400	2,600	2,800	3,000	3,200
Food Group	Food group amounts shown in cup (c) or ounce-equivalents (oz-eq), with number of servings (srv) in parentheses when it differs from the other units. See note for quantity equivalents for foods in each group. Oils are shown in grams (g) and teaspoons.
Fruits	1 c (2 srv)	1 c (2 srv)	1.5 c (3 srv)	1.5 c (3 srv)	1.5 c (3 srv)	2 c (4 srv)	2 c (4 srv)	2 c (4 srv)	2 c (4 srv)	2.5 c (5 srv)	2.5 c (5 srv)	2.5 c (5 srv)
Vegetables	1 c (2 srv)	1.5 c (3 srv)	1.5 c (3 srv)	2 c (4 srv)	2.5 c (5 srv)	2.5 c (5 srv)	3 c (6 srv)	3 c (6 srv)	3.5 c (7 srv)	3.5 c (7 srv)	4 c (8 srv)	4 c (8 srv)
Dark green veg.	1 c/wk	1.5 c/wk	1.5 c/wk	2 c/wk	3 c/wk	3 c/wk	3 c/wk	3 c/wk	3 c/wk	3 c/wk	3 c/wk	3 c/wk
Orange veg.	.5 c/wk	1 c/wk	1 c/wk	1.5 c/wk	2 c/wk	2 c/wk	2 c/wk	2 c/wk	2.5 c/wk	2.5 c/wk	2.5 c/wk	2.5 c/wk
Legumes	.5 c/wk	1 c/wk	1 c/wk	2.5 c/wk	3 c/wk	3 c/wk	3 c/wk	3 c/wk	3.5 c/wk	3.5 c/wk	3.5 c/wk	3.5 c/wk
Starchy veg.	1.5 c/wk	2.5 c/wk	2.5 c/wk	2.5 c/wk	3 c/wk	3 c/wk	6 c/wk	6 c/wk	7 c/wk	7 c/wk	9 c/wk	9 c/wk
Other veg.	4 c/wk	4.5 c/wk	4.5 c/wk	5.5 c/wk	6.5 c/wk	6.5 c/wk	7 c/wk	7 c/wk	8.5 c/wk	8.5 c/wk	10 c/wk	10 c/wk
Grains	3 oz-eq	4 oz-eq	5 oz-eq	5 oz-eq	6 oz-eq	6 oz-eq	7 oz-eq	8 oz-eq	9 oz-eq	10 oz-eq	10 oz-eq	10 oz-eq
Whole grains	1.5	2	2.5	3	3	3	3.5	4	4.5	5	5	5
Other grains	1.5	2	2.5	3	3	3	3.5	4	4.5	5	5	5
Lean meat And beans	2 oz-eq	3 oz-eq	4 oz-eq	5 oz-eq	5 oz-eq	5.5 oz-eq	6 oz-eq	6.5 oz-eq	6.5 oz-eq	7 oz-eq	7 oz-eq	7 oz-eq
Milk	2 c	2 c	2 c	3 c	3 c	3 c	3 c	3 c	3 c	3 c	3 c	3 c
Oils	15 g	17 g	17 g	22 g	24 g	27 g	29 g	31 g	34 g	36 g	44 g	51 g
Discretionary Calorie allowance	165	171	171	132	195	267	290	362	410	426	512	648

Source: U.S. Department of Agriculture, Center for Nutrition Policy and Promotion. MyPyramid, 2005.

Does supplementation improve an athlete's performance? According to the United States Olympic Committee on Sports Medicine, "there is no scientific evidence that intakes of vitamins and minerals greater than the recommended amounts will enhance performance." Supplementation during pregnancy and catastrophic illnesses, however, is beneficial.

Herbal Supplements

It is estimated that in the coming year, Americans will spend approximately 4.8 billion dollars on herbal supplements. Many consumers are unaware that herbal supplements do not fall under the control of the Food and Drug Administration (FDA). This means that *consumers have no guarantee as to how much of an active ingredient any tablet actually contains.* Products making claims for improved health, may be false.

One of the marketing appeals to the public is the phrase, "all natural." It is misleading to think that all natural means something is good for you. After all, poison ivy, spider venom, and snake venom are all natural. While some herbal supplements may prove beneficial, others can be harmful.

One herbal supplement that you should avoid is the herbal stimulant ephedra or ephedrine, also known as Ma Whang. Ephedra is a stimulant similar to amphetamines. Adverse effects include heart attack, stroke, seizures, dizziness, irregular heart beats, increased heart rate, increased blood pressure, and heart palpitations. Many fad diet products and protein drinks contain ephedra. As it increases the heart rate above normal levels, it raises one's metabolism, resulting in possible weight loss and extra stress on the body. Other products such as germander and pokeroot can hurt the liver (Kurtzweil, 1999).

If you, however, are convinced that herbal supplements are for you, educate yourself as to the potential benefits and/or hazards of each product. Some should be avoided, especially if you are hypertensive or present other health problems.

If you purchase herbal products, buy brand-name products made in this country. There are no guarantees about the conditions in which imported herbal preparations are grown, their purity, or composition. Always look for the word "standardized" on any herbal product. Remember, good health can best be attained through a well balanced diet along with regular exercise, not from pills or herbal supplementation.

Food for Performance

How Soon Can I Exercise after I Eat?

The question of how soon can a person participate in activity after he/she eats a meal is of concern for many. For example, coaches are concerned about scheduling meals before competitions so their players are not negatively affected by food intake. Many parents worry about children participating in swimming activities for fear of stomach cramps after a meal. In all cases, the underlying question or concern is how can an individual avoid digestive tract (i.e., stomach, gastrointestinal tract) discomfort during activity following a meal or food intake?

The answer is not clearly defined and is largely based on the individual. There appear to be several influencing factors. Discomfort appears to be related to: 1) the nature and intensity of the activity, 2) how soon the activity was begun following food intake, and 3) the nature and amount of food consumed.

The nature and intensity of activity seems to be directly related to how soon an activity can begin following a meal. In general, higher intensity activities will require greater amounts of time between food intake and the initiation of activity. Lower intensity activities will allow for shorter time periods. For example, a person wanting to run may need to wait several hours after a meal to avoid discomfort as compared to a person wanting to walk. The person wanting to walk may experience little, or no, discomfort walking shortly after a meal.

The nature and type of food consumed also appears to be related to discomfort. Foods, high in fat, proteins that are hard to digest, or extremely spicy foods may present more problems than foods high in carbohydrates, which are easily digested. Also, foods higher in fiber content are more likely to cause gastrointestinal distress.

Dietary Needs for the Physically Active

Clearly, nutrition and diet are related to physical performance, as well as recovery from physical activity. For example, individuals exercising more than an hour a day may need 70% of their calories to come primarily from complex carbohydrates as compared to the normal dietary recommendation of 60% of total calories consumed.

For organizational purposes, specific diet and nutritional needs are discussed under separate headers. It is important to recognize that while treated under separate header, many of these dietary issues are interwoven and may be addressed simultaneously through proper dietary and fluid intake. For example, the consumption of common, commercially-produced sports drinks may assist an individual in meeting carbohydrate, sodium, and fluid replacement needs.

Normally, active individuals who eat a variety of foods and maintain their body weight do not need vitamin and mineral supplementation. Individuals who are: 1) restricting calories in their diet, 2) are eating a lot of low micronutrient density foods, or 3) exercising and losing large amounts of weight, may find vitamin and mineral supplementation is warranted. In these types of situations a multivitamin/mineral supplement is recommended. Avoid using single nutrient supplements.

Carbohydrate Intake

Carbohydrate intake before, during, and after activity is directly related to blood glucose level, muscle glycogen levels, and physical performance. Carbohydrate intake is especially important for individuals or athletes participating in long-term activity. Low levels of blood glucose and muscle glycogen are directly related to fatigue, reduced power output, and other negative performance variables.

Individuals participating in events lasting longer than one hour should try to achieve increased glycogen storage prior to an event (especially endurance races). This procedure is called carbohydrate loading. Specific procedures for maximal carbohydrate loading have been identified and are discussed below under a separate header (see Carbohydrate Loading).

Individuals participating in continuous, long-term activities (lasting more than one hour), such as long distance running, will also benefit from carbohydrate consumption during activity. One of the more popular methods of carbohydrate supplementation is through the consumption of sports drinks. The American College of Sports Medicine (1996) recommends frequent (every 15 to 20 minutes), limited consumption (150 to 350 ml; 6 to 12 ounces) of a fluid containing 4 to 8% carbohydrates.

Simple carbohydrates, such as glucose or sucrose, or starch are recommended since they are easily absorbed. It should be noted that concentrations **greater than 8%** have been shown to *slow gastric emptying*. This finding would, of course, lead to greater dehydration risk. Precaution should be taken to avoid these higher levels of carbohydrate concentration in fluids consumed. Finally, to help prevent dehydration from occurring with carbohydrate supplementation, maintain the highest level of fluid volume in the stomach that can be comfortably tolerated.

Carbohydrate Loading

Carbohydrate loading is a procedure that combines dietary or nutritional manipulation with exercise to increase the amount of glycogen stored in the liver and muscles of the body. Carbohydrate loading is also referred to as *glycogen supercompensation*. If the procedure is properly followed, it has been shown to more than double the amount of stored glycogen in the active muscle tissues.

Increased glycogen storage has been linked to improved performance in endurance activities by reducing or slowing fatigue onset. The process of carbohydrate loading is extremely muscle tissue specific. Only muscles that are depleted through activity will store extra glycogen. As a result, individuals attempting to carbohydrate load need to carefully mimic their activity or sport during the depletion phase of the procedure. The two phases of the carbohydrate loading procedure are presented in Table 10-6.

It is important to recognize that carbohydrate loading has not been shown to benefit all types of activity. Clearly, *it is most beneficial when participating in intense endurance activities lasting longer than one hour.* Activities lasting less than 60 minutes do not require greater levels of stored glycogen. Individuals participating in activities lasting less than 60 minutes can meet their energy demands by following a normal diet.

Table 10-6 ■ Descriptive Phases of the Carbohydrate Loading Procedure

Depletion Phase
- **Day 1:** Deplete muscle glycogen in the active muscles by participating in 90 minutes or more of moderately intense activity.
- **Days 2, 3, 4:** Maintain a low-carbohydrate diet of less that 100 grams of carbohydrate intake per day. Eat foods high in protein and fat. Continue training regiment.

Carbohydrate Loading Phase
- **Days 5, 6, 7:** Maintain a high-carbohydrate diet of 400 grams or more per day. Eat a normal amount of protein and fat. Continue training regiment.
- **Day of Competition:** Eat a high-carbohydrate precompetition meal.

Source: Modified from McArdle, W., Katch, F. & Katch, V. (2001). *Exercise Physiology: Energy, Nutrition, and Human Performance* (5th ed.). Baltimore, MD: Lippincott Williams & Wilkins.

Fat Intake

Individuals participating in regular physical activity do not benefit, in terms of performance enhancement, from fat intake restriction. Additionally, no evidence has been offered to suggest that a diet high in fat intake enhances performance. Active individuals should maintain a normal diet with 20%–30% of their total caloric intake coming from fat.

Protein Intake

Individuals participating in regular physical activity may benefit from slightly higher protein intake. It is important to understand, however, that *muscle mass or gains in lean body weight cannot be attributed to high protein intake.* This finding contradicts the erroneous thinking of many that high-protein diets are required, for body builders and athletes require large amounts of strength.

A joint statement by the American College of Sports Medicine, the American Dietetic Association, and the Dietitians of Canada (2000) suggests a protein intake of approximately 1.2 to 1.4 grams per kilogram of body weight per day for endurance athletes, and as high as 1.6 to 1.7 grams per kilogram of body weight per day for strength-trained individuals. Recall, the recommended dietary intake of protein is .8 grams per kilogram of body weight per day.

Sodium Replacement

How much sodium is lost through sweating during strenuous activity? Are there physical risks if sodium levels are not replaced? How should sodium be replaced in the diet? What role does sodium play as it relates to performance? These are important questions that need to be addressed.

Sodium is related to performance in several ways. Perhaps, the most important is that adequate sodium intake will assist in water retention. This will help prevent a condition known as **hyponatremia**. Hyponatremia is a rare disorder and usually occurs in individuals who are participating in prolonged or long-term (i.e., several hours) activities while consuming large volumes of water and little sodium, during participation. As a result of their fluid intake behavior, electrolyte and sodium deficiencies are created. The low blood sodium concentrations associated with hyponatremia may lead to disorientation, confusion, and grand mal seizures.

Individuals participating in activity lasting longer than one hour should strongly consider the inclusion of sodium in their rehydration fluids. While drinking water will assist in the restoration of body sweating and lowering elevated plasma electrolyte concentrations, complete restoration of extracellular fluid volume cannot occur without sodium replacement (Lassiter, 1990; Takamata, Mack, Gillen, and Nadel, 1994).

Including sodium in any replacement fluids or foods consumed during long-term activity will help prevent hyponatremia onset. The recommended intake level is approximately .5 grams/liter of water (ACSM, 1996). Sodium replacement **does not** have to occur through oral rehydration. Research suggests that proper dietary intake, particularly from the meal immediately prior to activity, may be sufficient in meeting physiological needs.

Fluid Replacement

Proper hydration is another critical concern for the physically active individual. It is important to recognize that hydration levels before, during, and after activity are important. Adequate hydration, prior to participation in activity, helps to offset the risk of dehydration. Fluid consumption during activity helps to replace fluid loss occurring from sweating. Sweating is a body mechanism designed to help cool the body.

The rate of fluid loss is directly related to variables such as exercise intensity and environmental variables (i.e., temperature, humidity, wind speed). Individuals participating in high intensity activity, or in hot, humid environments are at greater risk of dehydration. Dehydration and heat-related disorders such as heat cramps, heat exhaustion, and heat stroke (see Chapter 13) are also more likely to occur in the unacclimated.

The risks associated with dehydration are numerous and dangerous. Included are:

- Impaired thermoregulation, leading to heat-related disorders,
- Hypertonicity of body fluids,
- Reduction in cardiac output during exercise.

Do not underestimate how much fluid can be lost from the body as a result of heavy sweating. Research findings reported by the American College of Sports Medicine (1996) suggests that for most people, voluntary drinking only replaces about two-thirds of the body water lost as sweat. Additionally, they indicate that it is common, even when fluids are available, for individuals to dehydrate by as much as 2%–6% of their total body weight. *Thirst should not be the stimulus to drink*. If a person waits to begin rehydration until he/she experiences thirst he/she has waited to long.

It is important to drink enough fluids after exercise to fully replace the volume lost during activity. Most individuals do not drink enough fluids during activity to balance or offset fluid losses occurring during activity.

The American College of Sports Medicine (1996) has provided guidelines to help limit dehydration risk. They recommend individuals consume approximately 500ml (approximately 17 ounces) of water about two hours prior to, and immediately before, activity. In general, two hours is enough time for the renal systems of most individuals to excrete excess ingested fluid.

During activity, supplemental consumption (150 ml or approximately 6 ounces) should occur about every 15 minutes. They recommend the consumed fluids be cooler than ambient temperature and be chilled to temperatures between 59 and 72 degrees Fahrenheit.

Vitamin and Mineral Supplementation

Does vitamin mineral supplementation improve athletic or physical performance? Even though many people believe that it does, the facts are that *no clinical research supports this finding*. Most likely any performance change resulting from vitamin or mineral supplementation can be explained as a placebo effect. While there is really no harm in an individual supplementing the diet with a multivitamin, the practice of megadosing vitamin and mineral intake may be harmful and should be considered contraindicated.

Caffeine

Common sources of caffeine include, but are not limited to, coffee, tea, and carbonated beverages (i.e., Surge, Mountain Dew). Caffeine is a central nervous system stimulant that serves to increase alertness and decrease fatigue. Large amounts of caffeine cause nervousness, irritability, increased heart rate, and headaches. It has been linked to fibro cystic breast disease in women. There is some evidence that caffeine enhances the use of fat during endurance exercise, and that caffeine may make more calcium available for muscular contraction.

Olympic officials consider caffeine a drug and large levels of consumption are restricted. An athlete who consumes more than 5–6 cups of coffee may find he/she tests drug positive for caffeine. Small amounts of caffeine (equivalent to 1–2 cups of coffee) are considered acceptable.

Understanding the New Food Label

The Nutrition Labeling and Education Act of 1990 (NLEA) requires nutrition labeling for most foods. Exceptions include meat and poultry, which are regulated by the U.S. Department of Agriculture (USDA). Additionally, the NLEA authorizes the use of nutrient content claims and appropriate FDA approved health claims. These claims are discussed below under a separate header.

In 1994, the original food label was revised (FDA, 1995). In 2006, it was revised again. Trans fat labeling is now required. These revisions stemmed from new regulations from the Food and Drug Administration, the Department of Health and Human Services, and the Food and Safety and Inspection Service of U.S. Department of Agriculture. The revisions were made to help clarify the food label so consumers could make informed decisions, hopefully leading to more healthy diets. Additionally, it is believed the new label will motivate food companies to offer better, more nutritional products.

The consumer benefits by having a label that is easy to read and understand. By developing an understanding of label features such as % Daily Values, Nutrient Claims, and Health Claims, consumers can make judgments that may help them meet dietary, weight management and other food oriented goals and objectives. For example, a food can claim to be lower in calories or fat than a similar product of similar serving if it shows the difference.

Individuals on special or restricted diets can benefit from the new label. For example, individuals presenting failing or failed kidney functions are restricted from protein, potassium and sodium. Individuals with hepatitis, cirrhosis and other liver diseases may need diets high in calories and low in protein. An individual presenting chronic constipation, irritable bowel syndrome, and diverticulosis may want a diet high in fiber. In each of these situations, the new labels make it easier for the consumer to quickly and accurately identify the nutritional contents and appropriateness of a product.

Health claims can be made as well. For example, a diet low in sodium may claim to help in the reduction of hypertension. This health claim can be made, however, only by diets that meet the definition of "low sodium" or those that are 20% or less of Daily Value for fat, saturated fat, and cholesterol per serving.

Serving size information is used to describe the amount of the product to which all-numeric information on the food label applies. It is reported metrically, such as in grams (g) or milliliters (ml), and in household measures, such as cups, tablespoons, teaspoons, etc. Serving sizes are similar in size to normal or actual amounts eaten by most individuals. Serving sizes must be similar from product to like product. This helps in making it easier for the consumer to compare products of like kind.

Not all foods are labelled. The NLEA exempts foods served for immediate consumption (i.e., cafeterias, airplanes, vendors), ready to eat foods prepared on site (i.e., bakery, deli), foods shipped and not sold in bulk to consumers, medical foods, and foods that contain no significant amounts of any nutrients such as coffee, tea, and spices.

% Daily Values

The term Daily Value is a new reference tool used to provide the amount of nutrients on the new food label. This helps consumers in determining the overall nutritional value of a particular food. For example, a hypertensive individual trying to limit fat, cholesterol and sodium intake can quickly identify the amounts of these substances in a product and determine whether it is appropriate for his/her dietary goals.

The amount of nutrients in a food may be expressed in two ways. First, in metric units, grams or milligrams, or secondly, as a percentage of the Daily Value (% Daily Value).

A 2,000-calorie a day diet serves as the basis for calculating % Daily Values. The government sets this standard. Individual dietary needs will vary in the actual number of calories consumed and/or needed. An active individual may require a caloric intake of 2500 calories or greater, while a sedentary individual may find a 2,000 calorie diet exceeds his/her needs.

The purpose of the standard is to allow the consumer to make an informed judgement. The idea is to consume 100% of the Daily Value of each nutrient each day by eating a variety of foods. By standardizing the diet, it better informs the consumer as to how a serving of food fits into his/her total daily diet. Meeting the % Daily Value serves to limit intakes of foods negatively associated with diseases, such as saturated fat and cholesterol. It also encourages the consumption of food positively associated with disease risk. For example, increased intake of fiber is associated with decreased risk of coronary heart disease or increased calcium consumption is related to lower risk of osteoporosis.

Health Claims

Health claims describe a relationship between a nutrient or food and the risk of a disease or health related condition. This allows consumers to know that if they see the claims they can believe them. They are not simply "marketing ploys" used to encourage sales. The FDA has authorized the use of 10 claims (FDA Consumer: On the Teen Scene: Food Label Makes Good Eating Easier, 1995). These 10 are the only claims that can be used in a label. The claims may show a link between:

1. **Calcium and a decreased risk of osteoporosis:** This claim can be made if a food contains 20% or more of the Daily Value for calcium per serving. Additionally, the calcium content must equal or exceed the food phosphorous content, and contain calcium that is easily absorbed and used by the body. Target groups most affected or in need of calcium must be identified. Finally, the need for exercise and proper diet must be indicated.

2. **Fat and an increased risk of cancer:** This claim can be made if a food meets the descriptive requirements for low-fat. Game and fish must meet the descriptive requirements for extra lean.

3. **Saturated fat and cholesterol and an increased risk of coronary heart disease:** This claim can be made if a food meets the descriptive requirements for low saturated fat, low-cholesterol, and low-fat. Game and fish must meet the descriptive requirements for extra lean.

4. **Fiber-containing grain products, fruits and vegetables and a decreased risk of cancer:** This claim can be made if a food contains a grain product, fruit, or vegetable and meets the descriptive requirements for low-fat (3 g or less per serving) and, without alteration, meets the descriptive requirements of being a good source for dietary fiber.

5. **Fruits, vegetables and grain products that contain fiber and a decreased risk of coronary heart disease:** This claim can be made if a grain product, fruit, or vegetable meets the descriptive requirements for low saturated fat (3 g or less per serving), low-cholesterol, and low-fat and contain without alteration, at least 0.6 g soluble fiber per serving.

6. **Sodium and an increased risk of hypertension or high blood pressure:** This claim can be made if a food meets the descriptive requirement for low sodium (i.e., 140 mg or less per serving. If the serving is 30 g or less or 2 tablespoons or less, 140 mg or less per 50 g of the food).

7. **Fruits and vegetables and a decreased risk of cancer:** This claim can be made if a fruit or vegetable meets the descriptive requirements for low-fat and, without alteration, is considered a good source for at least one of the following: dietary fiber or vitamins A or C.

8. **Folic acid and a decreased risk of neutral tube defect-affected pregnancy:** This claim can be made if a food in conventional form is naturally high in folic acid. Recommended daily consumption for women of childbearing age is 0.4 mg.
9. **Sugar alcohols and a reduced risk of dental caries**
10. **Soluble fiber from whole oats, as part of a diet low in saturated fat and cholesterol, and a reduced risk of coronary heart disease:** This claim can be made if a food contains soluble fiber from whole oats and is eaten in a diet low in saturate fat and cholesterol. Foods may include oats, oat bran, and whole-oat flour.

Health claims can be used only in specific situations, such as when the food contains appropriate levels of the stated nutrients. Any claim must be stated clearly so the consumer can easily understand the relationship between the nutrient and the disease. For example, "Diets low in saturated fat and cholesterol may reduce the risk of coronary artery disease," is an appropriate claim.

Nutrient Content Descriptors

Nutrient claims can be made when strict definitions set by the government are met. As is the case with Health Claims, Nutrient Claims should allow for consumer confidence. If a consumer sees a nutrient content claim he/she can believe it. For example, Nabisco offers a baked snack cracker called a Wheat Thin. The reduced fat Wheat Thin must have 25% or more reduction in fat when compared to the normal Wheat Thin to make the claim of reduced fat. In this example, the original Wheat Thin had 6 grams of fat and the reduced fat Wheat Thin has 4 grams of fat. Since they have a 30% reduction in fat Nabisco can make its claim. There are 12 core terms that are allowed (FDA, 1995). These include:

1. **Free:** Synonymous with such terms as without, no, and zero. Free implies that a product contains no amount, or an insignificant or physiologically inconsequential amount, one or more of these components:
   - fat
   - saturated fat
   - cholesterol
   - sodium
   - sugars
   - calories

For example, a fat-free single-item food must have 0.5 g or less fat per serving. A sugar-free item must have 0.5 g or less sugar per serving. Therefore, if the serving size can be made small enough, the serving can be labeled fat-free.

2. **Low:** Used to describe foods that can be eaten frequently and not exceed recommended dietary guidelines on one or more of the fat, saturated fat, cholesterol, sodium, sugars, and calories. Table 10-7 provides examples of "Low" nutrient content descriptors. Other terms that are synonymous with Low are Little, Few, and Low Source Of.

Table 10-7 ■ Examples of Low Nutrient Content Descriptors

Descriptor	Defining Criteria
Low-fat	3 g or less per serving
Low-saturated fat	1 g or less per serving
Low-sodium	140 mg or less per serving
Very low-sodium	35 mg or less per serving
Low-cholesterol	20 mg or less and 2 g or less of saturated fat per serving
Low-calorie	40 calories or less per serving

3. **Lean:** Fat content in meats, poultry, game, and seafood may be described by the term lean. By definition, lean is less than 10 g fat, 4.5 g or less saturated fat, and less than 95 mg cholesterol per serving and per 100 mg.
4. **Extra lean:** Similar to lean, the term extra lean is used to describe fat content in meat, poultry, game, and seafood. By definition, extra lean is less than 5 g fat, less than 2 g saturated fat, and less than 95 mg cholesterol per serving and per 100 g.
5. **High:** Represents a food containing 20% or more of the Daily Value for a particular nutrient in a serving. For example, a food claiming to be high in fiber must have 5 g or more of fiber per serving.
6. **Good source:** Represents a food that contains 10 to 19% of the Daily Value for a particular nutrient in a serving. For example, a food claiming to be a good source of calcium must have at least 100 mg of calcium per serving.
7. **Reduced:** Represents a food containing 25% or less of calories or a nutrient per serving than the reference food. For example, a food claiming to have reduced sodium must have at least 25% less sodium per serving than the reference food.
8. **Less:** Represents a food, which may or may not be altered, containing 25% or less calories or a nutrient per serving than the reference food. The term "fewer" is an acceptable alternative descriptor for less.
9. **Light:** Can have two meanings. First, it means one third fewer calories or half the fat of the reference food. In foods where 50% or more calories are from fat, the reduction must be 50% of the fat. Secondly, light can mean that the sodium content of a low-calorie, low-fat food has been reduced by 50% compared to the reference food.
10. **More:** Represents a food, which may or may not be altered, containing a nutrient of 10% or greater of the Daily Value compared to the reference food. For example, a food claiming to have more vitamin D must have at least 40 International Units more vitamin D than the reference food. Note, the label will indicate 10% more of the Daily Value for vitamin D.
11. **Healthy:** Describes a food low in fat, saturated fat, cholesterol, and sodium. Single-item foods must provide 10% or more of one or more of vitamins A or C, iron, calcium, protein, or fiber. Meal-type products must provide 10% or more of two or more of these vitamins, minerals, protein or fiber.
12. **Fewer:** Synonymous term with Less. The descriptive criteria are the same as those listed above for Less.

Laboratory Activities

CHAPTER 10

Name: _____ Class Time/Day: _____ Score: _____

LABORATORY 10-A

Food Labeling

■ **Purpose:** This laboratory examines selected food labels for purposes of identifying relative information regarding issues such as advertising, cost, and nutrient values.

■ **Precautions:** There are no known risks of participation.

■ **Equipment:** Food label worksheet and selected food items.

■ **Procedure:** The subject should select compatible food items for purposes of comparison and complete the attached worksheet. For example, brownies could be compared to reduced fat brownies. Compare findings.

■ **Scoring:** None

■ **Data/Calculations:**

Name: Date: /   /

Gender: Age: Height: Weight:

Food Alternatives

Nutrition Facts	
Serving Size	
Serving Per Container	
Amount Per Serving	
Calories	Calories from Fat
	% Daily Value*
Total Fat g	%
Saturated Fat g	%
Trans Fat g	%
Cholesterol	%
Sodium mg	%
Total Carbohydrate g	%
Dietary Fiber g	%
Sugars g	
Protein g	%
Vitamin A % Vitamin C %	
Calcium % Iron % Vitamin D %	
*Percent Daily Values are based on a 2,000 calorie diet. Your daily values may be higher or lower depending on your calorie needs.	

Nutrition Facts	
Serving Size	
Serving Per Container	
Amount Per Serving	
Calories	Calories from Fat
	% Daily Value*
Total Fat g	%
Saturated Fat g	%
Trans Fat g	%
Cholesterol	%
Sodium mg	%
Total Carbohydrate g	%
Dietary Fiber g	%
Sugars g	
Protein g	%
Vitamin A % Vitamin C %	
Calcium % Iron % Vitamin D %	
*Percent Daily Values are based on a 2,000 calorie diet. Your daily values may be higher or lower depending on your calorie needs.	

11
Principles of Weight Management

*Obesity is the second most preventable
cause of death in the United States.*
Center for Disease Control and Prevention

*People who are overweight or obese have a higher risk
for heart disease, high blood pressure, high cholesterol,
and other chronic diseases and conditions.*
Center for Disease Control and Prevention

*The increase in obesity in Arkansas is three times
the increase observed nationally.*
Arkansas Health Counts

■ Chapter Outline ■

Introduction
Understanding Body Fat
Understanding Obesity
Regional Body Fat Storage
Understanding Energy Balance
Understanding Energy Balance and Weight Loss
Causes of Obesity
    Labor-Saving Devices/Technology
    Genetics
    Family Lifestyle
    Childhood Fatness

Set Point Theory
Understanding the Role of Exercise in Weight
    Control
Spot Reduction
Behavior Modification and Successful Weight
    Management
Eating Disorders
    Anorexia Nervosa
    Bulimia
Practical Guidelines for Gaining Weight

■ Learning Objectives ■

The student should be able to:

- Describe and distinguish the three somatotyped body builds.

- Identify and describe the physiological differences and implications between essential and nonessential body fat.

- Identify and describe the physiological differences and implications between android and gynoid obesity.
- Demonstrate understanding of the concept of energy balance as it relates to weight gain, loss, or maintenance.
- Identify and demonstrate understanding of the factors related to obesity.
- Demonstrate understanding of the role of exercise in weight control.
- Demonstrate understanding of the concept of spot reduction as it relates to weight management and body shaping.
- Identify and describe lifestyle and behavior management strategies related to weight management.
- Identify and describe individual characteristics, and eating patterns and behaviors of the anorexic and/or bulimic individual.
- Identify and demonstrate understanding of practical guidelines for gaining weight.

■ Keywords ■

Android obesity	Energy balance	Metabolism
Anorexia nervosa	Energy expenditure	Mesomorph
Basal metabolism	Energy intake	Nonessential body fat
Body mass index	Essential body fat	Obesity
Bulimia	Food label	Set point theory
Calorie	Food log	Somatotypes
Creeping obesity	Gynoid obesity	Spot reduction
Ectomorph	Lean body mass	Total body metabolism
Endomorph		

Introduction

The human body is composed of fat, bone, muscle and other tissues such as teeth, hair, organ tissue and connective tissue. The relative percentage of each will vary from individual to individual and will influence each individual's somatotype. There are three somatotyped body builds. These include:

- Ectomorph (Thin)
- Mesomorph (Muscular)
- Endomorph (Fat)

Figures 11.1, 11.2, 11.3 illustrate each somatotype.

Factors that contribute to this variance include, but are not limited to, gender, heredity, and individual lifestyle. For example, sedentary individuals and/or those who consume eat excessive calories are more likely to present excessive body fat levels and an endomorphic somatotype. Individuals who manage their caloric intake and participate in regular physical activity are more likely to present body forms containing less fat and more lean body mass. Lean body mass is considered the fat-free mass of the body. Individuals presenting more lean body mass and muscle tissue are considered mesomorphic somatotypes.

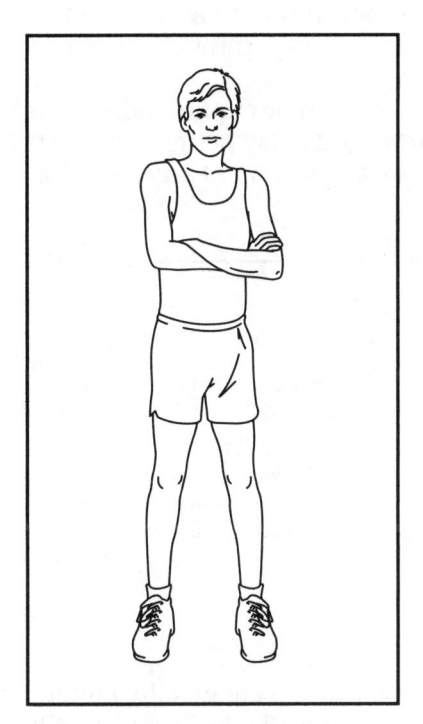

Figure 11.1 ■ Ectomorph Somatotype

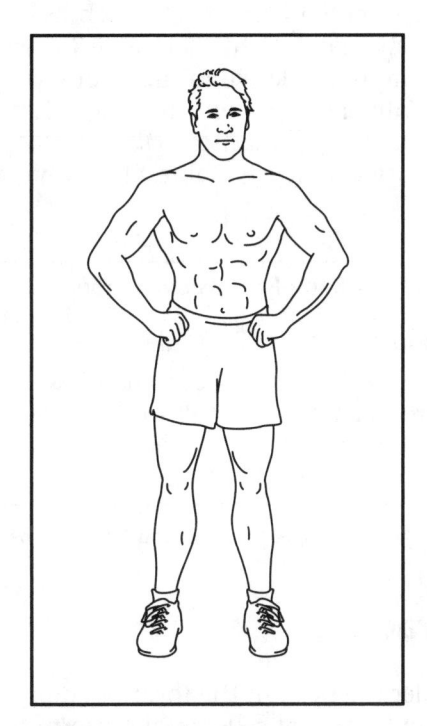

Figure 11.2 ■ Mesomorph Somatotype

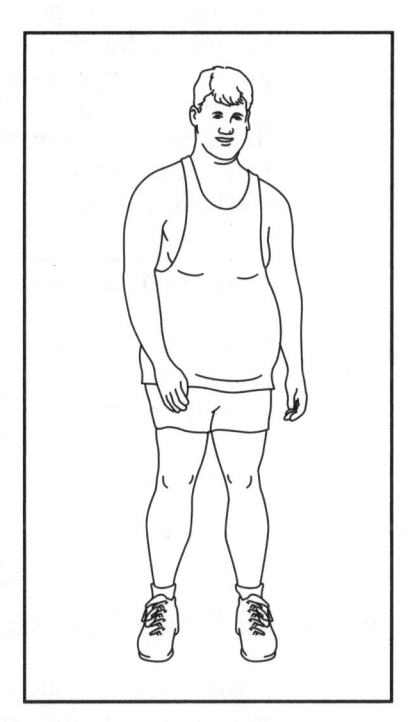

Figure 11.3 ■ Endomorph Somatotype

Understanding Body Fat

Body fat is a critical part of the human body. Body fat is typically categorized as either essential or nonessential. Essential fat should be considered as the minimal amount of fat that is needed by the body. The body uses fat to assist in temperature regulation, shock absorption, and organ protection. In addition, essential nutrients such as fat-soluble vitamins (i.e., A, D, E, and K) rely on fat to assist in nutrient regulation.

Nonessential fat results from excess caloric intake. This excess fat is stored in the body in the form of adipose tissue. The magnitude of storage determines an individual's level of fatness. This can range from excessively lean to morbidly obese.

Understanding Obesity

Obesity is the result of excess fat storage in the body. It results from an imbalance of energy intake and energy expenditure. In cases where energy intake is excessive, fat is stored, in triglyceride form, in adipose tissue. Obesity is a gender specific term identifying an above normal percentage of body fat. Exact levels vary, but most agree that for women, this level of overfatness is 30% and for men 25%.

Additionally, the level of acceptable fatness will vary depending on objectives. Acceptable levels of fatness associated with good health are higher than those associated with physical performance. In most cases, individuals, such as athletes, are found to seek and maintain lower levels of fatness. Excessive fat weight does not contribute to increased performance and may in some cases impair performance. Several factors contribute to this finding. For some sports, such as gymnastics and diving, altered physical appearance from excess fatness may in and of itself influence scoring. In other sports, such as boxing and wrestling, weight is used to standardize competitive classes. In all sports, however, excessive fat will influence oxygen consumption. Endurance oriented competitors such as cyclist and runners clearly stand to benefit by limiting excessive fat weight. Excessive fat weight on these individuals would lower their oxygen consumption relative to their body weight.

Excessive fat weight influences strength to weight ratios. Sports that require individuals to manage their weight, such as gymnastics, will find the participants may perform more efficiently by reducing excessive fat levels. Table 11-1 provides a classification of acceptable fat levels by gender.

Table 11-1 ■ Classification of Body Fatness by Gender

Body Fatness Classification	Male	Female
Essential Fat	Less than 5%	Less than 8%
Acceptable Fatness for Performance	5%–13%	12%–22%
Acceptable Fatness for Health	10%–25%	18%–30%
Overfatness	> 25%	> 30%

From: Wilmore, J., et. al. (1986). "Body Composition: A Round Table" in *The Physician and Sportsmedicine*, 14: 152.

Regional Body Fat Storage

Fat is stored, in cells under the skin, in the form of adipose tissue. There are literally billions of fat cells. Yet, the distribution of fat cells is not uniform throughout the body. Excessive cells in particular body regions contribute to more regional fat storage. Regional storage of fat appears to be related to genetics.

Regional storage in the abdomen and upper body (see Figure 11.4) is referred to as **android obesity**. Android obesity is related to higher risk of cardiovascular disease. **Gynoid obesity** is a term used to describe fat storage below the waist (see Figure 11.5). Men present android obesity more frequently than women.

Where fat is stored in the body appears to be related to morbidity and mortality. In fact, waist to hip circumference ratios are better predictors of coronary risk than body weight, body fat, or BMI.

It is important to recognize, however, that even though a genetic tendency toward obesity and distribution may exist, proper dietary and exercise interventions can and should alter these tendencies.

Figure 11.4 ■ Android Obesity

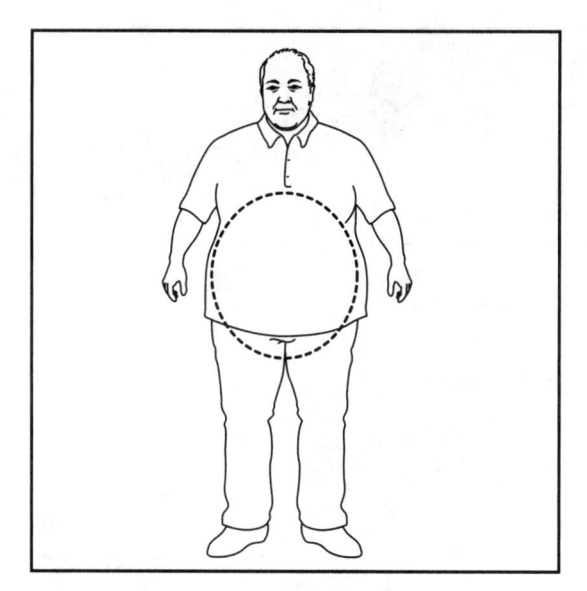

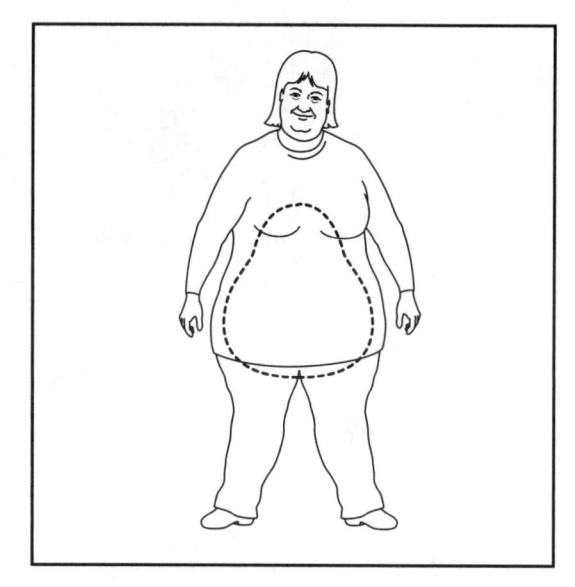

Figure 11.5 ■ Gynoid Obesity

Understanding Energy Balance

The concept of energy balance is used to explain weight gain, loss, or maintenance. The two variables that need to be considered are **energy intake** and **energy expenditure.** Energy intake is directly related to the type and quantity of food consumed. Energy expenditure is related to body metabolism. **Metabolism** is the rate at which our bodies burn energy or calories. The term calorie, which is technically inaccurate, has become the term used to express food energy. A kilocalorie is actually the true measure of energy in food.

Basal metabolism, or the number of calories expended at rest, and exercising or activity metabolism influences total body metabolism. Exercising or activity metabolism represents any energy expenditure over basal metabolism. Therefore, the more active an individual, the greater the exercising or activity metabolism.

How these two variables compare determines whether weight is gained, lost or maintained consistently (see Figure 11.6). In cases where energy intake exceeds energy expenditure, weight is gained. This is referred to as a positive caloric balance. An isocaloric balance exists if energy intake and expenditure equal. If an isocaloric balance exists, the body will remain constant. If, and only if, energy expenditure exceeds energy intake, can weight be lost. This situation is referred to as a negative caloric balance.

Energy intake and expenditure can be influenced by differing factors. For example, the amount and type of food an individual consumes can influence energy intake. High caloric foods, such as high fat foods and alcohol, and the consumption of large quantities of food, can lead to a positive caloric balance and body weight gain. Excessive energy expenditure from high levels of physical activity resulting from either occupation or exercise would lead to weight loss.

In terms of actual calories, one pound of body fat equals 3500 calories. As a result, if an individual would like to lose two pounds of body weight he/she will have to create a negative caloric balance that resulted in a 7000 caloric restriction. The actual rate of restriction can vary. In other words, one individual may elect to restrict 500 calories a day from his/her normal intake, whereas a second individual may elect to restrict 100 calories a day. Ultimately, both individuals would meet their weight loss objectives. The only difference is the first individual would meet the weight loss objective in less time.

In the opposite vein, the gradual increase in body fat known as "creeping" obesity is the result of a small positive caloric balance over time. Ultimately, this results in body weight

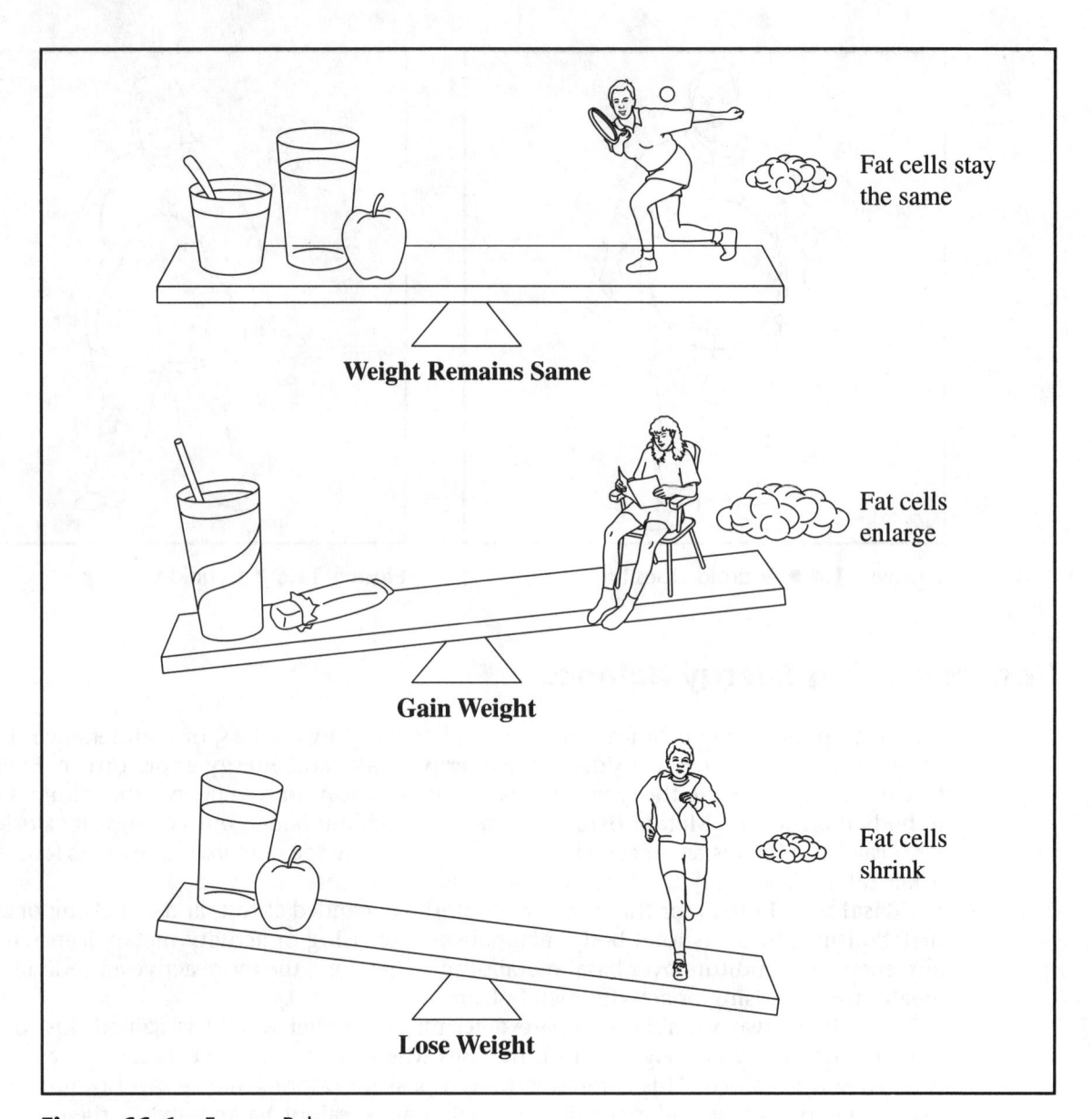

Figure 11.6 ■ Energy Balance

gain. **"Creeping" obesity** may stem from such lifestyle behaviors as decreased physical activity, decreases in basal metabolism with age, and changes in dietary behavior.

Aging has been associated with weight gain. This, in part, is the result of a limited decrease in basal metabolism that occurs with age. The primary influencing factor is the loss of muscle tissue. In simple, muscle tissue requires a greater number of calories to sustain than body fat. For many, activity levels are lowered as we age allowing for muscle atrophying to occur, subsequently, leading to less lean body mass.

Another variable that may influence creeping obesity is the type of food consumed. Diets high in fat lead to higher caloric intake and fat storage. Carbohydrates and proteins are more readily used by the body and less likely to be stored as fat. This, of course, helps in limiting fat storage and the potential for creeping obesity.

In other words, there is literally a hierarchy of nutrient utilization. *The body tends to metabolize carbohydrates and proteins before it metabolizes fat.* If a person has a positive caloric intake, limited fat metabolism easily leads to increased fat storage. If a person is going to have excessive caloric intake, it is much better for those calories to be in the form of carbohydrates or protein. Candidly stated, these nutrients are easier to metabolize and are less likely to be converted to fat storage. In addition, the body tends to store fat more easily than carbohydrates and proteins. Both of these findings strongly support limited fat intake as a measure of controlling body weight.

Understanding Energy Balance and Weight Loss

Once a person understands the concept of energy balance it is relatively easy to determine the number of calories that must be restricted to meet weight loss objectives. However, several important guidelines must be considered. First, any weight loss program should be designed to allow for a *1 to 2 pound body weight loss per week*. Any greater loss will result from lean body weight loss, not fat weight.

Also, many people will experience, in the early stages of their program, large weight loss that exceeds the recommended 2 pounds per week. In most cases, these can be attributed to water losses and do not represent losses in actual body fat or body composition. This is one of the factors that mislead individuals who try differing commercial weight loss programs. Diets that are wrongly interpreted as being highly successful may be illusionary. Results may be influenced by body water loss.

Another reason why individuals should restrict their weight loss goals to 1 to 2 pounds a week is to ensure the individual is maintaining an adequate diet, not deficient in nutrients. To lose two pounds a week, a person must restrict 1000 calories a day. That is an exceptionally high level of caloric restriction. Precaution to ensure a balanced diet is warranted. It should also be emphasized that dietary intake of less than 1000 kcal/day should only be undertaken under medical supervision.

Clearly, exercise should be considered as a means of assisting in increasing caloric expenditure. The relationship of exercise and weight reduction is discussed under a separate header.

Causes of Obesity

What causes obesity? Such a simple question, and yet, unfortunately, there is no simple answer. Many factors contribute to obesity. As a result, a complete and full understanding is not possible. It is possible, however, to discuss selected, common contributing factors. These are described below.

Labor Saving Devices/Technology

From earlier discussion, it is easy to see that obesity results from excess energy intake. Yet, this imbalance may result from a number of factors. For example, as technology has advanced many labor saving devices have been developed. We now ride mowers to cut our grass or use industrial equipment to dig our ditches. We cut trees with power saws, not handsaws. We use elevators instead of steps. In simple, we have made our lives more energy efficient. As a result, we have created a life that is more sedentary which results in limited energy expenditure. The end result, of course, is weight gain.

Genetics

Genetics is a contributing factor. Studies conducted on identical twins have illustrated this relationship. Identical twins share not only identical genetic codes, but research suggest they share similar tendencies in weight gain and fat distribution (Pochlman, 1986). This pattern is not as readily observed in fraternal twins. These findings contribute to the constant search by researchers to identify what has commonly become labeled the "fat gene."

Family Lifestyle

Family lifestyle will contribute to obesity. Children raised by parents who are overweight and sedentary tend to share similar characteristics. These findings are important and clearly illustrate the importance of parents modeling and living healthy, active lifestyles.

Childhood Fatness

There are limited times in an individual's life who a person actually develops fat cells. Two important times are (a) the first year of life and (b) from approximately age 10 through adolescence. After those times, unless extreme weight gains occur, the number of fat cells in the body remains relatively constant. Unfortunately, once a fat cell is formed it becomes a part of that person. Surgery is the only method known that can lower the number of cells. In simple, once a fat cell is formed, it is yours for life.

Weight loss and weight gain does not increase the number of fat cells. Changes in weight only influence the size of fat cells. Therefore, to allow a child to develop excess fat cells during those critical times will burden that individual for the remainder of his/her life. Those extra cells will always have the potential to store fat. Precaution to avoid over feeding the newborn and children during adolescence seems warranted.

Set Point Theory

Is there a body fat thermostat or body fatometer? Are we preprogrammed to remain at a certain body weight or body fatness level? Some evidence would suggest the answers to these questions are yes.

The phenomenon commonly referred to as "set point theory" suggests that every individual has a particular body fat level that the body tries to maintain. By altering an individual's appetite, hunger, satiety level, and metabolism, a person maintains a fairly constant body fat level.

For example, if a person attempts to lose weight through caloric restriction, his/her metabolism may slow. Physiologically, his/her body has recognized the reduction in energy intake and is adjusting by requiring a lower resting energy expenditure (basal metabolism). In simple, it is working more efficiently. It is conserving what energy or calories that are ingested and is making maximal use from them. This is particularly frustrating and challenging for any individual trying to lose weight through caloric restriction or diet. Another way this individual's body is likely to react is to raise the appetite, making it difficult to remain comfortable on similar food intake.

Set point theory has been supported by controlled research studies. Individuals placed on controlled diets that allowed for either weight loss or gain were found to gradually drift back to their predetermined weight or fatness level when the dietary control was removed.

So how do we set or adjust the set point? This is a highly desired answer. Unfortunately, it is not a simple one. No medicine or body fatometer is readily and easily adjustable. Clearly, dietary restriction has been shown not to lower the set point. If this were true, anyone who has lost weight through caloric restriction would easily be able to go to a caloric neutral level (i.e., no weight is lost or gained) and would have no trouble remaining at his/her new body weight. Sadly, this pattern rarely occurs.

Evidence would suggest that exercise, coupled with proper dietary intervention, has helped individuals to lower fat levels that the body can maintain. Aerobic activities have proven to be especially positive. Similarly, diets that are low in fat and high in carbohydrates have shown to be especially positive.

Diets high in fat, refined sugars, and artificial sweeteners have been shown to raise set point levels. Lastly, as suggested in the example above, severe caloric restrictions, such as those that occur during fasting or near fasting diets, have been shown to raise set points, as well as alter basal metabolisms.

Unfortunately, nicotine consumption and amphetamine usage have been shown to lower set points. Obviously, both of these are associated with negative health risks and should not be considered as options. Yet, the findings do help to understand why many individuals struggle with weight gain after the cessation of cigarettes or other forms of nicotine. Similarly, amphetamines, which serve as central nervous system stimulants, are highly addictive and are associated with a number of health risks.

Finally, it is important to understand that each individual will respond differently when trying to readjust his/her set point. Some will find a reasonably rapid response and will quickly move to a lower weight and be easily able to maintain it with continued activity and proper diet. Unfortunately, not everyone experiences this ease of adjustment and may find that change will take as long as a year. Patience is critical. Continued activity and dietary modification will pay off even for these individuals.

Understanding the Role of Exercise in Weight Control

The role of regular physical activity in weight reduction or management is well documented. Simply stated, regular exercise contributes to long-term weight reduction. Several factors contribute to this relationship. First, and perhaps most obvious, increased physical activity or exercise increases energy expenditure. The relationship between energy expenditure and weight loss has been discussed in detail under a separate header (see Understanding Energy Balance).

Additionally, regular exercise is extremely important in limiting the loss of lean body mass during weight reduction. If an individual attempts to lose weight only by caloric restriction, he/she will lose fat and lean body weight. By exercising while dieting, weight loss is limited to fat loss. Lean body mass is maintained.

This finding is important because basal metabolism is directly related to lean body weight. *As lean body weight is increased, basal metabolism is increased.* The increase in basal metabolism will assist in caloric expenditure and weight loss. It is estimated that for each additional pound of muscle tissue, basal metabolic rate increases by 30–50 calories per 24-hour period. An increase of one pound of body fat burns only 2 calories for every 24-hour period.

Another important consideration is that dieting lowers an individual's basal metabolism. Regular exercise, in and of itself, or coupled with dieting, increases metabolism. That is to say, that after an individual finishes his/her activity there is a period of time following activity that the body's metabolism remains elevated. As much as 70% of an individual's total energy expenditure is the result of basal metabolism. Any post exercise metabolism increase seems warranted.

In the opposite vein, if an individual attempts to lose weight only by caloric intake reduction, his/her body will respond by becoming more energy efficient and will lower basal metabolism. This will make it more difficult to lose weight.

Both aerobic activity and resistive training should be considered as a positive, effective weight management intervention. Recall that aerobic activity by itself, or in combination with caloric restriction, is helpful in establishing a new set point. The addition of resistive training into the exercise program will assist in developing lean body mass. In simple, as lean body mass is increased, basal metabolism will be increased. Therefore, more calories will be expended, assisting in body fat reduction.

Exercise has been shown to control many of the related health risks of obesity. These include, but are not limited to, hypertension, hypercholesterolemia, hyperlipidemia, and increased risk of coronary heart disease. Each is discussed in Chapter 4.

Exercise is related to decreased appetite in some individuals. This finding is especially positive for those attempting to lose weight. Unfortunately, this finding is not consistent throughout the population. Some find that increased energy expenditure will stimulate their appetite. Their body recognizes the increased energy expenditure and tries to replace the calories expended during activity.

Finally, the psychological and social implications of obesity are quite negative. Overweight individuals frequently present limited self-esteem and depression. Many feel or have felt some sense of social rejection either from friends or job interactions. Individuals who include regular exercise as part of their weight management program not only experience the physical benefits of activity but, for many, find a whole, fulfilled, new life and positive self-image. Simple day-to-day tasks become possible.

For example, normal weight individuals have never felt the frustration of not being able to find clothes that fit or not being able to wear the latest styles because of excessive weight. The normal weight individuals will never know the challenge of theater, airplane, or stadium seats that are too small. Normal weight individuals have probably never felt embarrassed to put on a bathing suit because of their physical appearance. They may have never felt the frustration of not being able to participate in sports or other physical activities because of excess weight. They do not know the rejection of being passed over in a job or job advancement because they don't "look the part."

Exercise is power. Power to take control of your body weight and your life. It can and will open up opportunities for everyone who takes advantage of it.

Spot Reduction

Individuals wanting to shape their bodies often attempt to lose fat regionally or in specific areas. This is referred to as **spot reduction.** For example, many believe that participating in an abundance of sit-ups will burn fat away from the stomach regions. Others buy special clothes or body wraps designed to melt fat away. Specific products are marketed as fat reducing lotions. Do these spot reduction methods work?

The simple answer is no. *Spot reduction is not possible.* In actuality, the human body loses the highest amount of fat from areas of highest fat storage. Fat cannot be burned off a specific area of the body by increased physical activity, even when the activity focuses on a specific area of the body. Wearing a special fat burning suit cannot melt it off. It does not melt off with the application of special lotions or herbs. Any such claims are made purely from a marketing standpoint. Physiologically, the body is not influenced to burn fat by such products.

How can the observed weight loss or body shape be explained. Unfortunately, many people notice changes in their body shape and this, in part, contributes to some of the misunderstanding. The example of the use of sit-ups can serve as an illustration. Participating in sit-ups will increase caloric expenditure, but will not cause specific fat utilization from the stomach region. Any noticeable change in that region would most likely be explained by muscle toning of the abdominal muscles.

Behavior Modification and Successful Weight Management

Individual lifestyle and behavior are directly related to weight management. Any changes in body weight must result from short and long-term changes. This is one of the reasons that dieting, in and of itself, rarely results in long-term weight loss. In order for an individual to successfully lose weight and maintain that weight loss for life requires lifestyle changes and behavior modification.

Managing body weight requires an individual to understand more than energy balance. Developing an understanding that weight is gained or lost depending on a positive or negative energy balance does not constitute effective treatment, nor will it lead to successful weight management. Successful weight management does not result simply by answering the question, "How many calories can I eat?"

To successfully manage weight, the relationships between (a) factors leading up to eating, (b) eating, and (c) the events following eating, must be understood. Behaviors can be changed, if they are understood and, when necessary, relearned (see Chapter 2). Maintaining a food diary (Laboratory 11-I) may prove especially useful in establishing an individual's dietary characteristics.

It is important to establish what events are associated with or lead up to eating. How did the person feel? What was he/she thinking? What was he/she doing at the time? Are other activities such as watching television associated with eating? The answers may lead to the identification of stimuli that a person relates to food consumption.

Additionally, it is important to establish eating behaviors? Is bingeing or over eating involved? Are meals frequently skipped? Does the individual eat a limited variety of foods? Is there a particular time and location where meals are consumed? Does the individual eat alone? The use of a food log can help to establish eating patterns.

Finally, an individual needs to fully understand the consequences and results of their eating behaviors. Is an eating disorder involved? Are they getting adequate nutrition? How are foods prepared?

If this level of understanding can be established, then it is possible for a person to successfully develop behavior modification strategies and coping skills to assist in managing weight. For example, a person can learn to avoid situations or individuals that encourage or are associated with overeating. An individual may find a history of eating while watching television and must learn to avoid snacking during those times. Individuals who frequently skip meals may find they tend to overeat and that they can avoid this type of negative behavior by altering their schedule to allow for regular meals. Simply stated, you cannot change or modify a behavior if you don't understand it. Remember that you are not simply trying to lose body weight but rather you are trying to alter an established lifestyle. Your objectives should not be focused on the short-term. Successful, long-term weight loss can result only from altered lifestyles that last a lifetime.

There are, however, a number of techniques that can be incorporated that may contribute to successful, safe, and long-term weight management (Dolgener and Hensley, 1998). These include:

- **Make a commitment to change:** This is, without question, the first and most important step when attempting to alter body weight. Success stems from changes, and these changes must be desired and adopted. They must be accepted as changes that will last a lifetime. Any other level of thinking may allow some short-term success, but over time, any and all gains will be lost. If a person is not willing to commit to, or accept long-term lifestyle changes, there is little chance of long-term success.
- **Establish realistic weight loss goals:** Body weight is not gained or lost overnight. Patience is critical. Unfortunately, many individuals establish unrealistic weight loss goals that simply are unachievable. Even though these individuals enter into their weight management programs with enthusiasm and purpose, they frequently experience failure in achieving these lofty goals resulting in program attrition. Slower, controlled programs that allow for a 1–2 pound weekly loss are recommended.
- **Exercise:** *Any weight management program relying completely on caloric restriction should be avoided.* These programs allow for body weight reduction that results from the loss of fat and lean body weight. As indicated above, the incorporation of activity into a weight management program will allow lean body mass to be maintained and any weight loss will result from fat weight loss.
- **Eat a variety of foods:** Many fad diets require the consumer to concentrate his/her caloric intake on certain foods or nutrients. These diets have appeared in a variety of formats and suggest special food properties that may assist in accelerating body fat utilization or fat burning. These "one and two food" diets, or high/low nutrient diets should be approached with caution. Can they be sustained for a lifetime? Do they allow for proper nutrition? How much do they cost? Are special products involved? Questions like these must be addressed if long-term results are to be expected.
- **Select and prepare foods wisely:** The nature of foods eaten can significantly impact the magnitude of calories associated with the foods. For example, selecting and consuming fresh fruit over canned fruit will lead to significantly lower caloric intake. Purchasing leaner meats, trimming fat, and removing skin can all lower fat and caloric values. Baking, broiling, or even boiling food as opposed to frying can significantly cut fat and caloric intake. Table 11-2 shows a comparison of a traditional daily diet and a modified, healthier diet. Clearly, a comparison of the daily totals presented in the Table illustrates the power of proper food selection in terms of total caloric and nutrient intake.
- **Develop healthy (low-calorie) eating patterns:** Successful weight management requires a lifestyle of consistent, healthy eating patterns. You cannot choose to eat healthy every now

and then and expect any level of sustained success. Individuals who successfully manage their weight frequently demonstrate similar eating patterns. For example, thinner individuals typically *eat slower* than their heavier counterparts. In simple, they know how to put the fork down. They know how to slowly savor and enjoy each bite. By controlling the rate at which they eat, they prevent gulping of food and over eating.

Learn to eat slow foods. For example, it requires more time to peel and eat an orange as compared to drinking a glass of orange juice. Soups take longer to eat than solid foods.

Individuals who successfully manage their weight do not just eat rabbit food. This mindset stems from a public misperception that in order for a food to be low in calories and low in fat, it has to be associated with a salad or it has to taste bad. Nothing could be further from the truth.

There are an unlimited number of foods that are healthy and meet the demands of a low fat, low calorie diet. In fact, many of the foods that we eat that contribute to poor dietary behavior are healthy foods. It is how we dress them that is problematic. For example, the typical bake potato is a perfect low-fat, low-calorie food choice. Yet, if we dress it with cheese, butter, or sour cream we have taken a 100-calorie food choice and created a several hundred-calorie food. To further compound the situation, the additional calories are mostly in the form of fat.

- **Avoid automatic eating:** People associate food with other aspects of their lives. These are learned relationships. For example, many individuals watch television while eating. As a result, a relationship between food and television is formed. This leads to unwarranted eating. For these individuals, each time they sit down to watch television, it presents a stimulus to eat. Unfortunately, if acted upon, many unnecessary and unwanted calories get consumed.

- **Stay busy:** Boredom, stress, depression, and other emotional states are related to eating. The process of preparing and consuming food fills time or helps to take a person's mind off of a problem. Hunger is not necessarily the stimulus for these behaviors. Rather, it is the need to be busy. If a person can stay busy or develop other coping skills, he/she may not get involved in unnecessary and unwanted food consumption. Food should not be considered a coping device and should never be used in that capacity. Don't let food become your friend or comforter.

- **Plan meals ahead of time:** *Do not grocery shop hungry.* Clearly, shopping while hungry leads to over and inappropriate purchasing. High calorie foods such as snack foods end up getting purchased to be eaten on the way home. When hungry, it is difficult to limit your food selections for a meal. Many foods look appealing. Careful consideration about the type and nature of the food gets lost in the simple desire to eat.

- **Do not serve more food than you should eat:** Learning to eat a proper proportion of any food is critical to successful weight management. Learn not only to plate a proper proportion, but to not eat beyond what is served. It is surprising how many calories are added to a diet as a result of tasting or nibbling while foods are being prepared. To help establish an understanding of food portions or serving size, Table 11-3 provides descriptive itemizations of food serving or portion sizes based on food groups and serving dishes or utensils.

- **Avoid negative social settings and social bingeing:** Food is a social item. For example, we associate it with weddings, parties, and football games. We prepare foods for those who are sick or have family members who are sick or experiencing other traumas in their lives. It becomes an item used to help express emotion. For those receiving the invitations to the socials or other generosities, they must develop dietary management skills. For example, eat a light meal or drink several glasses of water before going to a social event. This will minimize over eating. Avoid the high calorie, fatty appetizers such as cheeses and sausages. When nibbling, choose the broccoli and carrot sticks.

- **Avoid food raids:** Refrigerators, candy bowls, and cookie jars are objects of temptation. To help prevent raiding do not leave foods that can be easily snacked on readily available. Ideally, do not even purchase them. But if they are purchased, keep them out of sight and on the highest shelf. Make it difficult to get to them. Control temptation!

Table 11-2 ■ Comparison of a Traditional Daily Diet and a Healthy Choice Daily Diet

Traditional Breakfast	Calories	Protein	Fat	Carbohydrates
Fried Eggs (2)	183	12	14	1
Bacon (2 strips)	170	4	8	0
Hashbrowns (1 cup)	345	3	18	45
White Toast (1 slice—with marg.)	100	2	5	12
Orange Juice (½ cup)	55	0	0	14
Whole Milk (1 cup)	150	8	8	1
Totals	1003	29	53	83
Healthy Breakfast				
Branflakes (1 cup)	134	4	1	33
Banana (½)	52	1	0	13
Skim Milk (½ cup—for cereal)	43	4	0	6
Wheat Toast (1 slice)	65	2	1	12
Jelly (1 tsp)	17	0	0	4
Orange Juice (½ cup)	52	1	0	12
Skim Milk (1 cup)	86	8	0	12
Totals	449	20	2	92
Traditional Lunch				
McDonald's (Quarterpounder with cheese)	520	28	29	37
McDonald's (Supersized Fries)	540	8	26	68
McDonald's Apple Pie	497	13	11	89
Milkshake (Chocolate)	290	3	15	37
Dr. Pepper (12 oz)	156	0	0	40
Total	2003	52	81	271
Healthy Lunch				
Tuna Sandwich				
Chunklight Tuna (½ cup)	77	15	1	0
Whole Wheat (2 slices)	139	6	2	26
Lettuce (½ cup)	5	0	0	1
Tomato (½)	13	1	0	3
Fat-Free Mayo (1 tbsp.)	10	0	0	2
Skim Milk (8 oz)	86	8	0	12
Apple (2¾ inch diameter)	81	0	0	21
Nonfat Cottage Cheese (4 oz)	73	13	0	5
Totals	484	43	3	70
Traditional Dinner				
Roast Beef (3 oz)	375	17	33	0
Baked Potato (with skin)	212	5	0	49
Margarine (1 tbsp for potato)	90	0	10	0
Sweet Corn (canned—1 cup)	184	4	1	46
Dinner Roll (1)	85	2	2	14
Margarine (1 tbsp for roll)	30	0	3	0
Apple Pie (1 piece)	300	3	13	41
Ice Cream (Vanilla—½ cup)	150	3	8	15
Whole Milk (1 cup)	150	8	8	11
Total	1476	52	78	176
Healthy Dinner				
Chicken Breast (no skin)	142	27	3	0
Baked Potato (no skin)	156	3	0	36
Rye Crisps (2)	50	2	0	10
Green Beans (Fresh—1 cup)	50	2	0	12
Angel Food Cake (1 piece)	73	2	0	16
Strawberries (Sweet—1 cup)	100	1	1	25
Skim Milk (1 cup)	86	8	0	12
Total	657	45	4	111
Total—One Day Summary: Traditional	*4482*	*133*	*212*	*550*
Total—One Day Summary: Healthy	*1590*	*108*	*9*	*273*

Table 11-3 ■ Understanding Food Serving or Portion Sizes

Portion or Serving Size	Descriptive Comparison
The Bread, Cereal, Rice, and Pasta Group	
1 cup of potatoes, rice, pasta	Tennis ball, ice cream scoop
1 pancake	Compact disc (CD)
½ cup cooked rice	Cupcake wrapper full
1 piece of cornbread	Bar of soap
1 slice of bread	Audiocassette tape
1 cup of pasta, spaghetti, cereal	Fist
2 cups of cooked pasta	Full outstretched hand
The Vegetable Group	
1 cup green salad	Baseball or a fist
1 baked potato	Fist
¾ cup tomato juice	Small styrofoam cup
½ cup cooked broccoli	Scoop of ice cream or a light bulb
½ cup serving	6 asparagus spears; 7 or 8 baby carrots; 1 ear of corn
The Fruit Group	
½ cup of grapes (15 grapes)	Light bulb
½ cup of fresh fruit	7 cotton balls
1 medium size fruit	Tennis ball or a fist
1 cup of cut-up fruit	Fist
¼ cup raisins	Large egg
The Milk, Yogurt, and Cheese Group	
1½ ounces of cheese	9-volt battery; 3 dominoes
1 ounce of cheese	Pair of dice; thumb
1 cup of ice cream	Large scoop the size of a baseball
The Meat, Poultry, Fish, Dry Beans, Eggs, and Nuts Group	
2 tablespoons peanut butter	Ping-pong ball
1 teaspoon peanut butter	Fingertip
1 tablespoon peanut butter	Thumb tip
3 ounces cooked meat, fish, poultry	Palm, a deck of cards or a cassette tape
3 ounces grilled/baked fish	Checkbook
3 ounces cooked chicken	Chicken leg and thigh or breast
Fats, Oils, and Sweets	
1 teaspoon butter, margarine	Size of a stamp the thickness of your finger
2 tablespoons salad dressing	Ping-pong ball
1 ounce of nuts or small candies	One handful
1 ounce of chips or pretzels	Two handfuls
½ cup of potato chips, crackers or popcorn	One man's handful
⅓ cup of potato chips, crackers, or popcorn	One woman's handful
Serving Dishes/Utensils	
½ cup	Small fruit bowl; custard cup
1½ cups	Large cereal/soup bowl
1½ cups of pasta, noodles	Dinner plate not heaped
½ cup of pasta, noodles	Cafeteria vegetable dish

Source: Oregon State University Extension Home Economics, http://osu.orst.edu/dept/ehe/index2.html.

Eating Disorders

Two of the more common eating disorders found in the United States include anorexia nervosa and bulimia. Both conditions are found predominately in the female population and, if unaddressed, can result in extreme health risk, including death. Interestingly, despite being termed eating disorders, both stem more from inappropriate body perception rather than feelings and attitudes about food.

Typically, the anorexic or the bulimic individual is an adolescent, female member of a middle to upper class family with an extreme fear of becoming fat. In the case of the anorexic, the fear of becoming fat is actually greater than the fear of death. Yet, even though they share this fear, they are different eating disorders and present distinct characteristics. Broadly stated, the anorexic tends to be linked with starvation. The bulimic tends to present characteristics of gorging and then purging the food intake by vomiting. For reader ease, each is presented under separate headers.

Anorexia Nervosa

Anorexia nervosa is a psychosocial eating disorder that affects approximately 2% of all females. Statistically, 90–95% of all cases of anorexia nervosa effect females. Why this gender relationship exists is not completely understood.

Anorexia nervosa is a mental and a physical disease. Specific descriptive criteria as established by the American Psychiatric Association (1994) include:

- Sustained weight maintenance 15% below expected.
- Intense, inappropriate, unmanaged fear of fatness or weight gain despite presence of significant underweight conditions.
- Distorted body perception, including but not limited to, weight, size, and shape in the presence of serious weight reduction.
- In the case of post-menarcheal females, the absence of at least three menstrual cycles.

Anorexia nervosa is related to the individual, his/her family, and to social pressures. From a personal standpoint, the anorexic is generally extremely self critical, introverted, and has exceptionally low self-esteem. He/she frequently will deny his/her condition while at the same time present compulsive, obsessive behaviors related to food. He/she will be completely engrossed with food, meals, meal planning, grocery shopping, and other related behaviors.

As mentioned above, the typical anorexic is a member of a middle to upper class family. Additionally, this family is generally mother dominated.

Societal pressures supporting and promoting extreme thinness appear to influence and contribute to a distorted self-image. Even when gross leanness exists, these individuals continue to view their bodies as excessively fat and will starve themselves in an attempt to control their perceived fatness. Clearly, this distorted body perception must be viewed as life-threatening and should not go unattended.

Treatment of anorexia nervosa requires both medical and family intervention. Rarely will the anorexic seek assistance. In fact, in most cases, the anorexic will deny the existence of any disorder despite attempts of family, friends, and health care professionals to avail the condition. Deep, intense denial, secretive eating patterns, including starvation, excessive exercise, and laxative abuse are common behavior patterns demonstrated by the anorexic in an attempt to establish body thinness. Unless addressed, these behaviors will become life-threatening.

Medical intervention must include a number of different, and yet, critical disciplines. Intervention may require hospitalization. It may involve years of psychotherapy and nutritional counseling. Therapy can and has proven effective approximately 70% of the time (Hsu, 1988). Unfortunately, not everyone responds fully to treatment. It is estimated that up to 15% will become episodic and ultimately, will die from complications resulting from long-term starvation (Anderson, 1986). Timing of intervention appears related to reversal and cure. The sooner anorexia nervosa is treated the better the chances of successful intervention and the reversal of tissue and organ damage.

Untreated anorexia nervosa will lead to a variety of physical complications. If left untreated, these conditions become life threatening. Inadequate dietary intake contributes to nutrient deficiencies and associated complications. Electrolyte imbalances may lead to irregular or deadly heart rhythms and other complications. Dry skin and unusually fine hair growth results from fluid deficiency and the body's attempt to warm itself. Immunal system functions become compromised. Emotional and mental disorders become present, including mental confusion, lethargy, and depression. Muscular, neural, and skeletal degeneration leads to damaged tendons, nerves, and bones.

Bulimia

Bulimia is the most common of the eating disorders and is characterized by binge eating followed by purging. Purging is normally demonstrated in the form of self-induced vomiting. In addition, laxative and diuretic abuse may be present. Similar to the anorexic, in selected situations, excessive exercise and extreme dietary restrictions, including near starvation or starvation, may be present.

As with anorexia nervosa, bulimia appears to afflict the female population at a higher level of incidence than the male population. It is estimated that as many as 20% of the female college population will present, at some time, bulimic behavior. Only 5% of the male college students are thought to demonstrate, even on a limited basis, bulimic characteristics (Andersen, 1983; Borgen & Corbin, 1987; Schotte & Stunkard, 1987).

Physically, the anorexic and the bulimic differ. Whereas the anorexic presents a look of excessive thinness, the bulimic will either present a look of normal weight or slightly overweight. Anorexics may practice bulimic behaviors, but bulimics rarely develop starvation habits to the point of excessive weight loss.

From a personality prospective, the bulimics tends to seek social acceptance. They demonstrate bouts of severe depression, mood swings, and impulsive behaviors, including suicidal tendencies. In addition to bulimic characteristics, they may have lifestyles that include unhealthy abusive behaviors such as smoking, substance abuse, and improper and poor nutritional or dietary food intake. Descriptive criteria for bulimia include:

- Recurrent overeating or bingeing.
- Loss of control during bingeing.
- Recurrent, inappropriate compensatory behaviors to lose weight or prevent weight gain, including, but not limited to, self-induced vomiting, laxative and diuretic abuse, near starvation or starvation, and excessive exercise.
- Episodic recurrence of bingeing and purging, on average at least twice weekly for a period of three months.
- Intense, extreme, negative perception in regards to body shape and weight which may lead to emotional dysfunctions such as depression and violent recurrent mood swings.

The binge-purge cycle of the bulimic is recurrent and severe. Bingeing may be stimulated by some external life event, be premeditated, or result from personal uncontrolled compulsion. It is common for food intake to be extreme and include as many as 10,000 calories daily. Following a brief period of relief, the bulimic becomes overwhelmed with deep feelings of fear, shame, and guilt and begins purging to correct for the food intake and prevent weight gain. Shame may lead to secretive behaviors and attempts to hide the binge-purge cycle.

Recognition of the condition by the bulimic is delayed and/or denied, averaging five and one-half years from first onset of symptoms (Dolgener & Hensley, 1998). Treatment is similar to that used with anorexia nervosa. Medical intervention and psychotherapy are warranted. Treatment strategies include:

- Dietary and nutritional counseling.
- Developing an understanding of the complications and destructive nature of bulimia.
- Developing an understanding of proper weight management strategies.

Untreated bulimia may lead to a number of physical and emotional complications. Excessive vomiting may contribute to electrolyte imbalance, esophageal inflammation, gum damage, and tooth decay. Cardiac arrhythmias, amenorrhoea, and ulcers are prevalent. Clinical depression, anxiety, and other mood states may require antidepressive drugs and psychological counseling. Unlike anorexia nervosa, bulimia rarely requires hospitalization.

Practical Guidelines for Gaining Weight

Given that over one-half of the American population is overweight, it may come as some form of ironic surprise that some individuals desire to gain weight. In these cases, the motivations vary. It is not uncommon for thin, elderly individuals to seek additional weight or body mass. Many men would like to present a more muscular physique to improve their self-image. Excessively thin women may desire some weight gain in order to offer some improvement in their bodylines and curvature.

Precautions should be taken in how an individual attempts to gain weight. Simply attempting to create a lifestyle that includes a positive energy intake by overeating will result in an overall body weight gain that is the result of increases in body fatness only. A recommended and healthier approach would be to increase body weight by increasing lean body weight. This approach requires a higher caloric intake, as well as a regular muscular strength and endurance training program. Guidelines for implementing such a program and resistive training actives are described in Chapters 6 and 7. Following this approach will allow the body weight gain to be in the form of increased muscle mass and not body fat. There is no special product or easy method to increase one's lean body mass. Muscle cannot be purchased. Muscle has to be created. The key to successful muscle mass gain is proper diet and intense, vigorous resistive training.

Most individuals should be able to successfully gain muscle mass. Patience is required. Research would suggest, on average, men and women gain muscle mass at a rate of approximately .25 pounds per week. To allow for these gains, increases in daily caloric intake of 90–100 kcal are recommended. This increase should come in the form of complex carbohydrates. High carbohydrate intake is required to support increases in lean body mass. This finding tends to contradict the typical mindset. Many individuals falsely believe that to increase muscle mass they must increase protein intake. Most Americans consume about 100 grams of protein daily. This is an excessive level. For most, this excess may be as high as 60 grams of protein a day above the RDA. The current RDA recommendation for protein is 0.8 grams per kilogram of body weight.

These findings suggest no additional protein intake is required to support gains in lean body weight. Similarly, there is no evidence to suggest that protein supplements are any better than normal protein sources (i.e., meat). Finally, every effort should be made to avoid the temptation of increasing high-fat foods. Fatty food intake will not increase the rate of lean body weight gain.

Laboratory Activities

CHAPTER 11

Name: _____ Class Time/Day: _____ Score: _____

LABORATORY 11-A
Body Composition Assessment: Procedural Instructions

■ **Purpose:** This test determines estimated percent body fat using anthropometric skinfold measures. These procedures are to be used as required by Laboratories 11-B, 11-C, and 11-D.

■ **Precautions:** Some individuals might experience slight discomfort from their skin being pinched.

■ **Equipment:** Skinfold caliper

■ **Procedure:** Each site, as described below, should be identified and marked, if necessary. The skinfold should be firmly grasped between the thumb and index finger of the left hand. Lift the fat away from the body to ensure that muscle tissue has not been included. Open the tips of caliper and place the tips ¼ to ½ inch from the fingers of the left hand. Precaution should be taken not to place the caliper tips too deep or shallow. Inaccurate placement will result in false measurements. Measure only the true double fold thickness. Place the caliper perpendicular to the skinfold and upright, so the dial is easily visible. The dial should be read a few seconds after the caliper has been applied. Maintain constant pressure on the skinfold between the thumb and index finger while the dial is read. Measurements should be taken a minimum of three times or until consistent readings (< 2 mm difference) are obtained. Measurements should be taken at a minimum of 30 seconds apart. All measurements should be taken on the right side of the body. When measuring extremely obese individuals, two hands may be necessary to grasp the skinfold, while an assistant places and reads the skinfold caliper.

Description of Skinfold Sites

Chest: A diagonal fold taken half of the distance between the anterior axillary line and nipple for men and one-third of the distance from the anterior axillary line to the nipple for women (see Figure 11.7).

Triceps: A vertical fold on the posterior mid-line of the upper arm (over the triceps muscle), halfway between the acromion and olecranon processes; the elbow should be extended and relaxed (see Figure 11.8).

Axilla: A vertical fold on the midaxillary line at the level of the xiphoid process of the sternum (see Figure 11.9).

Subscapular: A fold taken on a diagonal line coming from the vertebral border to 1 to 2 cm from the inferior angle of the scapula (see Figure 11.10).

Abdominal: A vertical fold taken at a lateral distance of approximately 2 cm from the umbilicus (see Figure 11.11).

Suprailium: A diagonal fold above the crest of the ilium at the spot where an imaginary line would come down from the anterior axillary line (see Figure 11.12).

Thigh: A vertical fold on the anterior aspect of the thigh midway between the hip and knee joints (see Figure 11.13).

Source: Jackson, A. & Pollock, M. (1978). Generalized Equations for Predicting Body Density of Men. *British Journal of Nutrition, 40*: 497. And Jackson, A., Pollock, M., & Ward, A. (1980). Generalized Equations for Predicting Body Density of Women. *Medicine and Science in Sports and Exercise, 12*: 175.

■ **Scoring:** Percent body fat is estimated from body density. Different procedures and regression equations can be used when determining body density. Each regression equation used to determine body density is specifically related to variables such as gender, and the number and location of skinfold sites. Three and seven site models are provided on Laboratories 11-B, 11-C, and 11-D. When using a three site procedure, gender differences exist. Be sure to use the appropriate sites and refer to the appropriate Table when determining percent body fat from the sum of three scores. Females should use the procedures and sites described in Laboratory 11-B. Males should use the procedures and sites described in Laboratory 11-C. Both genders can use the 7 site procedures described in Laboratory 11-D. Fat weight, lean body mass, and desired body weight based on predetermined percent body fat can be computed using the equations provided.

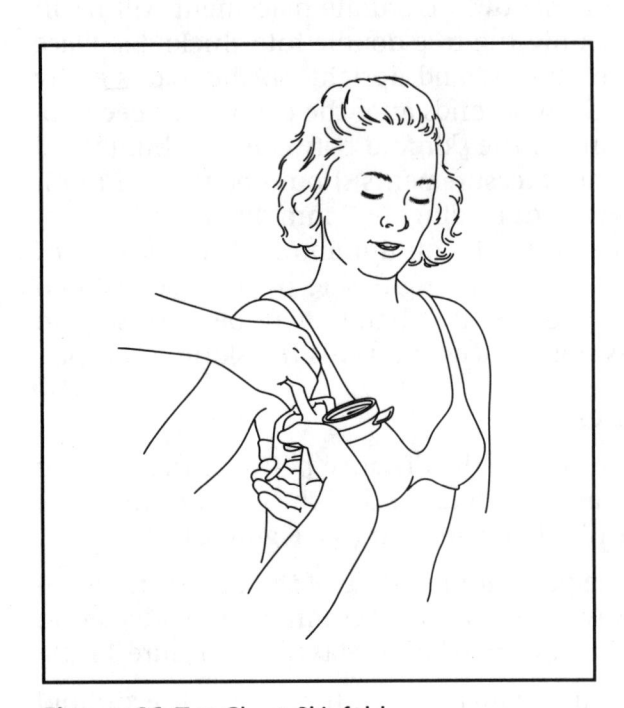

Figure 11.7 ■ Chest Skinfold

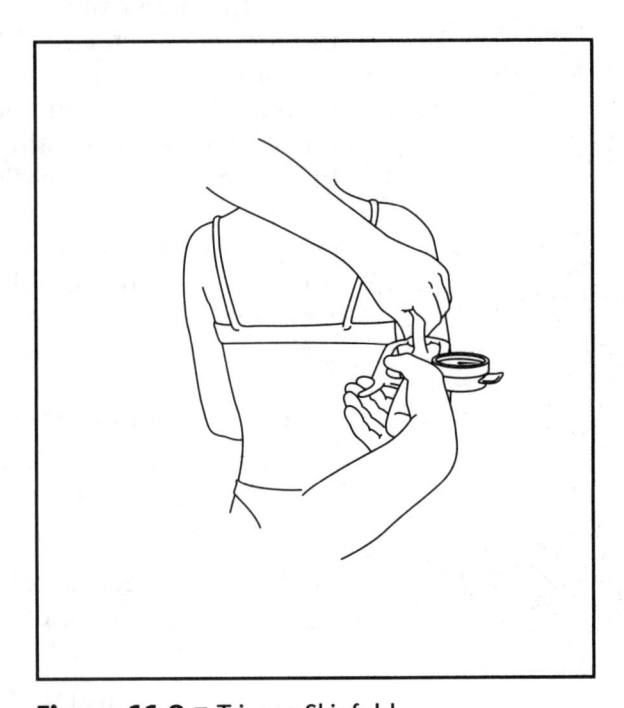

Figure 11.8 ■ Triceps Skinfold

Principles of Weight Management ■ 289

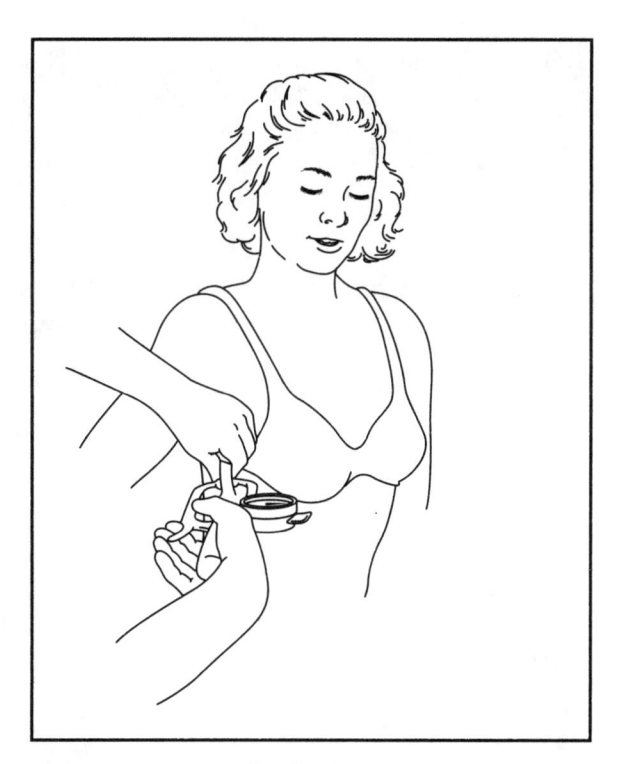

Figure 11.9 ■ Axilla Skinfold

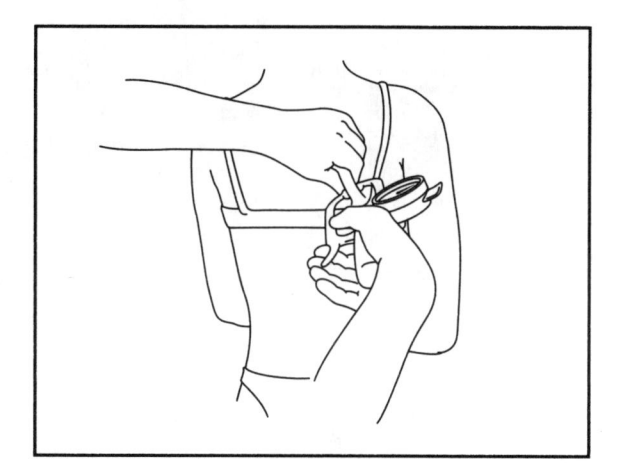

Figure 11.10 ■ Subscapula Skinfold

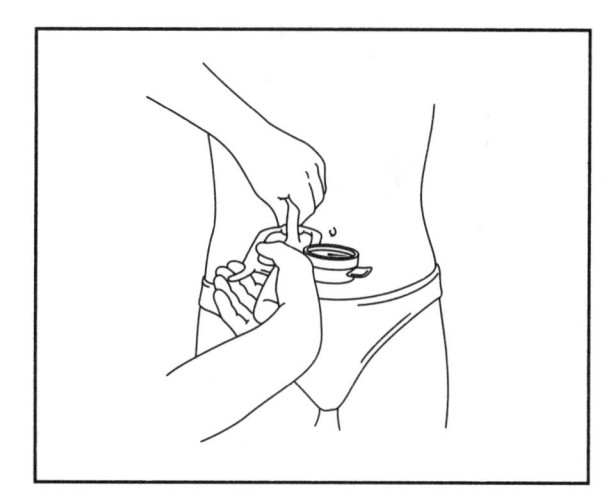

Figure 11.11 ■ Abdominal Skinfold

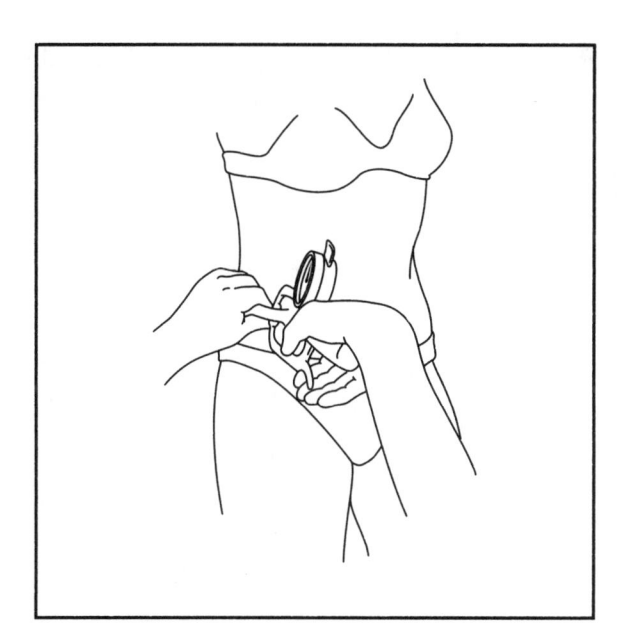

Figure 11.12 ■ Suprailium Skinfold

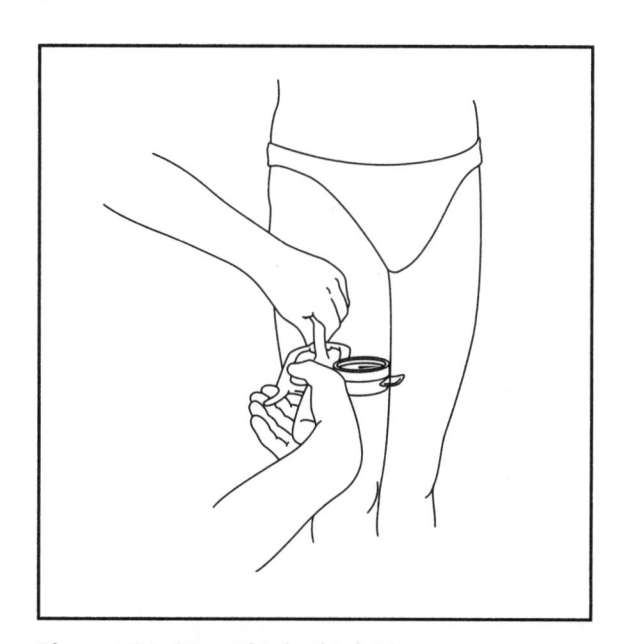

Figure 11.13 ■ Thigh Skinfold

Name: _____ Class Time/Day: _____ Score: _____

LABORATORY 11-B
Body Composition Assessment: Three Site Skinfold—Female

Sex: _____   Age: _____   Height: _____   Weight: _____

Skinfold Sites:

    Triceps = _____ mm

    Suprailium = _____ mm

    Thigh = _____ mm

    Sum of Three Sites = _____ mm

% Body Fat, % Body Fat Classification and Percentile Score:

Data Needed:

    Sum of three sites: _____

    Age: _____

    % Body Fat (Based on sum of 3 sites. See Table 11-5): _____

    % Body Fat Classification (see Table 11-4): _____

    % Body Fat Percentile Score (see Table 11-4): _____

Fat Weight and Lean Body Mass:

Data Needed:

    Body Weight (BW: dry scale weight): _____

    % Body Fat (% BF: Based on sum of 3 sites. See Table 11-5): _____

Formulas and Computations:

- Fat Weight (FW) = BW × % BF

    FW = _____ × _____

    FW = _____

- Lean Body Mass (LBM) = BW − FW

    LBM = _____ − _____

    LBM = _____

Ideal or Desired Body Weight:

Data Needed:

    Lean Body Mass (LBM): _____

    Ideal or Desired Percent Body Fat (IFP): _____

Formulas and Computations:

- Ideal Body Weight (IBW) = LBM / (1.0 − IFP)

    IBW = _____ / (1.0 − _____) = _____

    IBW = _____

Table 11-4 ■ Percent Body Fat Classification for Women

Classification	Percentile	20–29	30–39	40–49	50–59	60+
Excellent	90	14.5	15.5	18.5	21.6	21.1
	80	17.1	18.0	21.3	25.0	25.1
Above Average	70	19.0	20.0	23.5	26.6	27.5
	60	20.6	21.6	24.9	28.5	29.3
Average	50	22.1	23.1	26.4	30.1	30.9
	40	23.7	24.9	28.1	31.6	32.5
Below Average	30	25.4	27.0	30.1	33.5	34.3
	20	27.7	29.3	32.1	35.6	36.6
Poor	10	32.1	32.8	35.0	37.9	39.3

From: *ACSM's Guidelines For Exercise Testing and Prescription,* 6th Edition. 2000. Philadelphia: Lippincott Williams & Wilkins.

Table 11-5 ■ Percent Body Fat Values for Women Based on the Sum of Three Skinfolds (Triceps, Hip, and Thigh) and Age

Sum of 3 Skinfolds (mm)	Under 22	23–27	28–32	33–37	38–42	43–47	48–52	53–57	Over 58
23–25	9.7	9.9	10.2	10.4	10.7	10.9	11.2	11.4	11.7
26–28	11.0	11.2	11.5	11.7	12.0	12.3	12.5	12.7	13.0
29–31	12.3	12.5	12.8	13.0	13.3	13.5	13.8	14.0	14.3
32–34	13.6	13.8	14.0	14.3	14.5	14.8	15.0	15.3	15.5
35–37	14.8	15.0	15.3	15.5	15.8	16.0	16.3	16.5	16.8
38–40	16.0	16.3	16.5	16.7	17.0	17.2	17.5	17.7	18.0
41–43	17.2	17.4	17.7	17.9	18.2	18.4	18.7	18.9	19.2
44–46	18.3	18.6	18.8	19.1	19.3	19.6	19.8	20.1	20.3
47–49	19.5	19.7	20.0	20.2	20.5	20.7	21.0	21.2	21.5
50–52	20.6	20.8	21.1	21.3	21.6	21.8	22.1	22.3	22.6
53–55	21.7	21.9	22.1	22.4	22.6	22.9	23.1	23.4	23.6
56–58	22.7	23.0	23.2	23.4	23.7	23.9	24.2	24.4	24.7
59–61	23.7	24.0	24.2	24.5	24.7	25.0	25.2	25.5	25.7
62–64	24.7	25.0	25.2	25.5	25.7	26.0	26.7	26.4	26.7
65–67	25.7	25.9	26.2	26.4	26.7	26.9	27.2	27.4	27.7
68–70	26.6	26.9	27.1	27.4	27.6	27.9	28.1	28.4	28.6
71–73	27.5	27.8	28.0	28.3	28.5	28.8	29.0	29.3	29.5
74–76	28.4	28.7	28.9	29.2	29.4	29.7	29.9	30.2	30.4
77–79	29.3	29.5	29.8	30.0	30.3	30.5	30.8	31.0	31.3
80–82	30.1	30.4	30.6	30.9	31.1	31.4	31.6	31.9	23.1
83–85	30.9	31.2	31.4	31.7	31.9	32.2	32.4	32.7	32.9
86–88	31.7	32.0	32.2	32.5	32.7	32.9	33.2	33.4	33.7
89–91	32.5	32.7	33.0	33.2	33.5	33.7	33.9	34.2	34.4
92–94	33.2	33.4	33.7	33.9	34.2	34.4	34.7	34.9	35.2
95–97	33.9	34.1	34.4	34.6	34.9	35.1	35.4	35.6	35.9
98–100	34.6	34.8	35.1	35.3	35.5	35.8	36.0	36.3	36.5
101–103	35.3	35.4	35.7	35.9	36.2	36.4	36.7	36.9	37.2
104–106	35.8	36.1	36.3	36.6	36.8	37.1	37.3	37.5	37.8
107–109	36.4	36.7	36.9	37.1	37.4	37.6	37.9	38.1	38.4
110–112	37.0	37.2	37.5	37.7	38.0	38.2	38.5	38.7	38.9
113–115	37.5	37.8	38.0	38.2	38.5	38.7	39.0	39.2	39.5
116–118	38.0	38.3	38.5	38.8	39.0	39.3	39.5	39.7	40.0
119–121	38.5	38.7	39.0	39.2	39.5	39.7	40.0	40.2	40.5
122–124	39.0	39.2	39.4	39.7	39.9	40.2	40.4	40.7	40.9
125–127	39.4	39.6	39.9	40.1	40.4	40.6	40.9	41.1	41.4
128–130	39.8	40.0	40.3	40.5	40.8	41.0	41.3	41.5	41.8

Source: Corbin and Lindsey (1994). *Concepts of Fitness and Wellness with Laboratories,* Dubuque, IA: Brown & Benchmark. From Comprehensive Therapy 6(9): 12–27, 1980. The Laux Company, Inc. P.O. Box 700, Ayer, MA 01432

Name: _____ Class Time/Day: _____ Score: _____

LABORATORY 11-C

Body Composition Assessment: Three Site Skinfold—Male

Gender: _____   Age: _____   Height: _____   Weight: _____

Skinfold Sites:

　　Chest = _____ mm

　　Abdominal = _____ mm

　　Thigh = _____ mm

　　Sum of Three Sites = _____ mm

% Body Fat, % Body Fat Classification and Percentile Score:

Data Needed:

　　Sum of three sites: _____

　　Age: _____

　　% Body Fat (Based on sum of 3 sites. See Table 11-7): _____

　　% Body Fat Classification (see Table 11-6): _____

　　% Body Fat Percentile Score (see Table 11-6): _____

Fat Weight and Lean Body Mass:

Data Needed:

　　Body Weight (BW: dry scale weight): _____

　　% Body Fat (% BF: Based on sum of 3 sites. See Table 11-7): _____

Formulas and Computations:

- Fat Weight (FW) = BW × % BF

　　　FW = _____ × _____

　　　FW = _____

- Lean Body Mass (LBM) = BW − FW

　　　LBM = _____ − _____

　　　LBM = _____

Ideal or Desired Body Weight:

Data Needed:

    Lean Body Mass (LBM): _____

    Ideal or Desired Percent Body Fat (IFP): _____

Formulas and Computations:

- Ideal Body Weight (IBW) = LBM / (1.0 − IFP)

    IBW = _____ / (1.0 − _____) = _____

    IBW = _____

Table 11-6 ■ Percent Body Fat Classifications for Men

Classification	Percentile	20–29	30–39	40–49	50–59	60+
Excellent	90	7.1	11.3	13.6	15.3	15.3
	80	9.4	13.9	16.3	17.9	18.4
Above Average	70	11.8	15.9	18.1	19.8	20.3
	60	14.1	17.5	19.6	21.3	22.0
Average	50	15.9	19.0	21.1	22.7	23.5
	40	17.4	20.5	22.5	24.1	25.0
Below Average	30	19.5	22.3	24.1	25.7	26.7
	20	22.4	24.2	26.1	27.5	28.5
Poor	10	25.9	27.3	28.9	30.3	31.2

(Age column spans 20–29 through 60+)

From: *ACSM's Guidelines For Exercise Testing and Prescription,* 6th Edition. 2000. Philadelphia: Lippincott Williams & Wilkins.

Table 11-7 ■ Percent Body Fat Values for Men Based on the Sum of Three Skinfolds (Chest, Abdomen, and Thigh) and Age

Sum of 3 Skinfolds (mm)	Under 22	23–27	28–32	33–37	38–42	43–47	48–52	53–57	Over 58
8–10	1.3	1.8	2.3	2.9	3.4	3.9	4.5	5.0	5.5
11–13	2.2	2.8	3.3	3.9	4.4	4.9	5.5	6.0	6.5
14–16	3.2	3.8	4.3	4.8	5.4	5.9	6.4	7.0	7.5
17–19	4.2	4.7	5.3	5.8	6.3	6.9	7.4	8.0	8.5
20–22	5.1	5.7	6.2	6.8	7.3	7.9	8.4	8.9	9.5
23–25	6.1	6.6	7.2	7.7	8.3	8.8	9.4	9.9	10.5
26–28	7.0	7.6	8.1	8.7	9.2	9.8	10.3	10.9	11.4
29–31	8.0	8.5	9.1	9.6	10.2	10.7	11.3	11.8	12.4
32–34	8.9	9.4	10.0	10.5	11.1	11.6	12.2	12.8	13.3
35–37	9.8	10.4	10.9	11.5	12.0	12.6	13.1	13.7	14.3
38–40	10.7	11.3	11.8	12.4	12.9	13.5	14.1	14.6	15.2
41–43	11.6	12.2	12.7	13.3	13.8	14.4	15.0	15.5	16.1
44–46	12.5	13.1	13.6	14.2	14.7	15.3	15.9	16.4	17.0
47–49	13.4	13.9	14.5	15.1	15.6	16.2	16.8	17.3	17.9
50–52	14.3	14.8	15.4	15.9	16.5	17.1	17.6	18.2	18.8
53–55	15.1	15.7	16.2	16.8	17.4	17.9	18.5	19.1	19.7
56–58	16.0	16.5	17.1	17.7	18.2	18.8	19.4	20.0	20.5
59–61	16.9	17.4	17.9	18.5	19.1	19.7	20.2	20.8	21.4
62–64	17.6	18.2	18.8	19.4	19.9	20.5	21.1	21.7	22.2
65–67	18.5	19.0	19.6	20.2	20.8	21.3	21.9	22.5	23.1
68–70	19.3	19.9	20.4	21.0	21.6	22.2	22.7	23.3	23.9
71–73	20.1	20.7	21.2	21.8	22.4	23.0	23.6	24.1	24.7
74–76	20.9	21.5	22.0	22.6	23.2	23.8	24.4	25.0	25.5
77–79	21.7	22.2	22.8	23.4	24.0	24.6	25.2	25.8	26.3
80–82	22.4	23.0	23.6	24.2	24.8	25.4	25.9	26.5	27.1
83–85	23.2	23.8	24.4	25.0	25.5	26.1	26.7	27.3	27.9
86–88	24.0	24.5	25.1	25.7	26.3	26.9	27.5	28.1	28.7
89–91	24.7	25.3	25.9	26.5	27.1	27.6	28.2	28.8	29.4
92–94	25.4	26.0	26.6	27.2	27.8	28.4	29.0	29.6	30.2
95–97	26.1	26.7	27.3	27.9	28.5	29.1	29.7	30.3	30.9
98–100	26.9	27.4	28.0	28.6	29.2	29.8	30.4	31.0	31.6
101–103	27.5	28.1	28.7	29.3	29.9	30.5	31.1	31.7	32.3
104–106	28.2	28.8	29.4	30.0	30.6	31.2	31.8	32.4	33.0
107–109	28.9	29.5	30.1	30.7	31.3	31.9	32.5	33.1	33.7
110–112	29.6	30.2	30.8	31.4	32.0	32.6	33.2	33.8	34.4
113–115	30.2	30.8	31.4	32.0	32.6	33.2	33.8	34.5	35.1
116–118	30.9	31.5	32.1	32.7	33.3	33.9	34.5	35.1	35.7
119–121	31.5	32.1	32.7	33.3	33.9	34.5	35.1	35.7	36.4
122–124	32.1	32.7	33.3	33.9	34.5	35.1	35.8	36.4	37.0
125–127	32.7	33.3	33.9	34.5	35.1	35.8	36.4	37.0	37.6

Source: Corbin and Lindsey (1994). *Concepts of Fitness and Wellness with Laboratories,* Dubuque, IA: Brown & Benchmark. From Comprehensive Therapy 6(9): 12–27, 1980. The Laux Company, Inc. P.O. Box 700, Ayer, MA 01432

Name: _____ Class Time/Day: _____ Score: _____

LABORATORY 11-D
Body Composition Assessment: Seven Site Skinfold—Male and Female

Gender: _____ Age: _____ Height: _____ Weight: _____

Skinfold Measurements

Chest: _____ mm
Triceps: _____ mm
Axilla: _____ mm
Subscapular: _____ mm
Abdominal: _____ mm
Suprailium: _____ mm
Thigh: _____ mm

Sum of Seven: _____ mm

Body Density and % Body Fat (Note: Formulas and computations are gender specific)

Data Needed:

   Sum of seven sites: _____

   Age: _____

Males

- Body Density = 1.112 − .00043499 (sum of seven sites) + .00000055 (sum of 7 sites)^2 − .00028826 (age)

   Body Density = 1.112 − .00043499 (_____) + .00000055 (_____)^2 − .00028826 (_____)

   Body Density = _____

- % Body Fat = 4.95 / Body density − 4.50 × 100

   % Body Fat = 4.95 / (_____) − 4.50 × 100

   % Body Fat = _____

% Body Fat Classification (see Table 11-6): _____

% Body Fat Percentile Score (see Table 11-6): _____

Females

- Body Density = 1.0970 − .00046971 (sum of seven sites) + .00000056 (sum of 7 sites)^2 − .00012828 (age)

    Body Density = 1.0970 − .00046971 (_____) + .00000056 (_____)^2 − .00012828 (_____)

    Body Density = _____

- % Body Fat = 4.95 / Body density − 4.50 × 100

    % Body Fat = 4.95 / (_____) − 4.50 × 100

    % Body Fat = _____

% Body Fat Classification (see Table 11-4): _____

% Body Fat Percentile Score (see Table 11-4): _____

Fat Weight and Lean Body Mass:

Data Needed:

    Body Weight (BW: dry scale weight): _____

    % Body Fat (% BF: Based on sum of seven site computation): _____

Formulas and Computations:

- Fat Weight (FW) = BW × % BF

    FW = _____ × _____

    FW = _____

- Lean Body Mass (LBM) = BW − FW

    LBM = _____ − _____

    LBM = _____

Ideal or Desired Body Weight:

Data Needed:

    Lean Body Mass (LBM): _____

    Ideal or Desired Percent Body Fat (IFP): _____

Formulas and Computations:

- Ideal Body Weight (IBW) = LBM / (1.0 − IFP)

    IBW = _____ / (1.0 − _____) = _____

    IBW = _____

Name: _____ Class Time/Day: _____ Score: _____

LABORATORY 11-E
Body Composition Assessment: Body Mass Index (BMI)

■ **Purpose:** This test will determine body weight status, estimated percent body fat, and related health risk by determining and using body mass index.

■ **Precautions:** None

■ **Equipment:** Height and weight scales, cloth tape measure.

■ **Procedure:**

Step 1: The subject should accurately determine his/her height (inches), weight (pounds) and waist circumference (inches). To determine waist circumference, measure between the navel and the xiphoid process of the sternum.

Step 2: Determine Body Mass Index (BMI) using the following formula:
- BMI = Weight (lbs.) × 705 / Height (in) / Height (in).
- BMI = _____ × 705 / _____ / _____

Step 3: Determine disease risk and BMI rating using Table 11-8.

Step 4: Determine percent body fat (% BF) using the following equation (Deurenberg, Weststrate, & Seidell, 1991):
- % BF = 1.20 × BMI + (0.23 × Age) − (10.8 × Gender) − 5.4
  - where gender = 0 for women; 1 for men
- % BF = 1.2 × BMI + (0.23 × ____) − (10.8 × ____) − 5.4

Step 5: Determine percent body fat classification and percentile score using Tables 11-4 and 11-5 (see Lab 11-B) for women, and Tables 11-6 and 11-7 (see Lab 11-C) for men.

■ **Scoring:** BMI, disease risk and percent body fat should be computed using the appropriate equations.

■ **Data/Calculations:**

Weight: _____
Height: _____
Waist Circumference: _____

BMI: _____
BMI Rating: _____
Health Risk: _____

301

Percent Body Fat: _____

Percent Body Fat Percentile: _____

Percent Body Fat Classification: _____

Table 11-8 ■ Normative Values for Classifying Disease Risk Based on Body Mass Index (BMI) and Waist Circumference

	BMI, kg/m²	Disease Risk* Relative to Normal Weight and Waist Circumference**	
		Men, <= 102 cm (40 inches) Women, <= 88 cm (34½ inches)	Men, > 102 cm (40 inches) Women, > 88cm (34½ inches)
Underweight	< 18.5	...	...
Normal***	18.5–24.9	...	...
Overweight	25–29.9	Increased	High
Obesity, Class			
I	30.0–34.9	High	Very High
II	35.0–39.9	Very High	Very High
III	=> 40	Extremely High	Extremely High

* Disease risk for type 2 diabetes, hypertension, and cardiovascular disease. Ellipses indicate that no additional risk at these levels of BMI was assigned.
** A gender neutral value for waist circumference (> 100 cm) has also been suggested as an index of obesity.
*** Increased waist circumference can also be a marker for increased risk even in persons of normal weight.

From: *ACSM's Guidelines For Exercise Testing and Prescription,* 6th Edition. 2000. Philadelphia: Lippincott Williams & Wilkins.

Name: _____ Class Time/Day: _____ Score: _____

LABORATORY 11-F

Regional Fat Distribution: Waist-to-Hip Ratio

- **Purpose:** This laboratory will identify coronary risk by determining regional fat distribution using a waist-to-hip ratio.

- **Precautions:** None

- **Equipment:** Cloth measuring tape

- **Procedure:** The waist-to-hip ratio is determined by measuring minimal waist and maximal hip circumference. To determine the smallest circumference around the waist measure between the navel and the xiphoid process of the sternum (see Figure 11.14). In cases of extreme obesity where abdomen tissue may hang, measure the individual lying down. Determine maximal hip circumference around the hips and buttocks with the individual standing (see Figure 11.15).

- **Scoring:** Determine coronary disease risk by referring to Table 11-9. The waist circumference used singularly can also be used to determine disease risk (see Table 11-8)

Table 11-9 ■ Risk Classification by Gender and Waist-to-Hip Ratio (WHR)

Gender	Age	Low	Moderate	High	Very High
Men	20–29	< 0.83	0.83–0.88	0.89–0.94	> 0.94
	30–39	< 0.84	0.84–0.91	0.92–0.96	> 0.96
	40–49	< 0.88	0.88–0.95	0.96–1.00	> 1.00
	50–59	< 0.90	0.90–0.96	0.97–1.02	> 1.02
	60–69	< 0.91	0.91–0.98	0.99–1.03	> 1.03
Women	20–29	< 0.71	0.71–0.77	0.78–0.82	> 0.82
	30–39	< 0.72	0.72–0.78	0.79–0.84	> 0.84
	40–49	< 0.73	0.73–0.79	0.80–0.87	> 0.87
	50–59	< 0.74	0.74–0.81	0.82–0.88	> 0.88
	60–69	< 0.76	0.76–0.83	0.84–0.90	> 0.90

From: Heyward, V. & Stolarcyzk, L. (1996). *Applied Body Composition Assessment*. Champaign, IL: Human Kinetics.

- **Data/Calculations:** The waist-to-hip ratio is determined by dividing the waist measurement by the hip measurement.

Subject: _____ Date: _____

Gender: _____ Age: _____ Height: _____ Weight: _____

Waist Measurement: _____

Hip Measurement: _____

Waist-to-Hip Ratio: _____ / _____ = _____

Risk Classification by Hip-to-Weight Ratio: _____

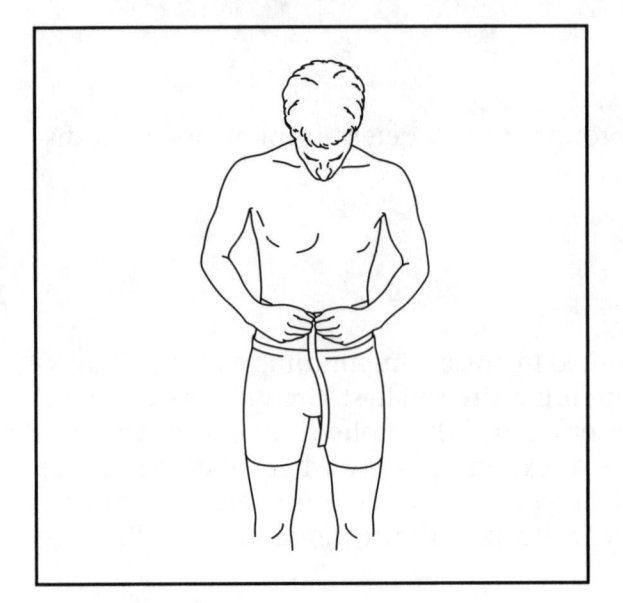

Figure 11.14 ■ Waist Measurement

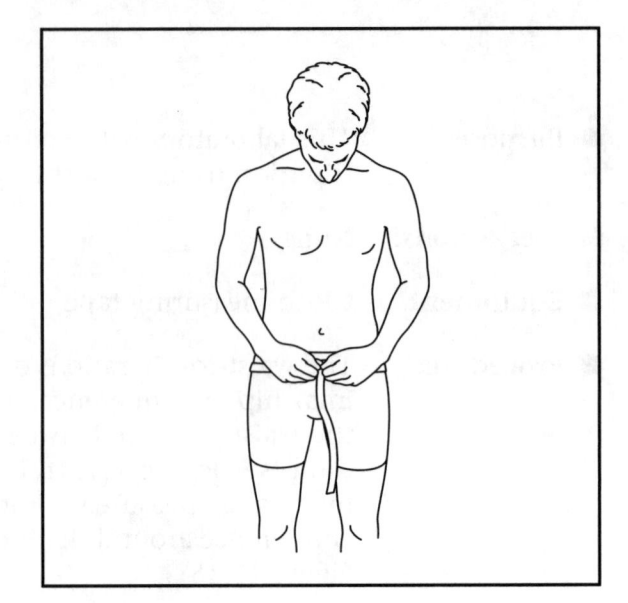

Figure 11.15 ■ Hip Measurement

Name: _____ Class Time/Day: _____ Score: _____

LABORATORY 11-G

Determining Basal Metabolic Rate

- **Purpose:** This laboratory will estimate basal metabolic rate.
- **Precautions:** None
- **Equipment:** Calculator, stedeometer, body weight scales
- **Procedure:** Determine estimated basal metabolic rate by completing the following steps.

Step 1: Determine standing height in inches and convert to height in centimeters.

Height (inches): _____

Conversion Formula: Height (cm) = Height (inches) × 2.54
Calculation: _____ = _____ × 2.54

Converted height (cm): _____

Step 2: Convert body weight in pounds to weight in kilograms

Body Weight (lbs): _____

Conversion Formula: Weight (kg) = Weight (pounds) × .454
Calculation: _____ = _____ × .454

Converted Body Weight (kg): _____

Step 3: Determine basal metabolic rate by fitting height (cm), weight (kg) and age (years) into the following equations.

Men:

Formula: BMR = 88.362 + (4.799 × height in cm) + (13.397 × weight in kg) − (5.677 × age in years)

Calculation: _____ = 88.362 + (4.799 × _____) + (13.397 × _____) − (5.677 × _____)

BMR (kcal per day) = _____

305

Women:

Formula: BMR = 447.593 + (3.098 × height in cm) + (9.247 × weight in kg) − (4.33 × age in years)

Calculation: _____ = 447.593 + (3.098 × _____) + (9.247 × _____) − (4.33 × _____)

BMR (kcal per day) = _____

■ **Scoring:** Individual basal metabolic rate may be estimated using the revised Harris-Benedict equations (Roza & Shizgal, 1984). These estimation equations are gender specific. Precaution should be taken to use the appropriate equation.

■ **Data/Calculations:**

Subject: _____ Date: _____

Gender: _____ Age: _____ Height: _____ Weight: _____

Estimated Basal Metabolic Rate: _____

Name: _____ Class Time/Day: _____ Score: _____

LABORATORY 11-H

Determining Estimated Daily Caloric Needs

- **Purpose:** This laboratory will estimate daily caloric needs based on basal metabolism and current physical activity levels.

- **Precautions:** None

- **Equipment:** Calculator, stedeometer, body weight scales.

- **Procedure:** Determine estimated daily caloric needs (Food and Nutrition Board, National Research Council, 1989).

Step 1: Determine basal metabolic rate by completing Lab 11-G.

Estimated BMR (kcal per day): _____

Step 2: Determine current activity status correction factor.

Activity Correction Factor	Description
1.4	Limited weekly physical exertion—No regular exercise program
1.6	Moderate activity—Regular submaximal exercise at least 3 days per week
1.8	Vigorous activity—Regular vigorous work related or exercise related activity 4 or more days per week

Step 3: Determine estimated daily caloric need.

Daily Caloric Need (kcal per day) = BMR (kcal per day) × Activity Correction Factor

Daily Caloric Need (kcal per day) = _____ × _____

- **Scoring:** Daily caloric need can be estimated using the procedures of the Food and Nutrition Board of the National Research Council (1989).

- **Data/Calculations:**

Subject: _____ Date: _____

Gender: _____ Age: _____ Height _____ Weight: _____

Estimated Daily Caloric Need (kcal per day): _____

Name: _____ Class Time/Day: _____ Score: _____

LABORATORY 11-I

Food Log

- **Purpose:** This laboratory will establish a dietary history through the use of a food log.

- **Precautions:** None

- **Equipment:** Pencil or pen.

- **Procedure:** Record your dietary history for one week. The food log record sheet should be copied as needed. **Document everything you eat or drink.** This should include not only foods that you plate, but foods that you may taste during cooking, pieces of candy or gum, anything that you consume. The rule should be, "if you swallow it, record it." Record all information immediately. Do not attempt to recall dietary behaviors at the end of the day. Record them as they occur. Take precaution to accurately report the amount consumed and how it was prepared (i.e., fried, broiled, skin on or off). Itemize foods containing multiple ingredients separately. For example, a bacon, lettuce and tomato sandwich might be itemized as: two pieces whole wheat bread, 3 slices of bacon, 1 slice of tomato, 2 leaves of iceberg lettuce, and 1 tablespoon of non-fat mayonnaise. Also, record the time of day, the stimulus to eat (i.e., hunger, lunch hour), the environment, and your emotional state when eating. Environmental considerations include such factors as, the location of your meal, and whether you ate alone or with others. In cases where meals were eaten with others, identify the person. Record any additional activities you were doing when eating (i.e., studying, watching television). Emotional considerations include personal feelings such as anger, frustration, and happiness. They may also include motivational behaviors such as predetermined rewards (i.e., eating a special treat) for accomplished goals.

- **Scoring:** Review the log to find patterns of dietary behavior. Are there particular foods you tend to abuse? Do you eat when you are emotionally upset? Do you find you eat more or less when you are eating with other people? Are there particular behaviors you associate with eating such as watching television? You may also enter the dietary log into any commercially available nutritional software package to determine nutritional information. Are you eating a recommended diet? Are there nutrient deficiencies in the diet?

■ Data/Calculations:

Subject: _____ Date: _____

Gender: _____ Age: _____ Height _____ Weight: _____

Food/Drink Consumed	Time	Descriptive Characteristics (amount, preparation)	Environment (Location, people, activity)	Emotional State (happy, sad, motivation to eat)

12

Low Back: Health and Fitness Management

Backache is second only to headaches as a common medical complaint.
Corbin and Lindsey, 1997

■ Chapter Outline ■

Introduction
The Lower Back: An Anatomical Review
    Components of the Vertebral Column
    Curvatures of the Vertebral Column
    Structure and Function of the Vertebral Column
Causes, Prevention, and Treatment of Low Back Pain
    Causes of Low Back Pain
    Prevention of Low Back Pain
        Lifting/Weight Belts
        Postural and Fitness Considerations
        General Guidelines
    Treatment of Low Back Pain
        Body Composition
        Cardiorespiratory Fitness
        Muscular Strength and Endurance

        Flexibility
Recommended Exercises for the Lower Back
    Low Back Exercises
        Prone Single Arm Lift
        Prone Double Arm Lift
        Prone Single Leg Lift (Extension)
        Kneeling Arm and Leg Extension
        Pelvic Tilt
        Curl-ups
        Bridging
    Additional Low Back Flexibility Exercises
    Contraindicated Low Back Exercises
        Curl-ups – Grasping behind the Head
        Double Leg Lifts
        Prone Double Leg Raise
        Simultaneous Arm and Leg Lifts
        Straight Leg Sit-ups

■ Learning Objectives ■

The student should be able to:

- Identify the relationship between lifestyle and wellness behaviors and low back pain.
- Identify the financial costs of low back pain.
- Identify and discuss the components of the vertebral column.
- Identify and discuss the curvature of the vertebral column.
- Identify and discuss the structural components of the vertebral column.

- Identify and discuss the function of the vertebral column.
- Identify and discuss personal characteristics, and physiological, occupational, and psychological factors related to low back pain.
- Identify and discuss the role of abdominal lifting belts in the prevention of low back pain.
- Identify and discuss the role posture and fitness in the prevention of low back pain.
- Identify and discuss recommended guidelines for preventing low back pain.
- Identify four health related fitness components and discuss their role in the treatment of low back pain.
- Identify specific fitness related activities that can assist in the prevention and rehabilitation of low back pain.
- Identify specific contraindicated exercises for the lower back and discuss the inherent risks of these activities.

■ Keywords ■

Abdominal ptosis	Low back pain	Sacral vertebrae
Cervical curve	Lumbar curve	Sciatica
Cervical vertebrae	Lumbar vertebrae	Thoracic curve
Coccygeal vertebrae	Osteoarthritis	Thoracic vertebrae
Coccyx	Pelvic curve	Vertebral column
Intervertebral discs	Sacral curve	Vertebral foramen
Lordosis		

Introduction

Low back pain is discussed in this text because of its relationship to lifestyle and wellness behaviors. It should be emphasized that making and living by proper lifestyle choices can prevent low back pain. Poor lifestyle choices, particularly sedentary lifestyle, contribute to the development of primary causative factors such as the loss of muscular strength and endurance and limited range of motion. The loss of muscular strength and endurance is especially related to low back pain when it occurs in the erector muscles of the back and the abdominal musculature. Similarly, inflexible or tight posterior thigh muscles (hamstrings) contribute to limited range of motion of the lower back and the potential for low back pain. Anspaugh, Hamrick, and Rosato (1991) have reported that 90% of all back problems occur in the lower region of the back known as the lumbar region.

Low back pain is the number one physical complaint by individuals age 25 to 60 in the United States. Headache is the only medical complaint more common than backache (Corbin & Lindsey, 1997). It is the most common cause of disability for individuals under the age of 45 (Oldridge & Stoll, 1997), as well as, the second most common ailment for job absenteeism for individuals age 30 to 60 (Donatelle, Snow, & Wilcox, 1999). It contributes to 25 % of days lost for the entire work force (Robergs & Roberts, 1997). Eighteen percent of the work force will present low back pain lasting at least one week annually (Park and Wagener, 1993). Fortunately, even without treatment intervention, over half (60%) of the work force is able to return to work within one week and almost all (90%) are able to return within six weeks (Plowman, 1992; Zammula, 1989).

Low back pain is estimated to affect 60–80% of the American and European population at some point in time (Nieman, 1999). Five percent of these individual conditions will progress to chronic low back pain (Frymoyer et. al., 1980). Twenty-six percent of teenagers report having experienced back pain (Corbin & Lindsey, 1997).

Low back pain does not discriminate by gender. It equally affects both men and women. While incidences have been reported in youth (Olsen, Anderson, Dearwater, et al., 1992), it is most commonly reported by individuals ranging in age between 25 and 60 (Plowman, 1992). It is the most frequent cause of activity limitation for individuals under the age of 45 (Donatelle, Snow, & Wilcox, 1999).

The financial costs of low back pain are staggering. Estimates suggest 50 billion dollars will be spent each year by government and industry (Donatelle, Snow, & Wilcox, 1999). These costs directly result from job absenteeism (and resultant lost output), disability payments, workmen's compensation, disability insurance, medical and legal fees, and other related factors. Approximately 7 billion dollars will be spent on disability compensation for low back pain claims alone. This represents nearly one-half of all worker's compensation spent annually (Robergs & Roberts, 1977). In most cases, the duration of job absenteeism is limited. Oldridge & Stoll (1997) report 75% of individuals presenting acute low back pain (less than 3 months duration) are back to work within four weeks.

The Lower Back: An Anatomical Review

Understanding the anatomical structures associated with the low back helps to develop a better understanding of the causes of low back pain, and the methods of preventing and treating low back pain. For reader ease, this discussion has been divided into sub headers.

Components of the Vertebral Column

The trunk of the body contains the low back region. The trunk is made up of the sternum, commonly known as the breastbone, ribs, and the vertebral column.

The vertebral column is also known as the spine. It consists of a series of bones called vertebrae. At birth, there are 33 separate vertebrae. These include seven cervical vertebrae (C1–C7), twelve thoracic vertebrae (T1–T12), five lumbar vertebrae (L1–L5), five sacral vertebrae, and four coccygeal vertebrae (see Figure 12.1). The cervical vertebrae are found in the neck region. The thoracic vertebrae are located in the thoracic (chest) region. The lumbar vertebrae are found in the lower back region.

Located between each of the cervical, thoracic and lumbar vertebrae are intervertebral discs. Intervertebral discs are composed of fibrcartilaginous tissue. This tissue acts as a shock absorber cushioning the vertebrae by bearing and distributing loads. Additionally, the discs separate the vertebrae, assist in restricting unwanted, excessive motion and prevent the bony vertebral structures from rubbing against each other. The union of the bony vertebrae and discs form a series of flexible joints.

As we mature, the **sacral vertebrae** and the **coccygeal vertebrae** will begin to fuse into two separate single bones. By adulthood, the five sacral bones have fused into a single wedge shaped bone known as the sacrum. Similarly, the four coccygeal bones fuse into the triangularly shaped **coccyx**.

In addition to the bony structure of the spine, there are numerous ligaments and muscles attached to the various bony processes projecting off the vertebrae. These act together to provide joint stability and allow for specific joint movements.

Curvatures of the Vertebral Column

At birth, the vertebral column when viewed laterally, or from the side, has one curve. This curve convexes posteriorly or backward away from the chest. As we mature, four curves will form; the vertebrae they include identify three of the four. These include the **cervical, thoracic, and lumbar curves.** The fourth curve, the **pelvic or sacral curve**, is formed by the shape of the sacrum and coccyx bones (see Figure 12.1).

The cervical curve begins to form when an infant begins to hold his/her head erect. This is the first of the secondary curves to form. This usually occurs somewhere around the third postnatal (after birth) month. This curve forms as a result of forces required to allow the young child to raise his/her head to look around. The neck extensor muscles are responsible for this movement.

Later, as we begin to stand and walk erect, the second secondary curve, or lumbar curve, begins to develop. The forces generated by the trunk and hip musculature allow for its formation. Both the cervical and lumbar curves, also known as the concave curves, bend anteriorly convex or toward a person's chest. The thoracic and sacral curve bends are referred to as convex curves and bend in the opposite direction or posteriorly convex.

Figure 12.1 ■ Components and Curvature of the Vertebral Column

Normally, there is no lateral (side to side) curvature associated with the vertebral column. When viewed from the back the spine should appear straight. If lateral curvature is present it is called scoliosis.

The curved shape of the vertebral column serves several functions. These include, but are not limited to, assisting to increase strength of the column, absorb shock, and protect the column from fracture.

Structure and Function of the Vertebral Column

The vertebral column serves a number of differing functions. Each, however, results from the structural characteristics of the vertebral column. One of the most obvious and visual functions of the vertebral column is to provide flexibility. This range of motion is a direct result from the vertebral column's make up. In total, at maturity, there are 26 movable parts. Interestingly, individual intervertebral joints allow for relatively limited movement. These joints are considered gliding (arthrodial) joints and allow limited movement in any direction. Yet, when these movements are combined throughout the whole column, the arrangement allows for a rather extensive range of spinal movement. It should be noted, however, that specific movements may vary by location or region. For example, the upper cervical vertebrae are considerably different from those allowed by the thoracic or lumbar vertebrae.

In addition to increased range of motion, this segmented structural arrangement allows the vertebral column to absorb vertical shock. During impact, the intervertebral discs flatten and bulge from their intervertebral spaces. This arrangement allows for some force amortization.

The seven cervical vertebrae serve two functions. First, they provide support for the head. Second, they act as a series of joints that allow for head movement. The first two cervical vertebrae differ from the other five. They are referred to as the atlas and axis, respectively. Together, they form a pivot joint, which allows the side-to-side rotation of the head. The movement of the head known as nodding occurs between the first cervical vertebrae or atlas and the occipital condyles of the occipital bone of the skull. Below the second cervical vertebrae or axis, the motions allowed by the remaining five cervical (C3–C7) vertebrae include: flexion, extension, lateral flexion, and axial rotation. The cervical aspect of the vertebral column is the most mobile of the spine.

The ribs attach to the twelve thoracic vertebrae. Together they form the thoracic cage. This bony structure serves to protect the vital organs of the body. Combined movements associated with the thoracic region include, torsal flexion and extension, lateral bending, and long axis twisting. Similar, but more restricted movements occur in the lumbar region.

Another important role of the vertebral column is to protect the spinal column. Vertebrae vary in size and shape depending on their region in the vertebral column. They all, however, share a similar characteristic known as a vertebral foramen. The **vertebral foramen** is an open, hollow space created by the bony vertebral arch and the body of the vertebrae. In the whole column, this hollow space forms a spinal canal that houses the spinal cord. This arrangement protects the spinal nerves with the hard skeletal bone of the vertebrae.

Numerous processes or bony protrusions form the shape of the differing vertebrae. The specific vertebral shape varies by region. Again, while recognizing specific structural difference, each process plays a similar, critical role. This role is to serve as a site for muscle and ligament attachment. Specific shapes of the processes vary according to need. For example, in the lumbar vertebrae, where the vertebrae are the largest and strongest, the spinous process is a large, thick, protrusion projecting nearly straight posteriorly. This large, structurally strong process serves as the attachment for the large, powerful back muscles.

Finally, the structural arrangement of the vertebral column provides support for the body. This is especially true for the thoracic area. Additionally, the curved arrangement of the spine allows for greater support of total body weight and assists in transmitting it to the lower body.

Causes, Prevention, and Treatment of Low Back Pain

Causes of Low Back Pain

Most low back pain occurs in the lumbar and sacral region. The most common specific site is in the region of the fourth and fifth lumbar (Plowman, 1992). The most common cause of low back pain is physical inactivity. Other factors related to back disorders include poor posture, faulty body mechanics, stressful living and working habits, weak musculature, specifically abdominal muscles, and poor flexibility in the lower back and hamstrings (Saunders, 1992). The following is an itemized list of plausible risk factors for low back pain (Fahey, Insel, & Roth, 1999; Robergs & Roberts, 1997).

- Personal Characteristics
  - Age > 34 years
  - Family history of back trauma
  - Low socio-economic status
  - Male gender
  - Smoking and associated chronic coughing
- Physiological Factors
  - Physical inactivity
  - Obesity
  - Low muscular strength relative to body weight especially in the abdominal, back, hips, and leg musculature
  - Limited flexibility, particularly in the low back and hamstring musculature
  - Degenerative disease
  - Poor posture when standing, sitting, or sleeping
- Occupational Factors
  - Low job satisfaction
  - Frequent or heavy lifting, twisting, bending, or standing up
  - High concentration demands
  - Physically hard work
  - Involve repetitive vibration affecting the whole body (i.e., truck driving)
  - Repetitive strain in forced positions over long time periods
- Psychological Factors
  - Depression
  - Anxiety

Interestingly, certain sport related movements and activities have been associated with increased risk of low back pain (Biering-Sorensen, et al., 1994). Relationships have been found when individuals are exercising or training excessively or when individuals are participating in activities that require loading or twisting movements.

For example, golf and tennis players have reported increased risks of structural injury such as disk herniation. Weight lifters and track athletes, such as shot putters and discuss throwers, have reported higher levels of back pain because of the excessive loading and twisting associated with their sport specific movements. Other sports, including but not limited to, rowers and gymnast, have reported higher incidence levels of low back pain.

Prevention of Low Back Pain

Lifting/Weight Belts

Lifting (abdominal) belts can be used to help prevent back injury. During heavy lifting, lifting belts have been shown to increase intraabdominal pressure and protect the lower back region (Harmon, E., et. al., 1989). This protection stems from a reduction in compressive forces on the vertebral discs when the belt is in use.

Precaution must be taken to rely on lifting belts only during heavy lifting. If belts are used routinely, they will contribute to weakened abdominal musculature and may, in time, contribute to increased risk of injury and low back pain. Additionally, wearing lifting belts provides a false sense of security. Many falsely believe they can safely lift heavier loads when wearing an abdominal belt. Finally, it has been shown that individuals presenting a history of low back injury are at greater risk of injury when wearing a belt (McGill, 2001).

Strengthening the back and abdominal musculatures will help protect the lower back region and lower the need for lifting belts. Strong back and abdominal muscles are capable of generating enough intraabdominal pressure to protect and support the vertebral column. A complete discussion on lifting belts can be found in Chapter 7.

Postural and Fitness Considerations

Many professionals consider muscle weakness and poor joint flexibility as the two primary factors related to low back pain. In fact, 80% of all low back pain problems are muscular in nature (Donatelle, Snow, & Wilcox, 1999). As a result, an understanding of the relationship between muscular weakness, especially in the abdominal and back muscles, and limited range of motion of the lower back and posterior leg or hamstring muscles seems appropriate.

Weakness in the erector muscles of the back and the abdominal musculature contributes to low back pain by allowing the pelvis to tilt forward creating a condition known as **lordosis** (see Figure 12.2). When the pelvis tilts forward, additional stress is placed in the lumbar region of the vertebral column leading to muscle fatigue, spasms, soreness, and/or injury. In extreme cases of pelvic tilt, the sacral bone or lumbar vertebra may press on spinal nerve roots leading to a painful condition known as **sciatica**. Depending on the amount of pressure, symptoms may include, but are not limited to, numbness, severe radiating pain, depressed reflexes, muscle spasms, and loss of function.

Strengthening the abdominal muscles will help to correct for **abdominal ptosis** (abdominal sagging) and prevent lordosis. This is because strong abdominal muscles will pull the lower pelvic area upward and tilt the pelvis backward reducing the stress placed on the lower vertebral column (see Figure 12.3).

The length of the hip flexors and the posterior thigh muscles (hamstrings) have also been linked to low back pain and lordosis. Like weak abdominal musculature, inflexible posterior thigh muscles (hamstrings) and short hip flexors tilt the pelvis forward. Increased range of motion in the hip flexors and hamstrings will correct for this improper pelvic alignment. Exercises designed to improve hamstring flexibility and hip flexor length are strongly recommended.

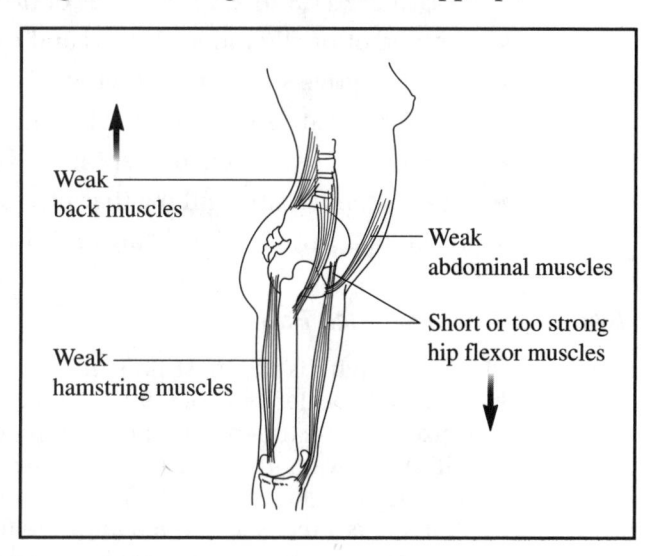

Figure 12.2 ■ Lordosis/Pelvic Tilt
Source: Modified from Corbin, C. & Lindsey, R. (1994). *Concepts of Fitness and Wellness*. Dubuque, Iowa: Brown and Benchmark.

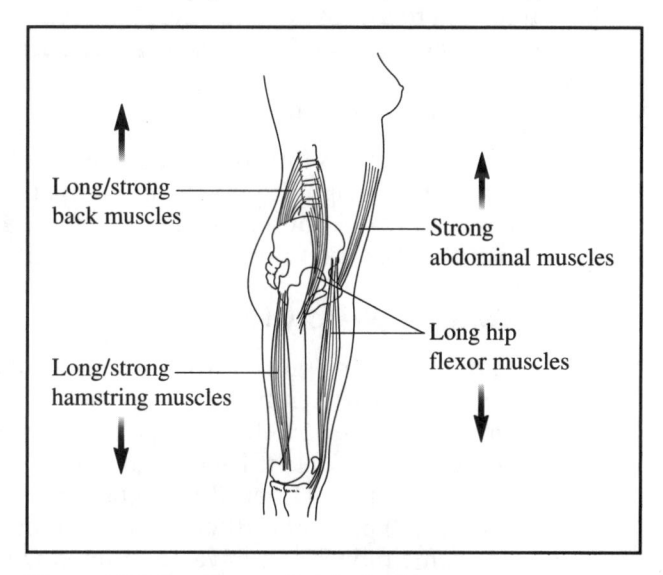

Figure 12.3 ■ Proper Pelvic Position
Source: Modified from Corbin, C. & Lindsey, R. (1994). *Concepts of Fitness and Wellness*. Dubuque, Iowa: Brown and Benchmark.

General Guidelines

In addition to maintaining good range of motion in the lower back and hamstring regions and a strong abdominal and hip flexor musculature, low back pain can be prevented by following some very simple guidelines. These include, but are not limited to:

- Maintain good posture or correct poor posture.
- Improve muscular strength and flexibility.
- Maintain normal body weight.
- Lift heavy objects by using the legs. **Bend your knees not your back.**
- Lift objects with the weight of the object close to your body.
- Never "twist" when carrying, handling, or transferring a heavy object.
- Avoid hyperextension of the back.
- Avoid "locking out" the knees (keep slightly bent).
- Avoid smoking. Smoking has been related to degenerative changes in the spine and increased risk (1.5 to 2.5 times that of non-smokers) of low-back pain.
- Limit emotionally induced stress and muscle tension.
- Use supportive seats when driving.
- Use a firm mattress and sleep with knee flexion.
- Sleep on your side. Avoid sleeping on your back or stomach.
- When sleeping, use a pillow that places the head in a neutral position.
- Avoid long periods of standing and sitting without breaks.

Treatment of Low Back Pain

Physical activity is the most nonsurgically recommended treatment for low-back pain (Cherkin, Deyo, Wheeler, & Ciol, 1995). In fact, by contrast, bed rest is usually not necessary and, if utilized as a treatment, should be limited to no more the 2–4 days. Any greater time of immobilization leads to weakened musculature and delayed recovery (U.S. Agency for Health Care Policy and Research, 1994).

Surgery is a realistic and reliable cure for only 1% of all back patients (Nachemson, 1985). This means that the key to low back pain rehabilitation and prevention is lifestyle related (Deyo & Bass, 1987). For example, negative lifestyle behaviors such as smoking, obesity, poor aerobic conditioning, poor muscular strength and endurance and limited flexibility are highly related to low back pain. Since the focus of this text is on the four health-related areas, these areas are discussed under separate headers below.

Body Composition

Low back pain is directly linked to excess levels in body fatness, and in the extreme case, obesity. Excess weight leading to abdominal ptosis can lead to lordosis and poor posture. In both cases, low back muscle fatigue, soreness, and injury can result. Programs designed to establish and maintain normal body weight are warranted.

Cardiorespiratory Fitness

Participation in regular aerobic exercise can contribute to both the prevention and treatment of low back pain. Aerobic activities such as walking, cycling, and swimming are highly recommended (Nutter, 1988). These particular activities offer excellent aerobic training stimulus with minimal stress on the back. Individual symptomatic response should be used to control exercise duration and intensity. Program objectives should include: 1) work within symptom limitations, 2) prevent further debilitation due to inactivity, and 3) improve functional capacity.

Some individuals have questioned whether jogging exposes the vertebral column to excessive levels of impact related force. These higher forces are thought to lead to early onset of osteoarthritis. **Osteoarthritis** is a degenerative joint diseases characterized by deterioration of articular cartilage. If osteoarthritis were to effect the joints of vertebral column it would lead to low back pain.

Research findings (Lane, et. al. 1986) suggest that running has no negative effect on the bone mineral content of the vertebral column. In fact, runners present as much as 40% higher levels of bone mineral content in the vertebral column than age matched nonrunners. These findings clearly suggest running should not be considered contraindicated.

Muscular Strength and Endurance

Participation in regular muscular strength and endurance activities designed to improve abdominal and back extensor musculature can contribute to both the prevention and treatment of low back pain. While there is no ideal set of activities, gravitational abdominal activities such as curl-ups, curl-ups with a twist, and pelvic tilts seem warranted. These particular activities will develop the abdominal musculature including the rectus abdominis, internal and external obliques, and the transverse abdominis.

In addition to abdominal activities, back extensor activities such as prone arm and leg lifts should be considered. It should be noted, however, that precaution is warranted. Avoid hyperextension of the lower back when participating in back extensor activities.

Specific resistive training activities focusing on the abdomen and back are presented in Chapter 7. Individuals presenting low back pain should perform all resistive training activities slowly and with precaution. Progress slowly and stay within symptom limitations. Programs emphasizing high repetition, low load are recommended. Strength programs emphasizing high load, low repetition are not warranted (McGill, 2001). Gravitational activities that do not require special resistive training equipment, and are designed to assist in the prevention and treatment of low back pain, are presented under separate headers below.

Flexibility

Poor flexibility in the lower back and hamstring muscles is directly linked to low back fatigues. Flexibility training programs designed to improve hip, and posterior and anterior thigh muscle flexibility are warranted. Back and trunk flexibility activities are appropriate when caution is used.

To prevent increased risk of injury, activities that include the spinal movements of flexion-extension, lateral bending, and axial twisting should be unloaded. Unwarranted spinal tissue loading during these types of movements may exacerbate the risk of injury. Specific flexibility activities focusing on the back, trunk, and upper thigh are presented in Chapter 9. Individuals presenting low back pain should perform all flexibility activities slowly and with precaution. Progress slowly and within symptom limitations.

Recommended Exercises for the Lower Back

Below are some recommended activities that can be used to develop muscular strength and flexibility to assist in the prevention and treatment of low back pain. For reader ease, subheaders have been used.

Low Back Exercises

The following gravitational activities are designed to assist in the prevention and treatment of low back pain. Because these activities rely completely on gravitational forces on body segments for external loading, resistive equipment such as free weights or progressive resistance equipment are not required.

Prone Single Arm Lift

Action

The subject should assume a prone position with the arms and legs fully extended. For subject comfort, a cushion may be placed under the forehead. To perform the prone single arm lift, the subject should raise one arm upward as high as possible, keeping the elbow extended and the forehead on the cushion. If a cushion is not used, the subject should keep his/her chin on the floor. To complete the movement, return the arm to its original position. Alternate arms and repeat. The subject should not hold his/her breath during the activity but should breathe freely with each repetition. The action of the prone single arm lift is illustrated in Figure 12.4.

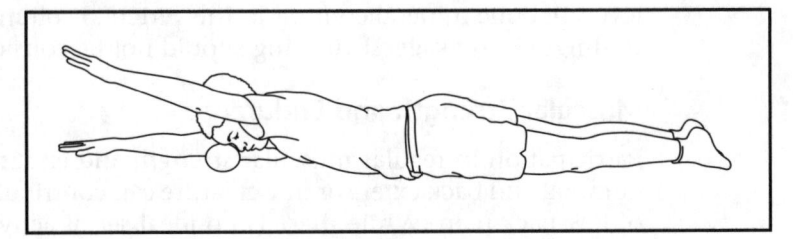

Figure 12.4 ■ Prone Single Arm Lift

Prone Double Arm Lift

Action

The subject should assume a prone position with the arms and legs fully extended. For subject comfort, a cushion may be placed under the forehead. To perform the prone double arm lift, the subject should raise both arms upward as high as possible, keeping the elbows extended and the forehead on the cushion. If a cushion is not used, the subject should keep his/her chin on the floor. To complete the movement, return the arms to their original position. The subject should not hold his/her breath during the activity, but should breathe freely with each repetition. The action of the prone double arm lift is illustrated in Figure 12.5.

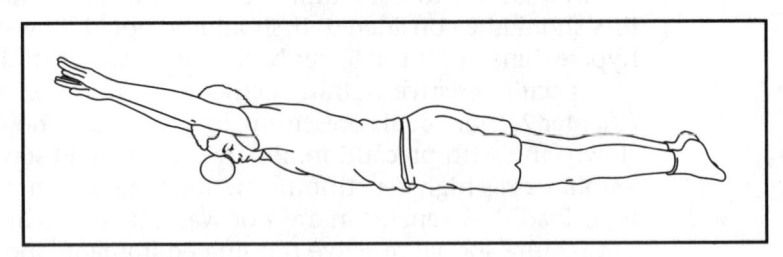

Figure 12.5 ■ Prone Double Arm Lift

Prone Single Leg Lift (Extension)

Action

The subject should assume a prone position with the arms and legs fully extended. For subject comfort, a cushion may be placed under the forehead. To perform the prone single leg lift, the subject should raise one leg as high as possible keeping the knee extended and the hips and upper body in contact with the floor. The forehead should remain stable on the cushion. For stability and comfort, the opposite arm should be repositioned so the arm is extended down toward the hip when the leg is being raised. If a cushion is not used, the subject should keep his/her chin on the floor during the leg extension movement. To complete the exercise, return the arm and leg to their original position. Alternate the arm and leg positions and repeat. The subject should not hold his/her breath during the activity but should breathe freely with each repetition. The action of the prone single leg lift (extension) is illustrated in Figure 12.6.

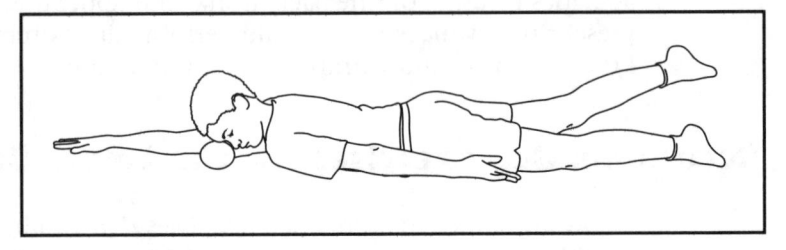

Figure 12.6 ■ Prone Single Leg Lift

Kneeling Arm and Leg Extension

Action

The subject should assume a kneeling position with the arms fully extended below the shoulders. To perform the kneeling arm and leg extension movements, the subject should raise and fully extend one leg. Simultaneously, the opposite arm should be raised and fully extended in front of the head. To complete the exercise, return the arm and leg to their original position. Alternate the arm and leg positions and repeat. The subject should not hold his/her breath during the activity, but should breathe freely with each repetition. The action of the kneeling arm and leg extension is illustrated in Figure 12.7.

Figure 12.7 ■ Kneeling Arm and Leg Extension

Pelvic Tilt

Action

The subject is placed in a supine position with the knees bent at approximately 90 degrees. The hands may rest comfortably on the hips or the arms may be fully extended by the hips. To perform the pelvic tilt exercise, press the low back region flat against the floor by contracting the abdominal muscles. Hold this position for several seconds and then relax the abdominal musculature and allow the pelvis to return to its original position. The subject's lower back should be fully flattened before the abdominal muscle is relaxed. The subject should not hold his/her breath during the activity, but should breathe freely with each repetition. The action of the pelvic tilt is illustrated in Figure 12.8.

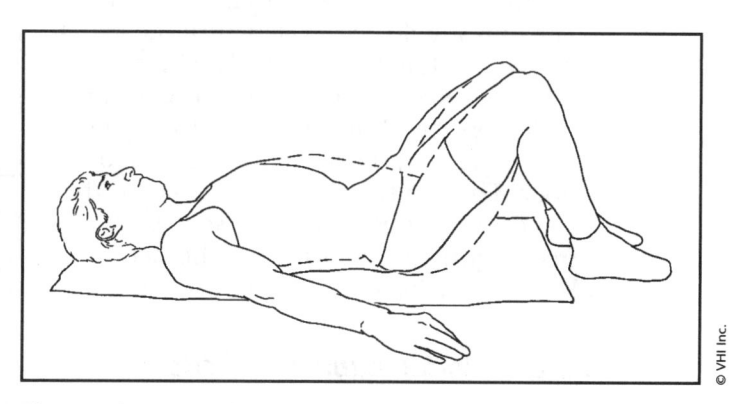

Figure 12.8 ■ Pelvic Tilt

Curl-ups

Action

The subject is placed, in a supine position, on his/her back with the arms and hands extended until the hands are touching the thighs. The legs should be bent at the knees so that the heels are 8–12 inches from the buttocks or the knees are bent at 90 degrees. An assistant may hold the ankles to keep the feet firmly on the ground and to provide support. A correct curl-up is performed when a subject curls-up, lifting his/her shoulders off the mat, while sliding his/her hands up his/her thighs until the hands touch the kneecaps. The lower back, buttocks, and feet should remain in contact with the mat. The trunk should be at approximately a 30-degree angle to the mat. To complete the curl-up, the subject returns to the mat and makes full contact with the back and shoulders. The subject's lower back should be fully flattened before beginning another curl-up. The subject should not hold his/her breath during this activity, but should breathe freely with each repetition. The action of the curl-up is illustrated in Figure 12.9.

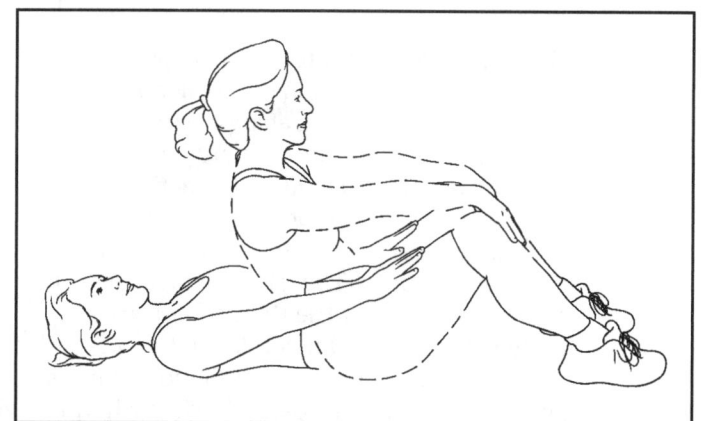

Figure 12.9 ■ Curl-Ups

Bridging

Action

The subject is placed, in a supine position, on his/her back with their arms and hands extended until the hands are touching his/her thighs. The legs should be bent at the knees so that his/her heels are 8–12 inches from the buttocks or his/her knees are bent at approximately 90 degrees. To perform the action of bridging, contract the gluteals and lift the hips and lower back off the floor. The hips should be elevated until the knees, hips, upper thighs, and trunk are inline. **Precaution should be taken to avoid arching or hyperextending the back.** To complete the movement, slowly return the hips to the floor. The subject should not hold his/her breath during this activity, but should breathe freely with each repetition. The action of bridging is illustrated in Figure 12.10.

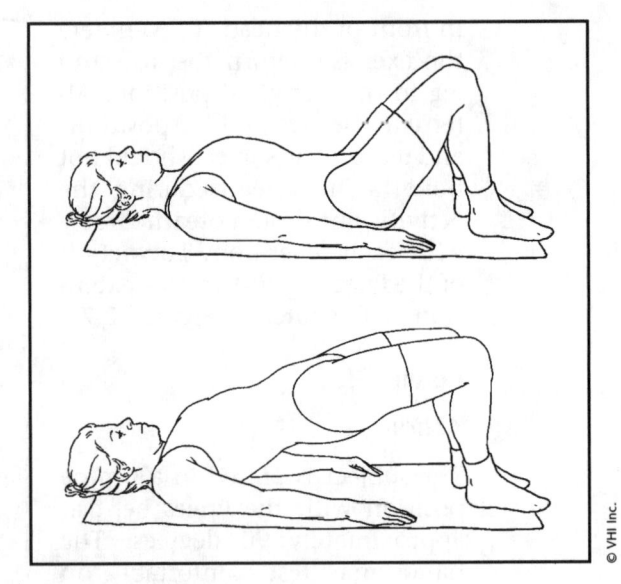

Figure 12.10 ■ Bridging

Additional Low Back Flexibility Exercises

The following flexibility exercises are recommended for the prevention and treatment of low back pain. Descriptive procedures for these activities are presented in Chapter 9.

- Cat Stretch (see Figure 9.21)
- Supine Single Leg Trunk Rotation (see Figure 9.19)
- Supine Double Leg Hip Rotation (see Figure 9.20)
- Single Leg Hip Flexion (see Figure 9.23)
- Double Leg Hip Flexion (see Figure 9.22)
- Hip Stretch (see Figure 9.18)
- Hamstring Stretch (see Figure 9.16 or 9.33)

Contraindicated Low Back Exercises

Curl Ups – Grasping behind the Head

Action

Curl ups are performed with a person lying in a supine position on his/her back. The legs should be bent at approximately 90 degrees. Unfortunately, many want to keep the legs fully extended. The action of the curl up is to contract the abdominal musculature and raise the head, shoulders, and trunk. The shoulder blades should be lifted off the floor to approximately a 30-degree angle. While this action is normally an acceptable abdominal activity, the inherent danger exists when individuals 1) *clasp their hands behind their heads* as they attempt to curl or situp or 2) *when they keep their legs fully extended*. The action of the curl-up while grasping behind the head is shown in Figure 12.11.

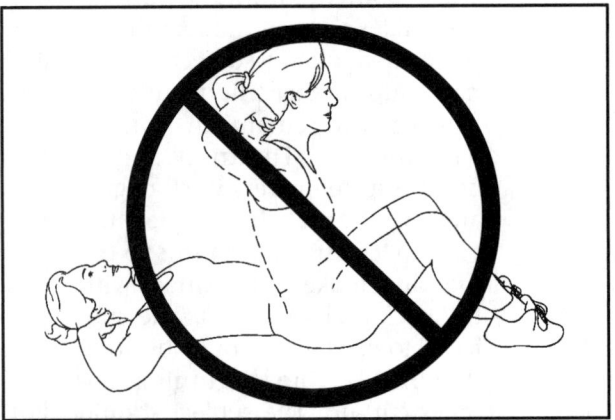

Figure 12.11 ■ Curl Ups - Grasping Behind the Head

Potential Risk

Curls-ups performed while grasping behind the head, place unwanted and unnecessarily high levels of strain on the cervical ligaments. Additionally, there is extreme risk of increased and potentially excessive pressure being placed on the cervical discs.

In addition, the action of curling up to an upright position with the legs fully extended places unwanted and unnecessary strain, particularly on the musculature, in the lower back region. This action also places unusual stress on the hip flexors, particularly the iliopsoas musculature. To eliminate this risk, curls-ups with the knees bent and the arms crossed across the chest are recommended.

Double Leg Lifts

Action

Double leg lifts are performed with the individual lying in a supine position on his/her back. Both legs are fully extended and lifted or raised several inches off the ground. The action of the double leg lift is shown in Figure 12.12.

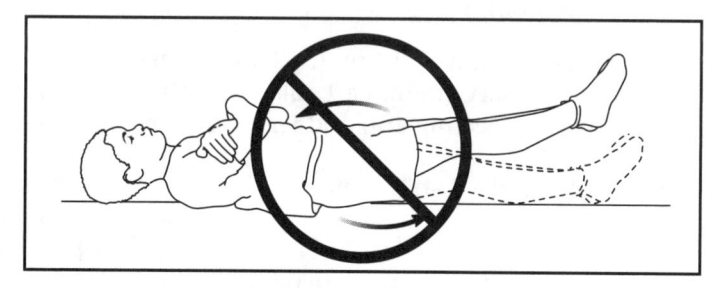

Figure 12.12 ■ Double Leg Lifts

Potential Risk

The action of lifting the legs arches the lower back and places unwanted and unnecessary strain, particularly on the musculature, in the lower back region. To eliminate this risk, single leg lifts are recommended.

Prone Double Leg Raise

Action

Reversed double leg raises are performed with the individual lying on his/her stomach. Both legs are fully extended and lifted or raised several inches off the ground. The action of the prone double leg raise is presented in Figure 12.13.

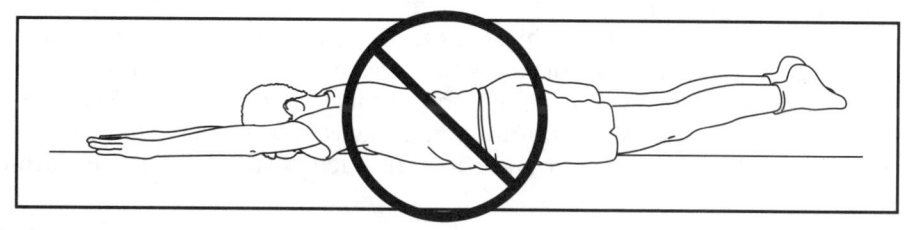

Figure 12.13 ■ Prone Double Leg Raise

Potential Risk

The action of lifting the fully extended legs off the ground hyperextends the back and places unwanted and unnecessary strain, particularly on the musculature, in the lower back region. To eliminate this risk, prone single leg lifts are recommended.

Simultaneous Arm and Leg Lifts

Action

Simultaneous arm and leg lifts are performed with the individual lying on his/her stomach. Both arms and legs are fully extended and lifted or raised several inches off the ground. The action of simultaneous arm and leg lifts are presented in Figure 12.14.

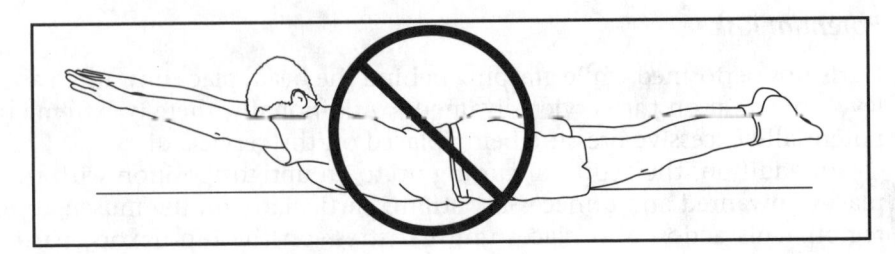

Figure 12.14 ■ Simultaneous Arm and Leg Lifts

Potential Risk

The action of lifting the legs and arms hyperextends the back and places unwanted and unnecessary strain, particularly on the musculature, in the lower back region. To eliminate this risk, kneeling arm and leg lifts are recommended.

Straight Leg Sit-ups

Action

Straight leg sit-ups are performed with the individual lying on their back with his/her legs fully extended. The arms and hands remain crossed across his/her chest as the subject sits up to an upright position. Alternatively, some individuals may choose to grasp their hands behind their heads. The action of the straight leg sit-up with hands grasped behind the head is presented in Figure 12.15.

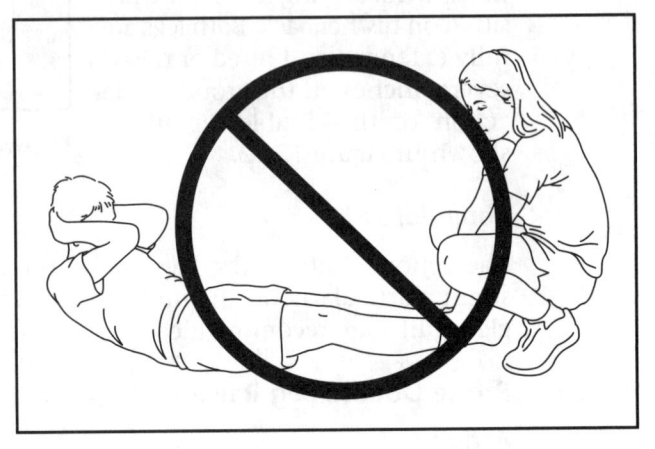

Figure 12.15 ■ Straight Leg Sit-Ups

Potential Risk

The action of sitting up to an upright position with the legs extended places unwanted and unnecessary strain, particularly on the musculature, in the lower back region. This action also places unusual stress on the hip flexors, particularly the iliopsoas musculature. In addition, straight legged sit-ups performed while grasping behind the head, place unwanted and unnecessarily high levels of strain on the cervical ligaments. There is extreme risk of increased and potentially excessive pressure being placed on the cervical discs. To eliminate this risk, curl-ups with the knees bent and the hands across the chest are recommended.

Laboratory Activities

CHAPTER 12

Name: _____ Class Time/Day: _____ Score: _____

LABORATORY 12-A

Low Back: Back-Extension

- **Purpose:** This test measures low back extension.

- **Precautions:** Individuals with a history of low back pain should consult with the instructor before participating. Individuals should warmup properly before participating.

- **Equipment:** Mat, yardstick.

- **Procedure:** Each subject should be allowed to warmup and become familiar with the back-extension test procedure. To measure back-extension, place the subject prone position, face down on the mat. The hands should be placed under the shoulders as if doing a push-up. By extending the arms, the subject should raise his/her trunk upward as high as possible from the floor while keeping the hips stationary to the floor (see Figure 12.16). An assistant may be used to keep the hips in contact with the floor. Precaution should be taken to raise the body with the use of the arms only. Contracting the musculature of the back should be avoided. The assistant should measure the vertical distance, in centimeters, between the floor and the suprasternal notch.

- **Scoring:** The distance, measured in centimeters, between the suprasternal notch and the floor represents the subject's score. Determine normative rating by using Table 12-1.

- **Data/Calculations:**

Name: _____   Date: / /

Gender: _____   Age: _____   Height: _____   Weight: _____

Back Extension Score: _____

Low Back Fitness Rating: _____

Table 12-1 ■ Normative Values for Back-Extension

Rating	Back Extension (inches)
Excellent	> 12
Good	10–12
Average	8–9
Fair	4–7
Poor	< 4

Source: Modified from Thygerson, A. (1989). *Fitness and Health: Lifestyle Strategies.* Boston, Ma: Jones and Bartlett Publishers.

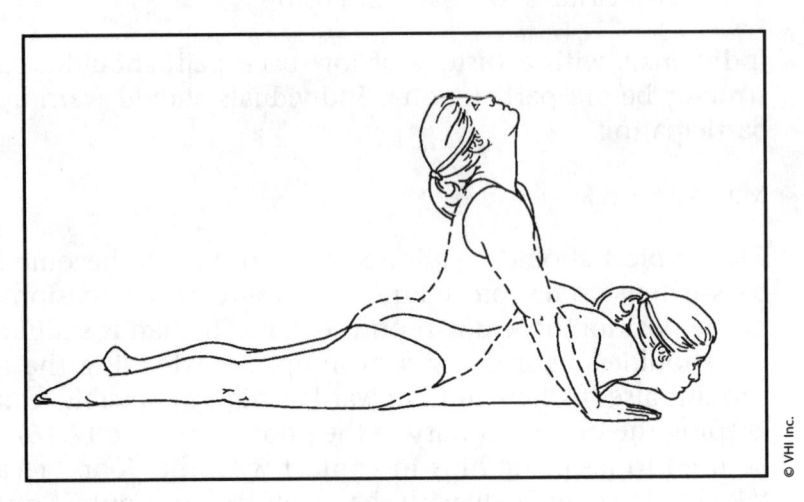

Figure 12.16 ■ Low Back: Back-Extension

Name: _____ Class Time/Day: _____ Score: _____

LABORATORY 12-B

Low Back: Hip and Lumbar Flexibility

- **Purpose:** This test measures hip and low back muscle flexibility.

- **Precautions:** Individuals with a history of low back pain should consult with the instructor before participating. Individuals should warmup properly before participating.

- **Equipment:** Mat, yardstick.

- **Procedure:** Each subject should be allowed to warmup and become familiar with the hip and lumbar flexibility test procedure. To measure hip and low back flexibility, place the subject on the mat with his/her knees bent (see Figure 12.17). Grasp the right knee with both hands and pull the knee tightly into the chest. While holding the knee against the chest, slowly straighten out the left leg. Precaution should be taken to ensure the right knee remains fixed against the chest. An assistant should measure the vertical distance, in inches, between the floor and the back of the knee of the straightened left leg (see Figure 12.18).

- **Scoring:** The distance, measured in inches, between the suprasternal notch and the floor represents the subject's score. Determine normative rating by using Table 12-2.

- **Data/Calculations:**

Name: _____   Date: ___/___/___

Gender: _____ Age: _____ Height: _____ Weight: _____

Hip and Low Back Flexibility score: _____

Low Back Fitness Rating: _____

Table 12-2 ■ Normative Values for Hip and Low Back Flexibility

Rating	Hip and Low Back Flexibility Score (inches)
Excellent	< 2
Good	2–4
Average	4–6
Fair	6–8
Poor	> 8

Source: Modified from Thygerson, A. (1989). *Fitness and Health: Lifestyle Strategies.* Boston, Ma: Jones and Bartlett Publishers.

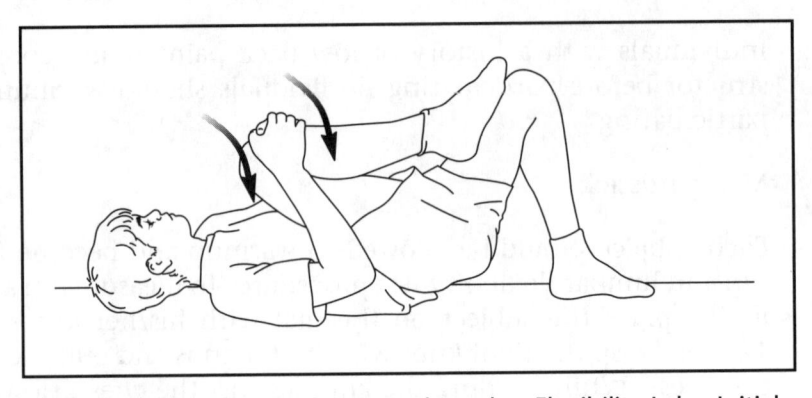

Figure 12.17 ■ Low Back: Hip and Lumbar Flexibility Lab - Initial Position

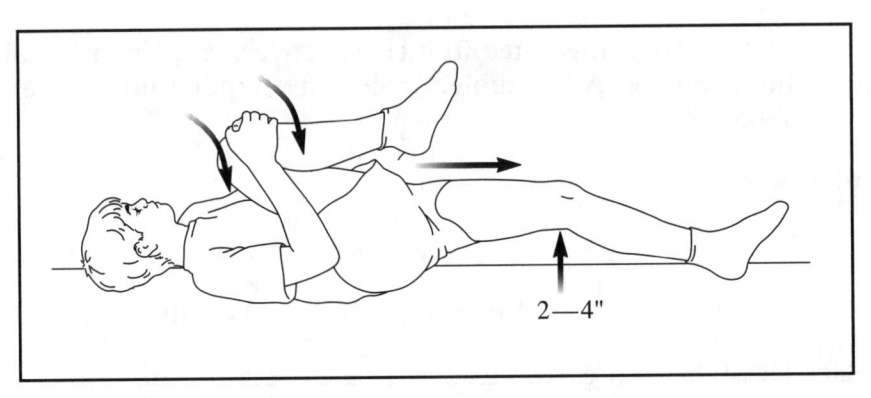

Figure 12.18 ■ Low Back: Hip and Lumbar Flexibility Lab - Final Position

13

Prevention and Treatment of Common Fitness Injuries

Those who do not find time for exercise will have to find time for illness.
Anonymous

■ Chapter Outline ■

Heat-Related Illness
    Heat Cramps
    Heat Exhaustion
    Heat Stroke
Prevention and Treatment of Heat-Related Illness
    Prevention
    Treatment
Prevention of Hypothermia: Exercising in Cold Weather
Prevention and Treatment of Common Fitness Injuries
    Shinsplints
    Muscle Cramps or Spasms
    Side Stitch
    Sprains
Strains
Contusion
Tendonitis and Bursitis
Muscle Soreness
Skeletal Fractures
    Stress Fractures
    Simple Fracture
    Compound Fracture
Skin Wounds
    Open Wounds
    Closed Wounds
Treatment and Management of Injuries Using RICE
Treatment and Management of Injuries Using Heat

■ Learning Objectives ■

The student should be able to:

- Identify and discuss methods of prevention and treatment of heat-related illness.
- Identify and discuss methods of treatment and prevention for hypothermia.
- Identify and discuss methods of treatment and prevention of fitness related injuries, including but not limited to, shinsplints, muscle cramps or spasms, side stitches, sprains, strains, contusions, tendonitis and bursitis, muscle soreness, and skeletal bone stress fractures.
- Discuss treatment and management of exercise related injuries using RICE.
- Discuss treatment and management of exercise related injuries using heat.

Keywords

Bursitis	Heat-related illness	Shinsplints
Closed wound	Heat stroke	Side stitch
Compound fracture	Hypothermia	Simple fracture
Contusion	Muscle cramps	Sprains
Cryotherapy	Muscle soreness	Strains
Heat cramps	Muscle spasms	Stress fractures
Heat exhaustion	Open wound	Tendonitis

Heat-Related Illness

Over-heating during an exercise bout can result in heat-related illnesses. In fact, overheating is the leading cause of noncardiovascular deaths in young athletes (Van Camp, Bloor, Mueller, et al., 1995). The Center for Disease Control and Prevention has suggested that the young, elderly, and those over exert themselves, at work, in play, or in hot environments present the greatest risk of heat-related illness. Other risks are associated with the nonacclimated, healthy adult and those who have consumed excessive levels of alcohol (Nieman, 1995).

Three of the major forms of heat related illnesses include heat cramps, heat exhaustion and heat stroke. These are presented, in order of severity (least to most), under separate headers below.

Heat Cramps

Heat cramping is the least serious of the heat-related disorders. It most frequently is associated with activities that involve prolonged, profuse sweating. Symptomatically, **heat cramps** present muscular pains and spasms. These symptoms are most commonly found in the active musculature.

Heat Exhaustion

Heat exhaustion involves general fatigue, dizziness, vomiting, untoward elevations in pulse, muscular weakness, and potential body collapse. During heat exhaustion, thermoregulatory mechanisms are functioning, but are not adequately meeting the cooling demands of the body.

Heat Stroke

Dangerously elevated body temperatures in excessive of 105° F characterize **heat stroke.** In this situation the thermoregulatory mechanisms of the body are non-functioning. Heat stroke requires immediate medical attention. It should be noted that heat stroke is life threatening. Heat stroke signs and symptoms include: paleness, elevated blood pressure, core body temperature >105 degrees, hot dry skin, cessation of sweating, sudden collapse with confusion or loss of consciousness, and the development of chill bumps while in a hot environment.

Prevention and Treatment of Heat-Related Illness

Prevention

The primary preventative behavior for heat-related illness is consumption of adequate fluids. Typically, water is sufficient to maintain adequate levels of hydration when a person is active for an hour or less. There are, however, occasions when electrolyte replacement drinks are recommended. If activity is to last longer than an hour and/or profuse sweating is anticipated, it may be advisable to consume a fluid such as "Gatorade" in conjunction with water. Any fluid consumed should be cool and have a sugar content of less than 8% so that it may quickly be absorbed into the system. Higher levels of glucose consumption may lead to slower absorption rates and dehydration. Consumption of extremely cold drinks should be avoided, since this behavior is associated with cardiac arrhythmias.

A general rule of hydration when attempting to prevent heat-related illnesses is to hydrate early. Don't wait until you are thirsty and don't wait to drink while you are thirsty. Sweat rates between 2 and 3 liters per hour have been reported during prolonged submaximal activity in hot and humid environments (Robergs and Roberts, 1997).

Thirst is not an accurate means for measuring or determining dehydration. You **do not** sense thirst until well after dehydration has occurred. Always remember that adequate fluid intake will minimize levels of dehydration, assist in body temperature regulation, and reduce cardiovascular stress. Proper procedures for fluid replacement are presented in greater detail in Chapter 10.

Treatment

Anyone experiencing heat-related illnesses should get in the shade, cool the body (possibly with wet towels, ice massage, or ice bath), and consume fluids. In the case of heat stroke, elevate the feet to assist in blood flow to the heart. This will help to reduce the risk of shock.

Humidity levels of 65% or higher greatly impair the body's ability to cool itself. The body normally cools itself by way of evaporation of sweat, but when humidity levels reach 75%, sweat evaporation is extremely limited. These values are important in areas that have extremely high humidity.

Should you plan to exercise in extreme weather conditions (hot, cold, or high humidity) it is advisable to acclimatize; that is, expose yourself to exercising in those environments in small amounts initially, gradually increasing exposure over several week's time.

Dress should be comfortable. Avoid dark, heavy clothing in hot weather, as well as rubberized suits. Many individuals falsely assume that additional caloric expenditure occurs by exercising in intense heat. This assumption is false, extremely dangerous and life threatening. When exercising in hot environments, every attempt to avoid extreme elevations in body temperature should be taken. Light colored clothing that allows for moisture to be wicked from the skin is highly recommended.

Shoes need not be the most expensive, but they should provide adequate support, cushioning and comfort. Any caps or hats should have mesh tops in order to allow body heat to escape.

Prevention of Hypothermia: Exercising in Cold Weather

Hypothermia occurs when the body looses its ability to produce heat. Normally, the hypothalamus has a set point of 98.6 °F. A body temperature of 95 degrees or less signals the onset of hypothermia. Unfortunately, many individuals are under the false assumption that air temperature must be freezing or below before hypothermia can occur. It is not uncommon for hypothermia to occur when air temperature is well above freezing. In addition to air temperature, other causes of hypothermia include: dampness, wind, and fatigue. Change in mental status, an abdomen that is cold to the touch, shivering, loss of coordination, and difficulty speaking are signs of hypothermia. In order to prevent the body from excessive cooling, it is important to dress properly. Covering the head and neck will prevent loss of body heat. Additionally, it is recommended to layer clothing, keep the trunk warm, and wear gloves or mittens.

Prevention and Treatment of Common Fitness Injuries

Injuries may occur no matter how carefully you plan your workout program. These injuries may occur in soft tissue (i.e., connective tissues, muscle cells) or skeletal tissue (i.e., bones). The most common causes of injuries include, but are not limited to, improper shoes and training surfaces, anatomical predisposition, beginning an activity program at a level that is too advanced, or trying to progress too quickly. The probability of injuries can be greatly reduced by adhering to the basic training principles (i.e., overload, progression, consistency, individuality, specificity, and safety). Additionally, proper warm-up and cool-down will assist in reducing the risk of injury.

Typically, injuries are classified as acute (traumatic/occurring suddenly) or chronic (from overuse/develops over time). Most injuries resulting from regular physical activity are chronic in nature. Common fitness injuries, their definitions, and suggested recovery procedures are listed below.

Shinsplints

Shinsplints may be caused from inappropriate footwear, poor training surfaces, and/or overuse that may occur during overtraining. Weak and/or inflexible muscles may also contribute. They result from disruption of the pereosteum and cortical bone of the long, shaft of the tibia. Shinsplints are characterized by pain in the anterior aspect of the lower leg, specifically, the soft tissue along the tibia or the large bone of the lower leg. One of the best methods of preventing shinsplints is to strengthen the anterior muscles of the lower leg through resistive dorsiflexion activities.

Rest, ice, compression, and elevation (RICE) should help in the treatment and recovery process. Increasing muscular strength, muscular endurance, and range of motion is also advisable.

Muscle Cramps or Spasms

Muscle cramps or spasms are sustained, involuntary, convulsive muscle contractions. Recommended procedures for alleviating muscle cramps include gradually stretching the cramping muscle and/or applying constant pressure to the cramping muscle. Caution should be taken to avoid kneading the cramping muscle. Kneading tissue may result in tissue damage.

Side Stitch

Many individuals incur exercise induced side aches commonly referred to as a "stitch in the side." The exact causative factor has not been identified. Factors thought to contribute to side stitches are gas in the large intestine, and diaphragmatic muscle spasms. Since the right side is the more common site of discomfort, it is believed the accumulation of blood in the liver may be a causative factor.

Treatment includes trunk movement and stretching, forceful ventilation, and reduction or cessation of activity. Normally, discomfort will resolve rapidly and allow the participant to return to activity.

Sprains

Sprains occur when ligaments are stretched beyond their capability. Because ligaments provide the main structural support and stability to the joints, once these ligaments experience damage, inelastic scar tissue forms preventing the ligament from regaining its normal tension.

To restore stability, muscles and tendons about the joint must be strengthened. The ankle is a common site for a sprain. RICE is an appropriate treatment.

Strains

A strain is the result of torn muscle fibers. Serious strains are often referred to as muscle pulls. Strains are one of the most common soft tissue injuries and occur most frequently in the hamstrings and quadriceps. They are not, however, limited to these locations.

Initial treatment includes RICE. In cases of severe injury, immobilization may be warranted. Anti-inflammatory drugs (i.e., aspirin) may be advised. After the initial inflammatory period has passed, heat, mild isometrics, range of motion activities and symptom limited isotonic activities may be introduced.

Contusion

A contusion is a direct blow to the outer surface of the body. The skin, however, will remain intact. Contusions are common injuries associated with contact sports. Contusions lead to hemorrhaging (bleeding) and are seen as a "bruise" and inflammation. Contusions vary in terms of seriousness depending on the magnitude of soft tissue damage.

Treatment includes limiting bleeding and inflammation by using the procedures of RICE. Tissue immobilization and blood aspiration may be warranted in severe contusions.

Tendonitis and Bursitis

Tendonitis indicates inflammation of a tendon (tissue connecting muscle to bone), while bursitis results from an inflammation in or around the bursa sacs of any given joint. Bursitis results in increased fluid collection in the lining of the bursa. This fluid accumulation adds to the pain and inflammatory processes. While these two injuries affect different tissues, recommended preventions and treatments are similar. Treatment recommendations include RICE and anti-inflammatory interventions.

Typically, the underlying cause for both tendonitis and bursitis is chronic in nature. Overuse, and/or over-training, are common causes. Additionally, anatomical limitations or equipment abnormalities, when used over time, may contribute. Acute trauma, however, may cause either condition.

Muscle Soreness

Muscle soreness may appear immediately after activity or as late as two days after activity. Overexertion is usually responsible for this discomfort. Gentle stretching and light, low intensity activity is recommended during the recovery period. A more specific discussion of muscle soreness can be found in Chapter 6.

Skeletal Fractures

Fractures to skeletal tissue occur in three forms. Included are stress, simple, and compound. Descriptive characteristics and recommended treatments vary according to the nature of the injury. Each is described under separate headers below.

Stress Fractures

Skeletal stress fractures result from chronic overuse (i.e., repetitive stress) not a traumatic force. In simple, they are small, microfractures occurring at the surface of the bone. They are characterized by a localized, point tenderness occurring at the site of injury. Common sites of injury are the weight bearing bones of the leg (tibia) or foot (tarsals or metatarsals).

Normally, the intensity of pain will increase post exertion or activity. It is unlikely that an individual exercising at moderate levels would develop a stress fracture. If a stress fracture is suspected, immediately begin rest and seek medical attention. Full fractures may develop if activity continues and injury care is not initiated. In some cases, a non-weight bearing activity, such as swimming or cycling, may be used to help limit loss in cardiorespiratory fitness.

Simple Fracture

Simple fractures of the skeletal system are disruptions in the bone resulting from traumatic forces. These types of forces are more often associated with sport-related activities that involve collision, as compared to health-related fitness activities. In the case of a simple fracture, the bone does remain under the skin. Simple fractures are characterized by pain, swelling, and disability. They require medical attention. Immobilization of the injured area will be required should a person need to be transported. Weight or load bearing of the injured area should be prevented.

Compound Fracture

Like simple fractures, compound fractures are disruptions in the bone resulting from a traumatic force. Compound bone fractures are open fractures resulting in exposure of the bone through the skin. As a result, compound fractures present much greater risk of infection. Pain, swelling, disability, and bleeding characterize them. They require medical attention. Bleeding must be controlled. Direct application of pressure and elevation of the injured area will help to control bleeding. **Precautions should be taken to prevent the transfer of blood-borne pathogens.** The nature of some injuries will prevent them from being elevated. Precaution is warranted. Application of sterile dressings and pressure are appropriate. Immobilization of the injured area will be required should a person need to be transported. Weight or load bearing of the injured area should be prevented.

Skin Wounds

Skin wounds are typically categories as either open or closed wounds. Descriptive characteristics and recommended treatments for each are described under separate headers below.

Open Wounds

Open wounds include skin wound injuries such as **punctures, lacerations and abrasions.** They are characterized by localized bleeding, swelling, discoloration (redness), pain and possible infection. In addition, open wounds may be associated with headache and mild fever. Immediate treatment includes controlling bleeding, and dressing the wound. Direct application of pressure and elevation of the injured area will help to control bleeding. **Precautions should be taken to prevent the transfer of blood-borne pathogens.**

Some injuries prevent elevation. Precaution is warranted. Application of sterile dressings should help control for infection. In cases of severe, deep, and/or large wounds, stitches and tetanus shots may be required. In these cases, medical evaluation and attention is warranted.

Closed Wounds

Closed wounds included skin wounds such as **blisters, corns, and sunburn.** They are characterized by pain, swelling, and possible infection. Treatment includes: cleaning and disinfecting the injured area, application of antibiotic ointments, and application of sterile dressing.

Treatment and Management of Injuries Using RICE

Cryotherapy, or the external application of cold, is one of the leading, readily available, immediate treatments for activity related injuries. When combined with rest, elevation, and compression, this intervention assists in controlling bleeding and inflammation by decreasing blood flow in the skin. Additionally, peripheral vasoconstriction occurs as cooled blood from the skin is circulated. The acronym **RICE** is used to reflect the treatment and is discussed below.

- **R—*REST:*** rest the injured site.
- **I—*ICE:*** apply ice immediately after an injury (acute or chronic). Icing decreases pain by slowing the speed of nerve transmissions. It promotes vasoconstriction, which reduces internal bleeding and swelling. If swelling is controlled, healing is expedited. Guidelines for icing include applying ice for at least 20 minutes followed by ice removal for at least 30 minutes. This will prevent the risk of frostbite and reflex vasodilation that will occur from more prolonged ice exposures. Ice as often as possible during the first 72 hours after an injury.
- **C—*COMPRESSION:*** wrap the site (roller bandage or ace bandage) in an effort to control swelling during the first 72 hours post injury.
- **E—*ELEVATION:*** elevate the injured area for the first 72 hours, above "heart" level if possible in order to reduce pain and further prevent swelling.

Treatment and Management of Injuries Using Heat

The use of heat is appropriate for most activity-related injuries after approximately 72 hours. Heat applications increase blood flow to an area (vasodilation) which results in increased swelling and a greater recovery time. As heat is applied, damaged tissue matter dissolves and is carried away in the blood stream.

Precaution should be taken to avoid heat application too early since it will increase blood flow, directly increasing the risk of local edema and hemorrhage. The rule of thumb should be to begin heat applications after swelling has reduced, normal pain-free range of motion has been restored, and the temperature of the injured area is normal.

References Cited

Chapter 1: Concepts of Health and Wellness

American Heart Association. (2001). *http://www.americanheart.org*

American Heart Association. (1998). *1997 heart and stroke statistical update.* American Heart Association.

Ardell, D. (1982). *Fourteen Days to a Wellness Lifestyle.* Mill Valley, CA: Whatever Publishing.

Dunn, H. (1961). *High-Level Wellness.* Arlington, VA: R.W. Beatty, 4.

LaFramboise, H. (1973). *Health policy: Breaking it down into more manageable segments. Journal of the Canadian Medical Association, 108* (Feb. 3), 388–393.

LaLonde, M. (1974). *A New Perspective on the Health of Canadians: A Working Document.* Ottawa, Canada: Ministry of National Health and Welfare.

National Center for Chronic Disease Prevention and Health Promotion. (2001). http://www.cdc.gov

Nieman, D. (1999). *Exercise Testing and Prescription: A Health-Related Approach,* (4th ed.). Mountain View, CA: Mayfield Publishing Company.

World Health Organization. (1947). *Constitution of the world health organization. Chronicle of the World Health Organization, 1*:29–43.

Chapter 2: Understanding and Changing Human Behavior

Cottrell, R., Girvan, J. & Mckenzie, J. (1999). *Principles and Foundations of Health Promotion and Education.* Needham, MA: Allyn and Bacon.

Hales, D. (2002). *An Invitation to Health,* Belmont, CA: Wadsworth Publishing.

Prochaska, J. (1979). *Systems of Psychotherapy: A Transtheoretical Analysis.* Homewood, IL: Dorsey Press.

Prochaska, J., Norcross, J., Fowler, J., Follick, M., & Abrams, D. (1992). *Attendance and outcome in a worksite weight control program: Processes and stages of change as process and predictor variables. Addictive Behaviors, 17,* 35–45.

Prochaska, J., & DiClemente, C. (1985). *Common processes of change for smoking, weight control, and psychological distress.* In Shiffman, S., & Wills, T. (Eds.), *Coping and Substance Abuse.* New York: Academic Press.

Prochaska, J., Norcross, J. & DiClemente, C. (1994). *Changing for Good: The Revolutionary Program that Explains the Six Stages of Change and Teaches You How to Free Yourself from Bad Habits.* New York: William Morrow and Company, Inc.

Chapter 3: Beginning a Health-Related Fitness Program

Holly, R. & Shaffrath, J. (2001). *Cardiorespiratory endurance,* In: *ACSM's Resource Manual for Guidelines for Exercise Testing and Prescription,* (4th ed.), Philadelphia, PA: Lippincott, Williams & Wilkins.

Dudley, G. & Ploutz-Snyder, L. (2001). *Deconditioning and bed rest: Musculoskeletal response,* In: *ACSM's Resource Manual For Guidelines For Exercise Testing and Prescription,* (4th ed.). Philadelphia, PA: Lippincott, Williams & Wilkins.

Robergs, R. & Roberts, S. (1997). *Exercise Physiology: Exercise, Performance, and Clinical Applications.* St. Louis, MO: Mosby.

Selye, H. (1956). *The Stress of Life,* New York, NY: McGraw-Hill.

Chapter 4: Understanding the Cardiovascular System

American College of Sports Medicine. (1998). *ACSM's Resource Manual for Guidelines for Exercise Testing and Prescription,* (3rd ed.). Philadelphia, PA: Williams & Wilkins.

American College of Sports Medicine. (2001). *ACSM's Resource Manual for Guidelines for Exercise Testing and Prescription,* (4th ed.). Philadelphia, PA: Lippincott, Williams & Wilkins.

American Heart Association. (1993). *1993 Heart and Stroke Facts.* Dallas, TX: American Heart Association.

American Society of Hypertension Public Policy Position Paper. (1992). *Recommendations for routine blood pressure measurement by indirect cuff sphygmomanometry. American Journal of Hypertension, 5:* 207–209.

Mangan, G., & Golding, J. (1984). *Psychopharmacology of Smoking.* London: Cambridge University.

Marks, B. (2001). *Tobacco exposure and chronic illness.* In: *ACSM's Resource Manual for Guidelines for Exercise Testing and Prescription, (4th ed.).* Philadelphia, PA: Lippincott, Williams & Wilkins.

Morris, J., Adam, C., Chave, S., Sirey, C., Epstein, L. & Sheehan, D. (1973). *Vigorous exercise in leisure-time and the incidence of coronary heart-disease. Lancet, 1,* 333–339.

Morris, J., Pollard, R., Everitt, M., Chave, Sheila & Semmence, A. (1980). *Vigorous exercise in leisure-time: Protection against coronary heart disease. Lancet, 2,* 1207–1210.

National High Blood Pressure Education Program. (1992). *Working Group Report on Primary Prevention of Hypertension. National Heart, Lung, and Blood Institute.* Hyattsville, MD: National Institutes of Health.

Powell, K., Thompson, P., Caspersen, C. & Kendrick, J. (1987). *Physical activity and the incidence of coronary heart disease. Annual Review of Public Health, 8,* 253–287.

Wilmore, J. & Costill, D. (1999). *Physiology of Sport and Exercise,* (2nd ed.). Champaign, IL: Human Kinetics.

Chapter 5: Principles of Cardiorespiratory Endurance

American College of Sports Medicine. (1990). *The recommended quantity and quality of exercise for developing and maintaining cardiorespiratory and muscular fitness in healthy adults.* (Position Stand of the American College of Sports Medicine). *Medicine and Science in Sports and Exercise, 22,* 265–274.

American College of Sports Medicine. (1998). *The recommended quantity and quality of exercise for developing and maintaining cardiorespiratory and muscular fitness in healthy adults.* (Position Stand of the American College of Sports Medicine). *Medicine and Science in Sports and Exercise, 30*(6), 975–991.

American College of Sports Medicine. (1998b). *ACSM's Resource Manual for Guidelines for Exercise Testing and Prescription,* (3rd ed.). Philadelphia, PA: Williams & Wilkins.

American College of Sports Medicine. (2000). *ACSM's Guidelines For Exercise Testing and Prescription* (6th ed.). Philadelphia, PA: Lippincott Williams & Wilkins.

American Society of Hypertension. (1992). *Recommendations for routine blood pressure measurement by indirect cuff sphygmomanometry.* (Public Policy Position Paper of the American Society of Hypertension). *American Journal of Hypertension, 5,* 207–209.

Blair, S., Kampert, J., Kuhl, H., Barlow, C., Macera, C., Paffenbarger, R., & Gibbons, L. (1996). *Influences of cardiorespiratory fitness and other precursors on cardiovascular disease and all-*

cause mortality in men and women. Journal of the American Medical Association, 276: 205–210.

Borg, G. (1983). *Perceived exertion: A note on history and methods. Medicine and Science in Sports and Exercise, 5,* 90–93.

Cantu, R. (1992). *Congenital Cardiovascular disease—the major cause of athletic death in high school and college. Medicine and Science in Sports and Exercise, 24:* 279–280.

Center for Disease Control and Prevention (1997). Atlanta: GA.

Coyle, E., Martin, W., Sinacore, D., Joyner, M., Hagberg, J., & Holloszy, J. (1984). *Time course of loss of adaptation after stopping prolonged intense endurance training. Journal of Applied Physiology, 57,* 1857–1864.

deVries, H. (1986). *Physiology of Exercise For Physical Education and Athletics* (4th ed.). Dubuque, IA: Wm. C. Brown.

Karlsson, J., Bonde-Petersen, F., Henriksson, J. & Knuttgen, H., (1975). *Effects of previous exercise with arms or legs on metabolism and performance in exhaustive exercise. Journal of Applied Physiology, 38,* 763–767.

Kraemer, W. (2000). *Physiological adaptations to anaerobic and aerobic endurance training programs.* In Baechle, T., & Earle, R. (Eds.) *Essentials of Strength Training and Conditioning,* (2nd ed.) Champaign, IL: Human Kinetics.

Hickson, R., & Rosenkoetter, M. (1981). *Reduced training frequencies and maintenance of increased aerobic power. Medicine and Science in Sports and Exercise, 13,* 13–16.

Hickson, R., Kanakis, C., Davis, J., Moore, A., & Rich, S. (1982). *Reduced training duration effects on aerobic power, endurance, and cardiac growth. Journal of Applied Physiology, 53,* 225–229.

Hickson, R., Foster, C., Pollock, T., Galassi, T., & Rich, S. (1985). *Reduced training intensities and loss of aerobic power, endurance and cardiac growth. Journal of Applied Physiology, 58,* 492–499.

Levine, B., Hanson-Zuckerman, J., & Cole, C. (2001). *Medical complications of exercise.* In American College of Sports Medicine. *ACSM's Resource Manual For Guidelines For Exercise Testing and Prescription* (4th ed.). Philadelphia, PA: Lippincott Williams & Wilkins.

McArdle, W., Katch, F. & Katch, V. (1991). *Exercise Physiology: Energy, Nutrition, and Human Performance* (3rd ed.). Philadelphia, PA: Lea & Febiger.

Mittleman, M., Maclure, M., Tofler, G., Sherwood, J. Goldberg, R., & Muller, J. (1993). *Triggering of acute myocardial infarction by heavy physical exertion: Protection against triggering by regular exertion. New England Journal of Medicine, 329:* 1677–1683.

Nieman, D. (1995). *Fitness and Sports Medicine: A Health-Related Approach,* (3rd ed.). Palo Alto, CA: Bull Publishing Company.

Pollock, M.L., Gettman, I., Milesis, C., Bah, M., Durstine, L. & Johnson, R. (1977). *Effects of frequency and duration of training on attrition and incidence of injury. Medicine and Science in Sports and Exercise, 9,* 31–36.

Powell, K., Thompson, P., Caspersen, C., & Kendrick, J. (1987). *Physical activity and the incidence of coronary heart disease. Annual Review of Public Health, 8:* 253–287.

Robergs, R. & Roberts, S. (1997). *Exercise Physiology: Exercise, Performance, and Clinical Applications.* St. Louis, MO: Mosby.

Siscovick, D., Weiss, N., Fletcher, R, et al. (1984). *The incidence of primary cardiac arrest during vigorous exercise. New England Journal of Medicine, 311:* 874–877.

Thompson, P. (1982). *Cardiovascular hazards of physical activity.* In *Exercise and Sport Sciences Reviews, 12,* 245–306, Terjung, R. (ed.), Philadelphia, PA: Franklin Institute Press.

Chapter 6: Principles of Muscular Strength and Endurance

American College of Sports Medicine. (2001). *ACSM's Resource Manual For Guidelines For Exercise Testing and Prescription* (4th ed.). Philadelphia, PA: Lippincott, Williams & Wilkins.

American College of Sports Medicine. (1993). *ACSM's Resource Manual For Guidelines For Exercise Testing and Prescription* (2nd ed.). Philadelphia, PA: Williams & Wilkins.

Anderson, T. & Kearney, J. (1982). *Effects of three resistance training programs on muscular strength and absolute and relative endurance. Research Quarterly for Exercise and Sport, 53,* 1–7.

Antonio, J., & Gonyea, W. (1993). *Skeletal muscle fiber hyperplasia. Medicine and Science in Sports and Exercise, 25* 1333.

Berger, R. (1982). *Applied Exercise Physiology.* Philadelphia, PA: Lea & Febiger.

Bowers, R., & Fox, E. (1992). *Sports Physiology* (3rd ed.). Dubuque, IA: William C. Brown.

Brooks, G., Fahey, T., & White, T. (1996). *Exercise Physiology: Human Bioenergetics and Its Applications.* Mountain View, CA: Mayfield Publishing Company.

Coggan, A., et. al., (1992). *Skeletal muscle adaptations to endurance training in 60-to70-yr old men and women. Journal of Applied Physiology, 72,* 1780.

Delorme, T., & Watkins, A. (1951). *Progressive Resistance Exercise.* New York: Appleton-Century-Crofts.

Dudley, G. & Ploutz-Snyder, L. (2001). *Deconditioning and Bed Rest: Musculoskeletal Response,* In: American College of Sports Medicine. *ACSM's Resource Manual For Guidelines For Exercise Testing and Prescription* (4th ed.). Philadelphia, PA: Lippincott, Williams & Wilkins.

Gonyea, W., Ericson, G., & Bonde-Peterson, F. (1977). *Skeletal muscle fiber splitting induced weight lifting exercises in cats. Acta Physiologica Scandanavica, 99,* 105–109.

Harris, R & Dudley, G. (2000). *Neuromuscular Anatomy and Adaptations to Conditioning.* In Baechle, T., & Earle, R. (Eds.) *Essentials of Strength Training and Conditioning,* (2nd Ed.) Champaign, IL: Human Kinetics.

Ho, K., Roy, J., Taylor, W., Heusner, W., Van Huss, W., & Carrow, R. (1977). *Muscle fiber splitting with weightlifting exercise. Medicine and Science in Sports and Exercise, 9*(1): 65.

Kraemer, W. (2000). *Physiological adaptations to anaerobic and aerobic endurance training programs.* In Baechle, T., & Earle, R. (Eds.) *Essentials of Strength Training and Conditioning,* (2nd Ed.) Champaign, IL: Human Kinetics.

Kraemer, W. & Fry, A. (1995). *Strength testing: Development and evaluation of methology.* In Maud, P. and Foster, C. (Eds.), *Physiological Assessment of Human Fitness,* Champaign, Il: Human Kinetics.

McArdle, W., Katch, F. & Katch, V. (1991). *Exercise Physiology: Energy, Nutrition, and Human Performance* (3rd ed.). Philadelphia, PA: Lea & Febiger.

McArdle, W., Katch, F. & Katch, V. (1996). *Exercise Physiology: Energy, Nutrition, and Human Performance* (4th ed.). Philadelphia, PA: Williams & Wilkins.

McArdle, W., Katch, F. & Katch, V. (2001). *Exercise Physiology: Energy, Nutrition, and Human Performance* (5th ed.). Baltimore, MD: Lippincott Williams & Wilkins.

McDonagh, M. & Davies, C. (1984). *Adaptive response of mammalian skeletal muscle to exercise with high loads. European Journal of Applied Physiology. 52:* 139–155.

Sola, O., Christensen, & Martin, A. (1973). *Hypertrophy and hyperplasia of adult chicken anterior latissimus dorsi muscle following stretch with and without denervation. Experimental Neurology, 41,* 76–100.

Stone, M., O'Bryant, H., & Garhammer, J. (1981). *A hypothetical model for strength training. Journal of Sports Medicine and Physical Fitness. 21,* 342–351.

Stone, M. & O'Bryant, H. (1984). *Weight Training: A Scientific Approach.* Minneapolis, MN: Burgess Publishing Company.

Powers, S. & Howley, E. (1990). *Exercise Physiology: Theory and Applications to Fitness and Performance.* Dubuque, IA: William C. Brown.

Wilmore, J. & Costill, D. (1999). *Physiology of Sport and Exercise,* (2nd ed.). Champaign, IL: Human Kinetics.

Chapter 7: Resistive Training Activities

Earle, R., & Baechle, T. (2000). *Resistive training and spotting techniques.* In Baechle, T., & Earle, R. (Eds.) (2000). *Essentials of Strength Training and Conditioning, (2nd Ed.)* Champaign, IL: Human Kinetics.

Harman, E. (2000). *The biomechanics of resistance exercise.* In Baechle, T., & Earle, R. (Eds.) (2000). *Essentials of Strength Training and Conditioning, (2nd Ed.)* Champaign, IL: Human Kinetics.

Fleck, S., & Kraemer, W. (1987). *Designing resistance training programs.* Champaign, IL: Human Kinetics.

Chapter 8: Principles of Flexibility

Alter, M. (1988). *Science of Stretching.* Champaign, IL: Human Kinetics.
American College of Sports Medicine. (1993). *ACSM's Resource Manual For Exercise Testing and Prescription* (2nd ed.). Philadelphia, PA: Williams & Wilkins.
American College of Sports Medicine. (2000). *ACSM's Guidelines For Exercise Testing and Prescription* (6th ed.). Philadelphia, PA: Lippincott Williams & Wilkins.
American College of Sports Medicine. (2001). *ACSM's Resource Manual For Exercise Testing and Prescription* (4th ed.). Philadelphia, PA: Lippincott Williams & Wilkins.
Bandy, W. & Irion, J. (1994). The effect of time on static stretch on the flexibility of the hamstring muscles. *Physical Therapy, 74,* 845–850.
Corbin, C. (1984). *Flexibility. Clinics in Sports Medicine, 3,* 101–117.
Holcomb, W. (2000). *Stretching and warm-up.* In Baechle, T., & Earle, R. (eds.), *Essentials of Strength Training and Conditioning* (2nd ed), Champaign, IL: Human Kinetics.
Komi, P. (1986). *The stretch-shortening cycle and human power output.* In Jones, N., McCartney, N. and McComas, R. (eds.), *Human Muscle Power* (pgs. 27–39).
Nieman, D. (1995). *Fitness and Sports Medicine: A Health-Related Approach* (3rd ed.). Palo Alto, CA: Bull Publishing Company.
Robergs, R. & Roberts, S. (1997). *Exercise Physiology: Exercise, Performance, and Clinical Applications.* St. Louis, MO: Mosby.
Sapega, A., Quedenfeld, T., Moyer, R. & Butler, R. (1981). *Biophysical factors in range-of-motion exercise. Physician and Sportsmedicine,* 9:57–65.
Smith, C. (1994). *The warm-up procedure: To stretch or not to stretch. A brief review. Journal of Sports Physical Therapy, 19:* 12–17.
Surburg, P. (1995). *Flexibility training: Program design.* In Miller, P., (ed.), *Fitness Programming and Physical Disability.* Champaign, IL: Human Kinetics.

Chapter 10: Principles of Nutrition

American College of Sports Medicine (1996). *Position Stand on Exercise and Fluid Replacement. Medicine and Science in Sports and Exercise, 28,* i–viii.
American College of Sports Medicine, American Dietetic Association & Dietitians of Canada (2000). *Joint Position Statement on Nutrition and Athletic Performance. Medicine and Science in Sports and Exercise, 32,* 2130–2145.
Hoeger, W. & Hoeger, S. (1999). *Principles and Labs for Physical Fitness.* Englewood, CO: Morton.
Insel, P. & Roth, W. (2002). *Core Concepts in Health (9th ed).* Boston, MA: McGraw-Hill.
Kurtzweil, P. (1999). *An FDA guide to dietary supplements.* FDA Consumer, Sept.–Oct. 1998. Publication No. (FDA) 99–2323.
Lassiter, W. (1990). *Regulation of sodium chloride distribution within the extracellular space.* In Seldin, D. & Giebisch, G. *The Regulation of Sodium and Chloride Balance,* New York: Raven Press, Inc.
McArdle, W., Katch, F. & Katch, V. (2001). *Exercise Physiology: Energy, Nutrition, and Human Performance* (5th ed.). Baltimore, MD: Lippincott Williams & Wilkins.
Mihoces, G. (1997). *Deaths raise suspicions. USA Today,* Dec. 18.
National Research Council, Food and Nutrition Board. (1989). *Recommended Dietary Allowances,* (10th ed). Washington, DC: National Academy Press.
Sizer, F., & Whitney, E. (1994). *Hamilton and Whitney's Nutrition: Concepts and Controversies.* St. Paul: West.
Takamata, A., Mack, C., Gillen, C., & Nadel, E. (1994). *Sodium appetite, thirst, and body fluid regulation in humans during rehydration without sodium replacement. American Journal of Physiology, 266,* R1493–R1502.
Thomas, D. (1997). *Nutrition.* In Howley, E., & Franks, D. *Health Fitness Instructor's Handbook* (3rd ed.). Champaign, IL: Human Kinetics.
US Food & Drug Administration. (1995). Publication No. BG 95-14.

US Food & Drug Administration. (1995). *On the teen Scene: Food label makes good eating habits.* FDA Consumer, Publication No. (FDA) 98-2294.

US Department of Health and Human Services, U.S. Department of Agriculture. *Dietary Guidelines for Americas 2005.* www.healthierus.gov/dietaryguidelines

Chapter 11: Principles of Weight Management

American Psychiatric Association, (1994). *Diagnostic and statistical manual of mental disorders,* Washington, DC: APA.

Andersen, A. (1986). Anorexia/Bulimia Association, inc. *Newsletter, 9:* 16.

Andersen, A. (1983). *Anorexia nervosa and bulimia. Journal of Adolescent Health Care, 4:* 15–21.

Borgen, J. & Corbin, C. (1987). *Eating disorders among female athletes. Physician and Sports Medicine, 15:* 89–95.

Deurenberg, P., Weststrate, J. A., & Seidell, J. C. (1991). *Body mass index as a measure of body fatness: age - and sex - specific prediction formulas. Journal of Nutrition, 65,* 105–114.

Dolgener, F. & Hensley, L. (eds.). (1998). *Personal Wellness.* Dubuque, IA: Eddie Bowers Publishing.

Food and Nutrition Board, National Research Council. (1989). *Recommended dietary allowances* (10th ed.). Washington, DC: National Academy press.

Hsu, L. (1988). *The outcome of anorexia nervosa: A reappraisal. Psychology and Medicine, 18,* 807–812.

Pochlman, E. (1986). *Genotype controlled changes in body composition and fat morphology following overfeeding in twins. American Journal of Clinical Nutrition, 43,* 723–730.

Roza, A. & Shizgal, H. (1984). *The harris-benedict equation reevaluated: Resting energy requirements and the body cell mass. American Journal of Clinical Nutrition, 40,* 168–182.

Schotte, D. & Stunkard, A. (1987). *Bulimia vs. bulimic behaviors on a college campus. Journal of the American Medical Association, 258:* 1213–1215.

Chapter 12: Low Back: Health and Fitness Management

Anspaugh, D., Hamrick, M., & Rosato, F. (1991). *Concepts and Applications of Wellness.* St. Louis, Mo.: Mosby.

Biering-Sorensen, F., Bendix, T., Jorgensen, K., Manniche, C., & Nielsen, H. (1994). *Physical activity, fitness and back pain.* In: Bouchard, C., Shephard, F. (eds.). *Exercise, fitness, and health: A consensus of current knowledge.* Champaign, IL: Human Kinetics.

Cherkin, D., Deyo, R., Wheeler, K. & Ciol, M. (1995). *Physicians views about treating low back pain: The results of a national survey.* Spine 20: 1–10.

Corbin, C. & Lindsey, R. (1997). *Concepts of Fitness and Wellness with Laboratories.* Boston, Ma: McGraw-Hill.

Deyo, R., & Bass, J. (1987). *Lifestyle and low back pain: The influence of smoking, exercise, and obesity. Clin. Res., 35;* 577A.

Donatelle, R., Snow, C. & Wilcox, A. (1999). *Wellness Choices For Health and Fitness.* Boston, MA: Wadsworth Publishing.

Fahey, T., Insel, P., and Roth, W. (1999). *Fit and Well: Core Concepts and Lab's in Physical Fitness and Wellness.* Mountain View, CA: Mayfield Publishing Co.

Frymoyer, J., Pope, M., Contanza, M, et.al. (1980). *Epidemiologic studies of low back pain. Spine. 5:* 419–423.

Harmon, E., et. al. (1989). *Effect of a belt on intra-abdominal pressure during weight lifting. Medicine and Science in Sports and Exercise, 21:* 605.

Lane, N. et. al. (1986). *Long distance running, bone density and osteoarthritis. Journal of the American Medical Association, 255:* 1147–1151

McGill, S. (2001). *Low back exercises: Prescriptions for the healthy back and when recovering from injury.* In: American College of Sports Medicine. *ACSM's Resource Manual For Guidelines For Exercise Testing and Prescription* (4th ed.). Philadelphia, PA: Lippincott Williams & Wilkins.

McGill, S. (1993). *Abdominal belts in industry: A position paper on their assets, liabilities, and use. American Industrial Hygiene Association Journal, 54:* 752–754.

Nachemson, A. L. (1985). *Advances in low-back pain. Clinical Orthopedics and Related Research, 200,* 266–278.

Nieman, D. (1999). *Exercise Testing and Prescription: A Health-Related Approach,* (4th ed.). Mountain View, CA: Mayfield Publishing Company.

Nutter, P. (1988). *Aerobic exercise in the treatment and prevention of low back pain. Occupational Medicine, 3:* 137–145.

Oldridge, N. & Stoll, J. (1997). *Low back pain syndrome.* In American College of Sport Medicine. *ACSM's Exercise management for persons with chronic disease and disabilities,* Champaign, IL: Human Kinetics.

Park, C. & Wagener, D. (1993). *Health conditions among the currently employed: United States 1998. National Center for Health Statistics, (PHS) 93-1412.* Washington, DC: Government Printing Office.

Plowman, S. (1992). *Physical activity, physical fitness, and low back pain. Exercise and Sport Sciences Reviews 20:* 221–242.

Robergs, R. & Roberts, S. (1997). *Exercise Physiology: Exercise, Performance, and Clinical Applications.* St. Louis, MO: Mosby.

Saunders, H. (1992). *For Your Back.* Minn. MN: Educational Opportunities.

U. S. Agency for Health Care Policy and Research. (1994). *Clinical Practice Guideline: Acute Low Back Problems in Adults.* Silver Spring, MD: Publications Clearinghouse.

Zammula, E. (1989). *Back talk: Advice for suffering spines. FDA Consumer,* April, pp. 28–35.

Chapter 13: Prevention and Treatment of Common Fitness Injuries

Nieman, D. (1995). *Fitness and Sports Medicine: A Health-Related Approach.* (3rd ed.). Palo Alto, CA: Bull Publishing Company.

Robergs, R. & Roberts, S. (1997). *Exercise Physiology: Exercise, Performance, and Clinical Applications.* St. Louis, MO: Mosby.

Van Camp, S., Bloor, C., Mueller, F., Cantu, R., & Olson, H. (1995). *Nontraumatic sports deaths in high school and college athletes. Medicine and Science in Sports and Exercise. 27:* 641–647.

Index

Note: Page numbers followed by f indicate figures; those followed by t indicate tables.

A

Abdominal belts, 152, 314
Abdominal machine, 165, 165f
Abdominal ptosis, 317
Abdominals, resistive training for
    machine, 165, 165f
    nonmachine, 192–193, 192f, 193f
Abdominal skinfold, 287, 289f
Abrasions, 337
Action stage, of behavior change, 41t, 42
Active flexibility, 196
Activity. *See* Exercise
Adaptation, 55–56
Adductor stretch, 230, 230f
    PNF, 238, 238f
Aerobic exercise. *See* Cardiorespiratory endurance exercise program
Age
    cardiovascular disease and, 82
    flexibility and, 198–199
    muscular strength and endurance and, 128–129
    weight and, 272
Agonist contraction, 199, 201–202
Amino acids, 247
    supplemental, 247–248
Amphetamines, weight and, 274–275
Android obesity, 82, 270, 271f
Ankle dorsi flexion, in flexibility assessment, 211–212, 212f, 212t
Ankle plantar flexion, in flexibility assessment, 209–210, 210f, 210t
Anorexia nervosa, 281–282
Anterior arm stretch, 234, 234f
Anterior foot and toes stretch, 227, 227f
Anterior lower leg stretch, 227–228, 228f
Anterior neck stretch, 232, 232f
Anterior shoulder stretch, 233, 233f
    PNF, 238, 238f
Anterior upper leg stretch, 236, 236f
Antioxidant vitamins, 248–249
Arm. *See also* Forearm; Upper arm
Arm curls
    dumbbell, 180–183, 181f-183f
    seated, 159, 159f
    standing cable, 160, 160f
Arm-leg lifts, simultaneous, 323–324, 324f
Arthritis, degenerative, 318

Assisted dips, 159, 159f
Athletic performance
    body fat and, 270
    nutrition and, 255–257
Atria, 77
Atrioventricular valves, 77
Atrophy, muscle, 128
    detraining and, 125
Autogenic inhibition, 201–202
Axilla skinfold, 287, 289f

B

Back. *See also under* Low back; Spine; Vertebrae
    resistive exercises for, 163–164, 163f, 164f
        with barbells, 177–178, 177f, 178f
        with dumbbells, 187–188, 188f
    stretching exercises for, 230–232, 230f–232f
        PNF, 237, 237f
Back bends, 226, 226f
Back extension, 164, 165f
Back pain. *See* Low back pain
Ballistic stretching, 200–201, 200t, 235
Barbell(s), 155–156. *See also* Resistive training
    exercises with, 170–178
Barbell bench chest press, 170, 170f
Barbell bent over row, 177, 177f
Barbell incline bench chest press, 170–171, 171f
Barbell inclined overhead press, 176, 176f
Barbell pull-over, 177–178, 178f
Barbell wrist curl, 174, 174f
Barbell wrist extensions, 175, 175f
Barriers, to change, 38
Basal metabolic rate, determination of, 305–306
Basal metabolism, 271
    body weight and, 275
    dieting and, 275
    set point and, 274–275
Behavior
    barriers for, 38
    determinants of, 37–39
    enabling factors for, 38
    predisposing factors for, 37
    reinforcing factors for, 38
Behavior change, 35–52
    action stage of, 41t, 42
    barriers to, 38
    behavior analysis for, 43–44
    contemplation stage of, 41, 41t
    efficacy and, 40
    goals and objectives for, 44

Behavior change, *continued*
    locus of control and, 40
    maintenance stage of, 41t, 42–43
    personal contract for, 44
    phases of, 40–43, 41t
    plan of action for
        implementation of, 45, 49–50
        preparation of, 44–45
        reevaluation and modification of, 45–46
    precontemplation stage of, 41, 41t
    preparation stage of, 41t, 42
    as process, 40, 41t
    readiness for, 51–52
    steps in, 43–46
    target behavior for, 43
    termination stage of, 41t, 43
    transtheoretical model for, 40–43, 41t
    in weight management, 276–278
Bench press, 156–157, 157f
    barbell bench, 170, 170f
    barbell incline bench, 170–171, 171f
    dumbbell, 179, 179f
    dumbbell incline, 179, 179f
    lying closed grip, 173–174, 174f
Bench press test, 143, 143f, 143t
Biceps stretch, 234, 234f
Bicuspid valve, 77
Binge-purge cycle, in bulimia, 282
Blisters, 337
Blood, oxygenation of, 77
Blood pressure
    classification of, 80t
    diastolic, 79, 80t
    elevated, 6
        cardiovascular disease and, 27t, 79–80
    measurement of, 80, 87–89, 87f
    systolic, 79, 80t
Body build, 269, 269f
Body building, 135. *See also* Resistive training
Body composition, fitness program for, 73
Body composition assessment
    body mass index in, 301–302, 302t
    skinfold measurements for, 287–288, 288f, 289f
        seven-site, 299–301
        three-site, 291–292, 292t, 293t, 295–296, 296t, 297t
    waist-to-hip ratio in, 303–304, 303t, 304f
Body fat, 269–270
    acceptable levels of, 270
    essential, 269
    gender differences in, 270, 270t
    nonessential, 269, 270
    regional storage of, 270, 271f
    skinfold measurement of, 287–288, 288f, 289f
    weight-to-strength ratio and, 270
Body mass index, 301–302, 302t
Body weight. *See* Weight
Breath control, in resistive training, 151–152
Bridges, 226, 226f
Bridging, 322, 322f
Bulimia nervosa, 281–282
Bursitis, 336

C

Caffeine, 259
Calcium, 249
    supplemental, 253
Calisthenics, 135
Caloric balance, 271–273, 272f
Caloric expenditure, exercise prescription for, 107, 108t
Caloric intake
    daily requirements for, 307
    energy expenditure and, 271–273, 272f
    for weight management, 279t
Calorie content, nutrient density and, 241
Carbohydrate loading, 256–257
Carbohydrates
    complex, 242–243
    food sources of, 242–243
    recommended intake of, 242, 242t
        for active persons, 256–257
        for weight management, 279t
    simple, 242
    utilization of, 272–273
Cardiac muscle, 123
Cardiac valves, 77
Cardiorespiratory endurance exercise program, 67–68, 93–109. *See also* Training
    benefits of, 95–96
        health- vs. fitness-related, 95, 95t
    components of, 96–105
    daily exercise session in, 105–106
    detraining and, 109
    exercise duration in, 102–103, 103t
    exercise frequency in, 96–97, 97t
    exercise intensity in, 97–102. *See also* Exercise intensity
    exercise modality in, 96
    exercise prescription for, 107
    heart rate determination for, 105
    improvement stage in, 103, 104t
    initial conditioning stage in, 103, 104t
    low back pain and, 318–319
    maintenance stage in, 104
    progression in, 103–104, 104t
    risks of, 107–109
    for weight loss, 107, 108t
Cardiorespiratory system, 75
Cardiovascular disease, 4–5, 77–83
    body fat and, 268
    exercise risk in, 107–109
    hypercholesterolemia/hyperlipidemia and, 80–81, 81t
    prevalence of, 79–80
    protective effects of exercise for, 83
    risk appraisal for, 91–92
    risk factors for, 27t, 78–82, 79t
    waist-to-hip ratio and, 270, 303–304, 303t, 304f
Cardiovascular system, 75–83
    structure and function of, 77
Carotid artery pulse, palpation of, 105, 115f
Cat stretch, 231, 231f
Cervical curve, 314, 314f
Cervical vertebrae, 313–314, 314f, 315
Chair dips, 190, 190f
Change. *See* Behavior change
Chest
    resistive exercises for
        with barbells, 170–171, 170f, 171f
        with dumbbells, 179–180, 179f, 180f
        with machines, 156–159, 156f-159f
    stretching exercises for, 233, 233f
        PNF, 237, 237f
Chest press, 156–157, 157f
    barbell bench, 170, 170f
    barbell incline bench, 170–171, 171f

Chest press, *continued*
    dumbbell, 179, 179f
    dumbbell incline, 179, 179f
    lying closed grip, 173–174, 174f
Chest skinfold, 287, 288f
Chest stretch, 233, 233f
    PNF, 237, 237f
Children, obesity in, 274
Cholesterol levels, 5–6, 27t
    cardiovascular disease and, 80–81, 81t
    fat intake and, 244–245
Cigarette smoking, 5
    cardiovascular disease and, 27t, 79
    weight and, 274–275
Circuit training, 134
Circulatory system
    pulmonary, 79
    systemic, 79
Closed hand push-ups, 191, 191f
Closed wounds, 337
Coccygeal vertebrae (coccyx), 313–314, 314f, 315
Cold injury, 334
Complete proteins, 247
Complex carbohydrates, 242–243
Compound fractures, 336–337
Concentric contraction, 126
Conditioning phase, of daily exercise session, 59, 106
Consent
    for fitness evaluations, 17–18
    for physical activities, 15–16
Consistency, in training, 57
Contemplation stage, of behavior change, 41, 41t
Contract, personal, 44
Contract-Relax, 201
Contusions, 335
Cool-down, 59, 106
Corns, 337
Coronary artery disease, 4–5, 77–83. *See also* Cardiovascular disease
Cramps
    heat, 333–334
    muscle, 335
Creatine, 248
Creeping obesity, 271–272
Crunches, 192, 192f
Crunch test, 147, 148f, 148t
Cryotherapy, 337
Curling bar, 171, 171f
Curling bench, 172, 172f
Curl-ups, 192, 192f, 321, 321f
    improper technique for, 322–323, 322f
Curl-up test, 147, 148f, 148t

D

Daily exercise sessions. *See also* Training
    in cardiorespiratory endurance exercise program, 59, 105–106
    conditioning phase of, 59, 106
    cool-down in, 59, 106
    elements of, 59, 105–106
    overtraining in, 59
Daily Value (%), 259–260
Death
    causes of, 4, 9t
    during exercise, 107–109
Deep knee squats/lunges, 224–225, 225f

Dehydration, 258, 333–334
Detraining effect, 57, 109
    in resistive training, 125
Diabetes mellitus, 5
    cardiovascular disease and, 82
Diastolic blood pressure, 79, 80t. *See also* Blood pressure
Diet. *See also* Food(s); Nutrition
    traditional vs. healthy choice, 279t
    for weight management, 279t
Dieting, 275. *See also* Weight management
    metabolism and, 275
Diet pills, 274–275
Dips, 190, 190f
    chair, 190, 190f
Disaccharides, 242
Diseases, lifestyle-related, 4, 9–10, 9t
Disuse, fitness reversibility and, 57, 109, 125
Double leg hip flexion, 231–232, 231f
Double leg lifts, 323, 323f
Dumbbell(s), 155–156. *See also* Resistive training
    exercises with, 178–189
Dumbbell bench press, 179, 179f
Dumbbell bent over row, 187, 188f
Dumbbell fly, 179, 179f
Dumbbell pull-over, 188, 188f
Dumbbell wrist curl, 185, 185f
Dumbbell wrist extensions, 185, 185f
Dynamic movements, muscular, 126
Dynamic stretching, 200–201, 200t, 235

E

Eating, after exercise, 255–256
Eating disorders, 281–283
Eccentric contraction, 126
Economic benefits, of physical fitness, 11
Ectomorph, 269, 269f
Efficacy, behavior change and, 40
Elastic elongation, 199
Elbow breadth, frame size and, 23t, 24f
Electronic heart rate monitors, 105, 119–120
Empty calories, 242
Enabling factors, 38
Endomorph, 269, 269f
Endurance. *See* Cardiorespiratory endurance exercise program; Muscular endurance
Energy balance, 271–273, 272f
    weight gain and, 272–273
    weight loss and, 273
Energy expenditure, 271
    exercise prescription for, 107, 108t
Energy intake, 271
Ephedra (ephedrine), 255
Essential amino acids, 247
Essential body fat, 269
Essential nutrients, 241–249
Exercise
    aerobic. *See* Cardiorespiratory endurance exercise program
    cardiovascular disease and, 83
    eating after, 255–256
    fitness-related benefits of, 95, 95t
    health-related benefits of, 95
    injuries and, 334–338
    lack of. *See* Inactivity
    power of, 6
    in weight management, 275–276, 277

Exercise(s)
    low back, 319–324, 327–330
    resistive. See Resistive training
    stretching. See Stretching
Exercise duration, 102–103, 103t
    energy expenditure and, 108t
Exercise frequency, energy expenditure and, 108t
Exercise intensity
    energy expenditure and, 108t
    heart rate reserve and, 98–99, 100, 100t, 101, 102t
    maximal heart rate and, 98–100, 101, 102t, 119
    overload and, 56
    rate of perceived exertion and, 100–101, 102t
Exercise participation
    medical examination for, 27t
    risk assessment for, 26t
Exercise prescription, 63
    for weight loss, 107
    worksheet for, 63
Exercise sessions. See also Training
    in cardiorespiratory endurance exercise program, 59, 105–106
    conditioning phase of, 59, 106
    cool-down in, 59, 106
    elements of, 59, 105–106
    overtraining in, 59
    warm-up in, 59, 106
Exercise testing
    medical examination for, 27t
    physician supervision for, 27t
    risk assessment for, 26t
Extension, 130
External locus of control, 40

F

Family history, cardiovascular disease risk and, 82
Family lifestyle, obesity and, 274
Fast-glycolytic muscle fibers, 127, 128
Fasting glucose, coronary artery disease and, 27t
Fast-oxidative-glycolytic muscle fibers, 127, 128
Fast-twitch muscle fibers, 128
Fat, body. See Body fat
Fats, 243–246
    food sources of, 244
    hydrogenated, 244–245
    recommended intake of, 242t, 244, 245t
        for active persons, 257
        for weight management, 279t
    saturated, 244–245
    unsaturated, 245–246
    utilization of, 272–273
Fat-soluble vitamins, 248
Fat substitute, 246
Fatty acids
    omega-3, 246
    omega-6, 246
    trans, 244–245
Feet, stretching exercises for, 226–227, 227f
Females. See Gender
Fiber, 243
Fitness, 9–11
    benefits of, 10–11, 95, 95t
    definition of, 10
    health-related components of, 10
    importance of, 9
    reversibility of, 57, 109, 125

Fitness evaluation
    informed consent for, 17–18
    medical examination for, 27t
    physician supervision for, 27t
    risk assessment for, 26t
Fitness injuries, 334–338
Fitness program. See also Training
    basic considerations for, 55
    for body composition, 73
    cardiorespiratory, 67–68
    cool-down in, 59
    daily exercise session in, 59, 105–106
    dropouts from, 58
    for flexibility, 71–72
    individualized, 58
    for muscular strength and endurance, 69–70
    overtraining in, 59–60
    training principles for, 55–58
    warm-up in, 59
    workout in, 59
Fitness-related benefits of activity, 95, 95t
Flexibility, 195–238
    active, 196
    benefits of, 196
    definition of, 196
    factors affecting, 196–199
    fitness program for, 71–72
    hip, assessment of, 329–330, 330f, 330t
    low back pain and, 319
    lumbar, assessment of, 329–330, 330f, 330t
    passive, 196
    stretching exercises for, 199–202. See also Stretching
Flexibility tests
    ankle dorsi flexion, 211–212, 212f, 212t
    ankle plantar flexion, 209–210, 210f, 210t
    long axis body rotation, 217, 218f, 218t
    shoulder and wrist elevation, 205, 206f, 206t
    sit and reach, 219, 220f, 220t
        modified, 213, 213t, 214f, 214t
    trunk and neck extension, 207, 208f, 208t
Flexion, 130
Fluid balance, 249
Fluid replacement, 258
Fly, 158, 158f
Food(s). See also Diet; Nutrient(s); Nutrition
    health claims for, 260–261
Food choices, for weight loss, 277–278, 279t
Food labels, 259–262
    misleading, 244
Food log, 309–310
Food servings
    number of, 253t
    size of, 253t, 280t
Foot plantar flexion, 169, 169f
Forearm, dumbbell exercises for, 185, 185f
Fractures, 336–337
Frame size, estimation of, 23t, 24f
Free weights. See also Resistive training
    barbells, 155–156, 170–178
    dumbbells, 155–156, 178–189
    pros and cons of, 155–156
French press
    barbell, 173, 173f
    dumbbell, 184, 184f
Fuel nutrients, 241
Full knee squats/lunges, 224–225, 225f
Full neck rolls, 225–226, 226f

G

Gender
    body fat and, 270t
    cardiovascular disease and, 82
    eating disorders and, 281
    flexibility and, 198–199
    muscular strength and endurance and, 128
General Adaptation Syndrome, 55
Genetic factors, in obesity, 273
Glucose intolerance, cardiovascular disease and, 82
Gluteals, resistive training for, 165–167, 166f, 167f
Glycogen storage, carbohydrate loading and, 256–257
Golgi tendon organs, 198
    autogenic inhibition and, 201–202
Grains, 243
Grips, in resistive training, 152–153
Gynoid obesity, 82, 270, 271f

H

Hamstring stretch, 237, 237f
Hand grips, in resistive training, 152–153
Hard/easy training, 58
HDL cholesterol, 27t, 81, 81t. *See also* Cholesterol levels
Health
    components of, 7–8
    definition of, 6–7
    vs. fitness, 95
    intellectual, 7–8
    mental, 7
    physical, 7
    social, 7
    spiritual, 8
    vs. wellness, 8
Health care society, vs. health prevention society, 6
Health claims, on food labels, 260–261
Health Field Concept, 8
Health problems
    lifestyle-related, 4, 9–10, 9t
    preventable, 4
Health questionnaire, 29–34
Health-related benefits of activity, 95
Health screening, routine, 39t
Healthy choice diet, 279t
Healthy People 2000, 10
Heart, structure of, 77
Heart attack, during exercise, 107–109
Heart disease, 4–5, 77–83. *See also* Cardiovascular disease
    risk factors for, 27t
Heart rate
    determination of, 105
    maximal
        determination of, 99
        exercise intensity and, 98–100, 101, 102t
Heart rate monitors, 105, 119–120
Heart rate reserve, exercise intensity and, 98–99, 100, 100t, 101, 102t
Heat, therapeutic, 337–338
Heat cramps, 333–334
Heat exhaustion, 333–334
Heat-related illness, 333–334
Heat stroke, 333–334
Herbal supplements, 255
High blood pressure, 6
    cardiovascular disease and, 27t, 79–80
High-density cholesterol, 81, 81t. *See also* Cholesterol levels

High nutrient density, 241
Hip flexibility test, 329–330, 330f, 330t
Hip sled, 165–166, 166f
Hip stretch, 230, 230f
Hold-Relax, 201
Hurdler's stretch, 224, 224f
Hydrogenated fats, 244–245
Hypercholesterolemia/hyperlipidemia, 5–6, 27t
    cardiovascular disease and, 80–81, 81t
    fat intake and, 244–245
Hyperplasia, muscle, 128
    overload and, 124
Hypertension, 6
    cardiovascular disease and, 27t, 79–80
Hypertrophy, muscle, 128
    gender differences in, 128
    overload and, 124
Hyponatremia, 257–258
Hypothermia, 334

I

Illness, lifestyle-related, 4, 9–10, 9t
Inactivity, 5
    cardiovascular disease and, 27t, 81, 109
    exercise risk and, 107–109
Inclined bent knee sit-ups, 193, 193f
Incomplete proteins, 247
Individualized training, 58
Informed consent
    for fitness evaluations, 17–18
    for physical activities, 15–16
Injuries, 334–338
    prevention of, 58
    stretching, 198
Insoluble fiber, 243
Intellectual health, 7
Intensity. *See* Exercise intensity
Internal locus of control, 40
Intervertebral disks, 314
Iron, 249
Isokinetic training, 130, 134. *See also* Resistive training
Isometric contraction, 126
    in proprioceptive neuromuscular facilitation, 201–202, 201f
Isometric training, 129, 131. *See also* Resistive training
Isotonic training, 129–130, 131–134. *See also* Resistive training

J

Joints, structure of, 198

K

Kneeling arm and leg extension, 320–321, 321f
Knee squats/lunges, deep, 224–225, 225f
Knee wraps, in resistive training, 152

L

Labels, food, 244, 259–262
Lacerations, 337
Lateral lower leg stretch, 228, 228f
Lateral neck stretch, 232, 232f
Lat pull down, 163, 163f
LDL cholesterol, 27t, 81, 81t. *See also* Cholesterol levels

Leg. *See also* Lower leg; Upper leg
    resistive exercises for, 167–169, 167f–169f
Leg abduction, 166, 166f
Leg adduction, 168–169, 169f
Leg curl, prone, 167–168, 168f
Lifestyle diseases, 4, 9–10, 9t
Lifestyle self-assessment, 19–23
Lifting belts, 152, 316
Lipid levels, 5–6, 27t
    cardiovascular disease and, 80–81, 81t
    fat intake and, 244–245
Lipoproteins, 81, 81t. *See also* Cholesterol levels; Lipid levels
Load, in resistive training, 131
Locus of control, 40
Long axis body rotation test, 217, 218f, 218t
Lordosis, 317, 317f
Low back exercises, 319–324, 327–330, 327–338
    contraindicated, 322–324, 322f–324f
Low back extension test, 327, 328f, 328t
Low back pain, 311–330
    causes of, 315–316
    financial impact of, 313
    muscle weakness and, 317, 317f
    prevalence of, 313
    prevention of, 316–318
    treatment of, 318–319
Low-density cholesterol, 81, 81t. *See also* Cholesterol levels
Lower back. *See also* Back; Spine; Vertebrae
    anatomy of, 313–315, 314f
    resistive exercises for, 164, 164f
    stretching exercises for, 230–232, 230f–232f
        PNF, 237, 237f
Lower leg. *See also* Leg
    resistive exercises for
        with barbells, 178, 178f
        with dumbbells, 188–189, 189f
        with machines, 169, 169f
    stretching exercises for, 227–229, 228f, 229f
Low nutrient density, 241
Lumbar curve, 314, 314f
Lumbar flexibility test, 329–330, 330f, 330t
Lumbar vertebrae, 313–314, 314f, 315
Lunges, deep knee, 224–225, 225f
Lying barbell triceps extension, 172–173, 173f
Lying closed grip bench press, 173–174, 174f
Lying dumbbell triceps extension, 184, 184f

M

Maintenance stage, of behavior change, 41t, 42–43
Males. *See* Gender
Ma Whang, 255
Maximal heart rate
    determination of, 99
    exercise intensity and, 98–100, 101, 102t, 119
Medical examination, for exercise testing/participation, 27t
Medical/health questionnaire, 29–34
Men. *See* Gender
Mental health, 7
Mesomorph, 269, 269f
Metabolic rate, determination of, 305–306
Metabolism, 271
    body weight and, 275
    dieting and, 275
    set point and, 274–275
Minerals, 249

    supplemental, 253–255
        athletic performance and, 258
Mitral valve, 77
Modified sit and reach test, 213, 213t, 214f, 214t
Monosaccharides, 242
Monounsaturated fats, 245
Mortality
    causes of, 4, 9t
    exercise-related, 107–109
Muscle
    cardiac, 123
    dynamic movements of, 126
    size of, 128
    skeletal, 123
    smooth, 123
    static movements of, 126
Muscle atrophy, 128
    detraining and, 125
Muscle contraction, 125–126
    concentric, 126
    eccentric, 126
    isometric, 126
        in proprioceptive neuromuscular facilitation, 201–202, 201f
Muscle cramps, 335
Muscle elongation
    elastic, 199
    plastic, 199
    temperature and, 199
Muscle fibers, 126–128
    exercise-induced changes in, 131
    fast-glycolytic (Type IIb), 127, 128
    fast-oxidative-glycolytic (Type IIa), 127, 128
    fast-twitch (Type II), 128
    slow-twitch (Type I), 127
Muscle hyperplasia, 128
    overload and, 124
Muscle hypertrophy, 128
    overload and, 124
Muscle soreness, 129, 336
    proprioceptive neuromuscular facilitation and, 202
Muscle spasms, 335
Muscle spindles, 198
Muscle temperature, flexibility and, 199
Muscle tension, Golgi tendon organs and, 198
Muscle weakness, low back pain and, 317, 317f
Muscular endurance
    curl-up test for, 147, 148f, 148t
    definition of, 123
    factors affecting, 128–129
    low back pain and, 319
    vs. muscular strength, 123
    1-minute bent-knee sit-up test for, 139, 140f, 140t
    push-up test for, 145–146, 146f, 146t
    resistive training for. *See* Resistive training
Muscular hypertrophy, gender differences in, 128
Muscular power, resistive training for, 132, 132t
Muscular strength
    bench press test for, 143, 143f, 143t
    definition of, 123
    factors affecting, 128–129
    low back pain and, 319
    vs. muscular endurance, 123
    resistive training for. *See* Resistive training
    typical gains in, 131
    upper leg press test for, 141–142, 142f, 142t
Myocardial infarction, during exercise, 107–109
MyPyramid Food System, 250–252, 251f

N

National Cholesterol Education Program (NCEP), 244
Neck, stretching exercises for, 232–233, 232f, 233f
Neck extension, in flexibility assessment, 207, 208f, 208t
Neck rolls, full, 225–226, 226f
Negative reinforcement, 38
Neutral grip, 153
Nonessential body fat, 269, 270
Nutrient(s)
    essential, 241–249
    on food labels, 259–262
    fuel, 241
    recommended intake of, 241, 242t, 250–252, 250t–252t
        for active persons, 256–258
            estimation of, 307
        serving size and, 253t
Nutrient claims, on food labels, 260–261
Nutrient content descriptors, 261–262, 261t
Nutrient density, 241
Nutrient utilization, hierarchy of, 272–273
Nutrition, 239–264. *See also* Diet; Food(s)
    performance and, 256–258
    in weight management, 277–278
Nutritional labels, 259–262
Nutritional supplements, 253–255

O

Obesity, 5, 268. *See also* Weight
    android, 82, 270, 271f
    cardiovascular disease and, 27t, 82
    causes of, 273
    childhood, 274
    creeping, 271–272
    energy balance and, 271–273, 272f
    family lifestyle factors in, 274
    genetic factors in, 273
    gynoid, 82, 270, 271f
    labor saving devices/technology and, 273
    low back pain and, 318
    set point theory of, 274–275
Olestra (Olean), 246
Omega-3 fatty acids, 246
Omega-6 fatty acids, 246
1.5-mile run test, 117
1-minute bent-knee sit-up test, 139, 140f, 140t
Open wounds, 337
Osteoarthritis, 318
Overhead press
    barbell, 175, 175f
    machine, 161, 161f
Overload, 56
    progressive, 56
    in resistive training, 124
    in stretching, 199
Overtraining, 59–60

P

Pain, back. *See* Low back pain
Passive flexibility, 196
Pelvic curve, 314, 314f
Pelvic tilt, 321, 321f
Percent daily value, 259–260
Performance
    body fat and, 270
    nutrition and, 256–258

Personal contract, 44
Personal exercise prescription, 63
Physical activity. *See* Exercise
Physical fitness. *See* Fitness
Physical health, 7
Physical inactivity, 5
    cardiovascular disease and, 27t, 81, 109
    exercise risk and, 107–109
Physician supervision, for exercise testing, 27t
Plantar arch stretch, 226–227, 227f
Plastic elongation, 199
Plough, 224, 224f
Plyometrics, 134–135
PNF. *See* Proprioceptive neuromuscular facilitation (PNF)
Polysaccharides, 242
Polyunsaturated fats, 246
Portion size, 253t, 280t
Positioning, in resistive training, 152–153
Positive reinforcement, 38
Posterior arm stretch, 234, 234f
Posterior lower leg stretch, 228–229, 229f
Posterior neck stretch, 232–233, 233f
Posterior shoulder stretch, 233–234, 234f
Posterior upper leg stretch, 236–237, 237f
Potassium, 249
Precontemplation stage, of behavior change, 41, 41t
Predisposing factors, 37
Pre-exercise self-assessment, 25–26
Pregnancy, flexibility in, 199
Preparation stage, of behavior change, 41t, 42
Prevention
    primary, 39
        routine health screening for, 39t
    secondary, 39
    tertiary, 39
Primary prevention, 39
Principle of adaptation, 55–56
Principle of consistency, 57
Principle of disuse, 57
Principle of hard and easy, 58
Principle of individuality, 58
Principle of overload, 56, 124
    in resistive training, 124
    in stretching, 199
Principle of progressive overload, 56
Principle of reversibility, 57, 109, 125
Principle of safety, 58
Principle of specificity, 57–58
    in resistive training, 124–125
    in stretching, 199
Progressive overload, 56
Progressive resistive exercise training, 129–134. *See also* Resistive training
Pronated grip, 152
Prone double arm lift, 320, 320f
Prone double leg raise, 323, 323f
Prone leg curl, 167–168, 168f
Prone position, in resistive training, 153
Prone single arm lift, 319–320, 320f
Prone single leg lift, 320, 320f
Proprioceptive neuromuscular facilitation (PNF), 201–202, 201f, 202f
    stretching exercises for, 235–238, 235f–238f, 236t
Protein, 246–248
    complete, 247
    food sources of, 246, 247
    functions of, 246
    incomplete, 247

Protein, *continued*
    recommended intake of, 242t, 247
        for active persons, 257
        for weight management, 279t
    utilization of, 272–273
Ptosis, abdominal, 317
Pull-ups, 192, 192f
    reversed closed-grip, 189, 189f
Pulmonary circulation, 79
Pulmonary valve, 77
Pulse, palpation of, 105, 115f
Pulse pressure, 79
Puncture wounds, 337
Push-ups, 191, 191f
    closed hand, 191, 191f
Push-up test, 145–146, 146f, 146t

R

Radial artery pulse, palpation of, 105, 115f
Range of motion, 197. *See also* Flexibility
Rate of perceived exertion, 100–101, 102t
Reciprocal inhibition, 202
Refined grains, 243
Reflex, stretch, 198, 200
Rehydration fluids, 258
Reinforcing factors, 38
Repetition maximum (RM), 131
Resistive training, 123–125. *See also specific exercises*
    for abdomen, 165, 165f
    for back, 163–164, 163f, 164f
    back injury in, 316–317
    basic techniques of, 129–136
    benefits of, 123
    in body building, 135
    body positioning in, 153
    breath control in, 151–152
    calisthenics in, 135
    for chest, 156–159, 156f–159f
    circuit training in, 134
    detraining and, 125
    free weights in, 155–156
    for gluteals, 165–167, 166f, 167f
    grips in, 152–153
    for hypertrophy, 132t, 133
    inter-set/inter-session rest periods in, 133
    isokinetic, 130, 134
    isometric, 129, 131
    isotonic (progressive), 129–130, 131–134
    knee wraps in, 152
    load in, 131
    low back pain and, 319
    for lower legs, 169, 169f
    machines in, 154–155, 155t
        exercises for, 156–169
    muscle fiber changes in, 131
    for muscular endurance, 132, 132t
    for muscular power, 132, 132t
    for muscular strength, 132, 132t
    overload in, 124
    plyometrics in, 134–135
    practical guidelines for, 133–134, 135–136
    principles of, 130–134
    program for, 69–70
    repetition maximum in, 131
    for shoulders, 161–163, 161f–163f
    specificity of, 124–125
    spotting in, 153–154, 156
    sticking point in, 156
    strength gains in, time course of, 130–131
    training volume in, 131
    for upper arms, 159–161, 159f–161f
    for upper legs, 167–169, 167f–169f
    Valsalva maneuver in, 151–152
    weight belts in, 152, 316–317
    weight control and, 275
Respiratory system, structure and function of, 77
Reversed closed-grip pull-ups, 189, 189f
Reversibility
    of fitness, 57, 109
    of muscular strength/endurance, 125
RICE, 335, 337
Risk assessment, for exercise testing/participation, 26t
Risk factors, for cardiovascular disease, 78–82, 79t
Rockport Walking Test, 113
Routine health screening, 39t

S

Sacral curve, 314, 314f
Sacral vertebrae (sacrum), 313–314, 314f, 315
Safety precautions, 58
Saturated fat, 244–245
Sciatica, 317
Screening, routine health, 39t
Seated arm curls, 159, 159f
Seated barbell curl, 172, 172f
Seated dumbbell curl, 182, 182f
    using curling bench, 183, 183f
Seated lateral raise, 162, 162f
Seated leg curl, 168, 168f
Seated leg extension, 167, 167f
Seated leg press, 166–167, 167f
Seated overhead dumbbell press, 186, 186f
Seated position, in resistive training, 153
Seated posterior deltoid, 163, 163f
Seated rowing, 164, 164f
Seated thigh dumbbell curl, 182–183, 183f
Seated triceps extension, 160, 160f, 173, 173f, 184, 184f
Secondary prevention, 39
Sedentary lifestyle, 5
    cardiovascular disease and, 27t, 81, 109
    exercise risk and, 107–109
Selye's General Adaptation Syndrome, 55
Semilunar valves, 77
Serum cholesterol/lipids, 5–6, 27t
    cardiovascular disease and, 80–81, 81t
    fat intake and, 244–245
Servings
    number of, 254t
    size of, 253t, 280t
Set point theory, 274–275
Shinsplints, 335
Shoulder
    resistive exercises for
        with barbells, 175–176, 175f, 176f
        with dumbbells, 186–187, 186f, 187f
        with machines, 161–163, 161f–163f
    stretching exercises for, 233–234, 233f, 234f
        PNF, 238, 238f
Shoulder and wrist elevation, in flexibility assessment, 205, 206f, 206t
Side stitch, 335
Simple carbohydrates, 242

Single leg hip flexion, 232, 232f
Sit and reach test, 219, 220f, 220t
    modified, 213, 213t, 214f, 214t
Sitting position. *See under* Seated
Sit-ups
    inclined bent knee, 193, 193f
    straight leg, 324, 324f
Skeletal muscle, 123. *See also* Muscle
Skinfold measurement, 287–288, 288f, 289f
    seven-site, 299–300
    three-site, 291–292, 293t, 295–296, 296t, 297t
Skin wounds, 337
Slow foods, 278
Slow-twitch muscle fibers, 127
Smoking, 5
    cardiovascular disease and, 27t, 79
    weight and, 274–275
Smooth muscle, 123
Social health, 7
Social readjustment rating scale, 24t
Sodium, 249
    replacement of, 257–258
Soft tissue, structure of, 198
Soluble fiber, 243
Somatotypes, 269, 269f
Soreness, muscle, 129
Specificity
    in resistive training, 124–125
    in stretching, 199
    in training, 57–58
Sphygmomanometer, 80, 87f
Spinal curves, 314, 314f
    abnormal, 317, 317f
Spine. *See also under* Back; Low back; Vertebrae
    range of motion of, 315
    structure and function of, 313–315, 314f
Spiritual health, 8
Sports drinks, 256
Sports performance
    body fat and, 270
    nutrition and, 256–258
Spot reduction, 276
Spotting, in resistive training, 153–154, 156
Sprains, 335
Squats, deep knee, 224–225, 225f
Standing barbell curl, 171, 171f
Standing barbell heel raise, 178, 178f
Standing barbell upright row, 176, 177f
Standing cable arm curl, 160, 160f
Standing dumbbell curl, 180–181, 181f
Standing dumbbell heel raise, 188–189, 189f
Standing dumbbell lateral row, 186–187, 186f
Standing dumbbell upright row, 187, 187f
Standing hammer curl, 181, 181f
Standing position, in resistive training, 153
Standing straight legged straddle toe touch, 225, 225f
Standing straight legged toe touch, 225, 225f
Standing triceps extension, 161, 161f
Standing upright cable row, 162, 162f
Static contraction, 126
Static movements, muscular, 126
Static stretching, 200, 200t
Static stretching exercises, 223–234
    contraindicated, 224–226
    guidelines for, 223, 223t
    recommended, 226–234
    sequence of action for, 223t

Sticking point, 156
Straight leg sit-ups, 324, 324f
Strains, 335
Strength. *See* Muscular strength
Strength-to-weight ratio, 270
Strength training. *See* Resistive training
Stress, cardiovascular disease and, 82
Stress fractures, 336
Stretching. *See also specific exercises*
    ballistic, 200–201, 200t, 235
    contract-relax in, 201
    dynamic, 200t, 201, 235
    elastic elongation in, 199
    guidelines for, 223, 223t
    hold-relax in, 201
    injuries in, 198
    low back pain and, 319
    overload in, 199–200
    plastic elongation in, 199
    proprioceptive neuromuscular facilitation and, 201–202, 201f, 202f, 235–238, 235f–238f
    specificity in, 199
    static, 200, 200t, 226–234
        exercises for, 223–234
    warm-up for, 199
Stretch-reflex mechanism, 198, 200
Subscapular skinfold, 287, 289f
Sudden death, during exercise, 107–109
Sugars. *See also* Carbohydrates
    simple, 242
Sunburn, 337
Supinated grip, 153
Supine double leg trunk rotation, 231, 231f
Supine position, in resistive training, 153
Supine single leg trunk rotation, 230–231, 230f
Supplements
    herbal, 255
    nutritional, 253–255
Suprailium skinfold, 288, 289f
Systemic circulation, 79
Systolic blood pressure, 79, 80t. *See also* Blood pressure

T

Temperature, muscle, flexibility and, 199
Tendonitis, 336
Termination stage, of behavior change, 41t, 43
Tertiary prevention, 39
Thigh skinfold, 288, 289f
Thirst, dehydration and, 333–334
Thoracic cage, 315
Thoracic curve, 314, 314f
Thoracic vertebrae, 313–314, 314f, 315
3–mile walk/run test, 119–120
Tissue elongation
    elastic, 199
    plastic, 199
    temperature and, 199
Toe stretch, 227, 227f
Toe touch
    standing straight legged, 225, 225f
    standing straight legged straddle, 225, 225f
Total cholesterol, 80–81
Total health-fitness profile, 65–66
Training. *See also* Workouts
    adaptation in, 55–56
    consistency in, 57

Training, continued
    hard/easy, 58
    individualized, 58
    overload in, 56
    overtraining and, 59–60
    principles of, 55–58
    progressive overload in, 56
    resistive. See Resistive training
    safety precautions in, 58
    specificity of, 57–58
Training volume, in resistive training, 131
Trans fatty acids, 244–245
Transtheoretical model, of behavior change, 40–43, 41t
Triceps extension
    lying barbell, 172–173, 173f
    lying dumbbell, 184, 184f
    seated, 160, 160f
    seated barbell, 173, 173f
    seated dumbbell, 184, 184f
    standing, 161, 161f
Triceps skinfold, 287, 288f
Triceps stretch, 234, 234f
Tricuspid valve, 77
Trunk, stretching exercises for, 230–232, 230f–232f
Trunk and neck extension, in flexibility assessment, 207, 208f, 208t

U

Unrefined grains, 243
Unsaturated fats, 245–246
Unsoluble fiber, 243
Upper arm, resistive exercises for
    with barbells, 171–174, 171f–174f
    with dumbbells, 180–185, 180f–185f
    with machines, 159–161, 159f–161f
    nonweight/nonmachine, 189–191, 189f–191f
Upper back. See also Back; Spine; Vertebrae
    resistive exercises for
        with barbells, 177–178, 177f, 178f
        with dumbbells, 187–188, 188f
        with machines, 163–164, 163f, 164f
    stretching exercises for, 230–232, 230f–232f
Upper leg. See also Leg
    resistive exercises for, 167–169, 167f–169f
    stretching exercises for, 229–230f, 229f, 230f
        PNF, 236–237, 236f, 237f
Upper leg press test, 141–142, 142f, 142t

V

Valsalva maneuver, 151–152
Valves, cardiac, 77
Variable resistance machines, 154–155, 155t. See also Resistive training
    exercises for, 156–169
Ventricles, 77
Vertebrae, 313–315, 314f. See also under Back; Low back; Spine
    structure and function of, 313–315, 314f

Vertebral foramen, 315
Vertical chest press, 157, 157f
Vertical pec, 158, 158f
Vitamins, 248–249
    supplemental, 253, 255
        athletic performance and, 258
VO_2max
    exercise intensity and, 101, 102, 102t
    improvement in, 96–97
    normal values for, 114t
    1.5-mile run test for, 114t
    Rockport Walking Test for, 113–114

W

Waist circles, 226, 226f
Waist circumference, body mass index and, 301–302, 302t
Waist-to-hip ratio, 270, 303–304, 303t, 304f
Warm-up, 59, 106
    for stretching, 199, 223
Water balance, 249
    rehydration for, 258
Water-soluble vitamins, 248
Weekend Warriors, 57, 97
    exercise risk for, 107–109
Weight, frame size and, 23t, 24f
Weight belts, 152, 314
Weight gain, guidelines for, 283
Weight loss
    exercise prescription for, 107, 108t
    rate of, 273
Weight management, 267–310
    behavior modification in, 276–278
    energy balance and, 271–273
    exercise in, 275–276
    recommended dietary intake for, 279t
    spot reduction in, 276
    weight gain and, 283
    weight loss and, 275–278
Weight tables, 23t
Weight-to-strength ratio, 270
Wellness, 8–9
    choice of, 4
Whole grains, 243
Women. See Gender
Workouts. See also Training
    in cardiorespiratory endurance exercise program, 59, 105–106
    conditioning phase of, 59, 106
    cool-down in, 59, 106
    elements of, 59, 105–106
    overtraining in, 59
    warm-up in, 59, 106
Wrist curls
    barbell, 174, 174f
    dumbbell, 185, 185f
Wrist elevation, in flexibility assessment, 205, 206f, 206t
Wrist extensions
    barbell, 175, 175f
    dumbbell, 185, 185f